Best Wishes
to
Mike

[signature]
11/17/05

CARDIAC SAFETY OF NONCARDIAC DRUGS

CARDIAC SAFETY OF NONCARDIAC DRUGS

PRACTICAL GUIDELINES FOR CLINICAL RESEARCH AND DRUG DEVELOPMENT

Edited by

JOEL MORGANROTH, MD
IHOR GUSSAK, MD, PhD, FACC

eResearch Technology Inc.,
Philadelphia, PA; Bridgewater, NJ; Peterborough, UK

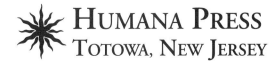

HUMANA PRESS
TOTOWA, NEW JERSEY

© 2005 Humana Press Inc.
999 Riverview Drive, Suite 208
Totowa, New Jersey 07512
www.humanapr.com

For additional copies, pricing for bulk purchases, and/or information about other Humana titles, contact Humana at the above address or at any of the following numbers: Tel.: 973-256-1699; Fax: 973-256-8341, E-mail: humana@humanapr.com; or visit our website at www.humanapress.com.

Production Editor: Mark J. Breaugh.

Cover design by Patricia F. Cleary.

This publication is printed on acid-free paper. ∞
ANSI Z39.48-1984 (American National Standards Institute) Permanence of Paper for Printed Library Materials.

Printed in the United States of America. 10 9 8 7 6 5 4 3 2 1

eISBN: 1-59259-884-6

Library of Congress Cataloging-in-Publication Data

Cardiac safety of noncardiac drugs : practical guidelines for clinical

research and drug development / edited by Joel Morganroth, Ihor Gussak.

    p. cm.

 Includes bibliographical references and index.

 ISBN 1-58829-515-X (alk. paper)

 1. Cardiovascular toxicology. 2. Heart--Effect of drugs on. 3.

Drugs--Side effects--Testing. 4. Electrocardiography. I. Morganroth, Joel.

II. Gussak, Ihor.

 RC677.C36 2005

 616.1'07--dc22

                            2004014055

DEDICATION

To our families, without whose support our professional activities would be diminished:

To my Wife Gail,
and Children Jason, Jennifer, and Jessica,
and to my Parents Ben and Grace

JOEL MORGANROTH

To my Wife Hiie,
and Children Maria and Georg,
and to my Parents Bohdan and Maria

IHOR GUSSAK

PREFACE

It is generally easy to define the efficacy of a new therapeutic agent. However, what is even more difficult and more
challenging yet more important is to define its safety when
administered to millions of patients with multi-faceted diseases, co-morbidities, sensitivities and concomitant medications. The commonest cause of new drug discontinuations,
cause for disapproval from marketing and removal from the
market after approval is a drug's effect on cardiac repolarization which is essentially identified by increasing the duration
of the QTc interval duration on the standard 12-lead electrocardiogram (ECG).

*Cardiac Safety of Noncardiac Drugs: Practical Guide-
lines for Clinical Research and Drug Development* is
designed to present the current preclinical, clinical, and regulatory principles to assess the cardiac safety of new drugs
based primarily on their effects on the ECG. Practical guidance to define cardiac safety at all stages of clinical research
and drug development are featured and discussed by internationally recognized experts with academic, industrial, and
regulatory experience. Each chapter contains the best available evidence, the author's personal opinions, areas of con-
troversy, and future trends. Although some of the areas are
highly specialized, this book has been designed for a broad
audience ranging from medical and graduate students to clinical nurses, clinical trial coordinators, safety officers, data
managers, statisticians, regulatory authorities, clinicians, and
scientists.

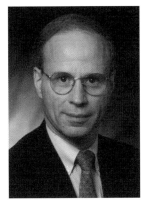

Joel Morganroth, MD

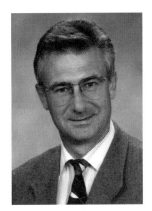

Ihor Gussak, MD, PhD

The book is organized in a practical and easy to assimilate manner, with each chapter
focusing on a particular aspect of cardiac safety. Part I contains an historical overview
from a clinical and regulatory prospective. Part II is devoted to preclinical and
pharmacogenomic aspects of cardiac safety in clinical research and drug development.
Part III includes clinical methodologies and technical aspects of assessing cardiac safety
of investigational drugs with the main focus on cardiac repolarization, especially as
defined by the duration of the QTc interval. Part IV provides a comprehensive review of
the application of electrocardiology in clinical research, including fundamentals of ECG
interpretation in clinical trials, cardiac safety assessment in all phases of drug development, statistical analysis plans for ECG data obtained in formal clinical trials, and practical interpretation of the results. Finally, Part V presents a broad spectrum of domestic
and international regulatory aspects in assessing the cardiac safety in clinical research and
drug development.

The editors of *Cardiac Safety of Noncardiac Drugs* wish to recognize the significant contribution made by all of the contributing authors. The book is the result of a collaboration that has brought together the skills and perspectives of researchers, scientists, and clinicians. Finally, we hope that the book will become a primary reference for drug developers in all therapeutic areas as well as academicians consulting in this arena.

Joel Morganroth, MD
Ihor Gussak, MD, PhD

CONTENTS

Part IV. Application of Electrocardiology in Clinical Research

Part V.   Regulatory Considerations

CONTRIBUTORS

AMY M. ANNAND-FURLONG, MS • *Senior Vice President, Regulatory Compliance, eResearchTechnology Inc., Philadelphia, PA, USA*

CHARLES ANTZELEVITCH, PhD, FACC, FAHA • *Executive Director and Director of Research, Gordon K. Moe Scholar, Experimental Cardiology Program Director, Masonic Medical Research Laboratory, Utica, NY, USA; Professor of Pharmacology, Upstate Medical University, Syracuse, NY*

FABIO BADILINI, PhD • *Chief Scientist, AMPS-LLC, New York, NY, USA*

MARTIN P. BEDIGIAN, MD • *Clinical Research and Development, Novartis Pharmaceuticals, East Hanover, NJ, USA*

ARTHUR M. BROWN, MD, PhD • *Professor, Physiology and Biophysics, Case Western Reserve University, MetroHealth Campus, Chairman and CEO, ChanTest, Inc., Cleveland, OH, USA*

BARRY D. BROWN, MS • *Product Integration Manager, Mortara Instrument, Inc., Milwaukee, WI, USA*

ROBERT BROWN • *Senior Vice President, eResearchTechnology Inc., Philadelphia, PA, USA*

JEAN-PHILIPPE COUDERC, PhD, MBA • *Assistant Professor of Medicine (Cardiology), Assistant Director of Heart Research Follow-up Program, University of Rochester Medical Center, Rochester, NY, USA*

GERALD A. FAICH, MD, MPH, FISPE • *President, Pharmaceutical Safety Assessments, Inc., Narberth, PA, USA*

SCOTT GRISANTI • *Senior Vice President, Business Development and Chief Marketing Officer, eResearch Technology Inc., Philadelphia, PA, USA*

IHOR GUSSAK, MD, PhD, FACC • *Vice President, Global Medical Affairs, eResearchTechnology Inc., Bridgewater, NJ; Clinical Associate Professor of Medicine, UMDNJ-Robert Wood Johnson Medical School, New Brunswick, NJ; Associate Editor, Journal of Electrocardiology, Bridgewater, NJ, USA*

ALAN S. HOLLISTER, MD, PhD • *Clinical Pharmacology Unit Director, GlaxoSmithKline, Philadelphia, PA, USA*

RICHARD JUDSON, PhD • *Chief Scientific Officer, Senior Vice President, Research & Development, Genaissance Pharmaceuticals, New Haven, CT, USA*

ROBERT S. KASS, PhD • *David Hosack Professor of Pharmacology, Chairman, Department of Pharmacology, Columbia University College of Physicians and Surgeons, New York, NY, USA*

ROBERT KLEIMAN, MD, FACC • *Senior Director of International Cardiology, eResearchTechnology Inc., Philadelphia, PA, USA*

RAYMOND JOHN LIPICKY, MD • *Director, LIPICKY LLC, Gaithersburg, MD; Former Director, Cardio-Renal Drug Products Division, Food and Drug Administration, USA*

JEFFREY S. LITWIN, MD, FACC • *Senior Vice President and Chief Medical Officer, eResearchTechnology Inc., Philadelphia, PA, USA*

PIERRE MAISON-BLANCHE, MD • *Hopital Lariboisiere, Paris, France*

TIMOTHY H MONTAGUE, MS • *Statistical and Data Sciences, GlaxoSmithKline, Collegeville, PA, USA*

JOEL MORGANROTH, MD • *Chief Scientist, eResearchTechnology Inc., Clinical Professor of Medicine, University of Pennsylvania School of Medicine, Philadelphia, PA, USA*

JUSTIN L. MORTARA, PhD • *Vice President of Sales and Marketing, Mortara Instrument Inc., Milwaukee, WI, USA*

ARTHUR J. MOSS, MD, FACC • *Professor of Medicine (Cardiology), Director of Heart Research Follow-Up Program, University of Rochester Medical Center, Rochester, NY, USA*

JEANNE M. NERBONNE, PhD • *Alumni Endowed Professor, Department of Molecular Biology and Pharmacology, Washington University Medical School, St. Louis, MO, USA*

NENAD SARAPA, MD • *Director, Clinical Pharmacology, La Jolla Laboratories, Pfizer Inc., San Diego, CA, USA*

RASHMI R. SHAH, MD, BSc, MBBS, FRCP, FFPM • *Senior Clinical Assessor, Medicines and Healthcare products Regulatory Agency, London, UK*

ANNETTE STEMHAGEN, DrPH, FISPE • *Vice President, Strategic Development Services, Covance Inc., Radnor, PA, USA*

WOJCIECH ZAREBA, MD, PhD • *Associate Professor of Medicine (Cardiology), Director of Clinical Research, Cardiology Unit, Associate Director of Heart Research Follow-up Program, University of Rochester Medical Center, Rochester, NY, USA*

I INTRODUCTION

1

Cardiac Safety of Noncardiac Drugs
Historical Recollections

Raymond John Lipicky, MD

CONTENTS

INTRODUCTION

This chapter is a set of recollections that would be difficult to document because they are based on my experience as a Food and Drug Administration (FDA) regulator and a pharmacologist with a special interest in cardiac repolarization. As is the common precedent, this is not related to considerations of antiarrhythmic drugs. Rather, this focus is upon drugs that have not been developed for the express purpose of modifying the behavior of cardiac ion channels, but as we all know many unexpectedly do.

My personal recollections about the "QT" and torsades de pointes (TdP), start somewhere in the early 1980s regarding the drug lidoflazine, and in this instance my recollections are very vague. Lidoflazine, an anti-anginal calcium channel blocker was being considered (for symptomatic relief of angina) in the early 1980s. The initial principal issue was an unusually high incidence of atrial fibrillation as an adverse effect. There was, as I remember, neither QT discussion nor argument, but then (after initial deliberations were concluded) it became recognized, by an isolated publication and anecdote that TdP was associated with lidoflazine as well as prolongation of the QT_C interval. The role of this latter observation played in final decision making is not within my recollection (so, it must not have been important).

The next event I recall was a meeting held in Philadelphia (*1*) in 1992 to discuss cardiac repolarization with special emphasis on the clinical significance of QT interval measurements. The major unstated question was "how much QT prolongation was acceptable?"

From: *Cardiac Safety of Noncardiac Drugs:*
Practical Guidelines for Clinical Research and Drug Development
Edited by: J. Morganroth and I. Gussak © Humana Press Inc., Totowa, NJ

At that meeting, I declared that any QTc interval prolongation was "bad," even 5 ms. Bad was used in the sense that such a finding raised some element of uncertainty and by inference imparted a mortality risk for a new drug, and that risk could be critical in determining the approvability of a nonantiarrythmic drug, especially if the indication was simply symptom relief. Others said that there must be some degree of prolongation of the QTc interval that would not be important enough to impact on the drug's approvability, of course, trying to define an acceptable risk vs benefit ratio. No person, however, had data (including me) that could be brought to bear on either point of view. The debate and search lives on, although 5 ms as a cut-off has been declared invalid by recent decision making (6 ms must be acceptable, see moxifloxacin).

There are hundreds of references that could be cited and dozens of conferences that could be referenced regarding cardiac repolarization and regulatory inferences but, in my opinion, they all add little to my considerations here, although they do represent a large database of opinions as well as new important data, some of which are represented elsewhere in this book.

What I think has been established is that the QT_C interval duration itself is not a sufficient condition to cause TdP. It is necessary as one component of making the diagnosis, else the ventricular arrhythmia is called multiform or polymorphic ventricular tachycardia. Nonetheless, we also know that persons with hereditary defects of the IK_r cardiac ion channel can have (although some do not) a prolonged QTc interval (presumably from in-utero), but can go decades without developing TdP. Some additional factor (other than the absence of currents mediated by the IK_r channel) is necessary to set off this ventricular tachyarrhythmia. We also now know that those patients who actually have a short QT interval duration on the basis of a hereditary defect in cardiac ion channels may also be at risk for a ventricular arrhythmia (2–4). There seems to be no reason to only be concerned with QT_C prolongation, except that it has been historically associated with TdP.

Since the early 1990s, astemizole, cisapride, grepafloxacin, terfenadine, and terodiline (all of which prolonged the QTc interval duration) were withdrawn from the market because of drug-induced TdP, not because they affect the QT interval. Yet, other drugs such as bepridil, moxifloxacin, and newer antiarrhythmic drugs have been approved for marketing despite known effects on increasing QTc interval duration with some having known TdP associated with their use before approval. These decisions were primarily based on an analysis of the risk vs benefit of a drug. Such assessment is a difficult task and subject always to increasing knowledge and experience. The following nonexhaustive set of examples outline some of the issues, as I remember them, involved in such regulatory assessment. Bear in mind that decisions made were in the context of what was known or believed to be known at the time and only those aspects that have a relationship to QT issues are included. The examples are not organized chronologically, because regulatory actions were taken at various times in relationship to when factual information first became available.

DISCUSSION

Assessment of the Risk–Benefit Ratio

Bepridil Approved 1990 —Still on the Market

Bepridil, a calcium channel blocker, is an example of a regulatory judgment that, loosely interpreted, means if a drug has unusual benefits despite demonstrated increased risk for mortality and, especially if there is no other member of the pharmacological class available for patients, that marketing approval can be achieved. Bepridil was at the time of approval known to produce dose-related increases in QT_C duration (about 8% or 30 to 70 ms change from baseline), as well as other ventricular arrhythmias. Moreover, in French post-marketing experience, Bepridil was known to produce TdP (over an 8 yr duration 124 verified cases were reported).

In more than one trial, bepridil demonstrated anti-anginal efficacy based on symptom-limited exercise tolerance trials. Approval, however, hinged entirely upon one trial in which randomized patients, who were intolerant to or continuing to have symptoms at maximum doses of diltiazem, were shown to respond better to bepridil when compared either to placebo or diltiazem. Thus, it was judged that bepridil was shown to have superior efficacy compared to other approved therapies and such alternatives were not available. Thus, bepridil was approved as a second line agent, approval, reserved for use when all others failed (in such a circumstance it was "better" than nothing because nothing else was available) despite its liability of known QTc prolongation and known TdP and known other ventricular arrhythmias.

MOXIFLOXACIN APPROVED IN 1999—STILL ON THE MARKET

Moxifloxacin, a fluroquinolone antibiotic with a clear dose-related increase in QTc duration and a placebo-corrected mean change from baseline of 6 ms at 400 mg per day was approved. Its short-term use (up to 14 d) for a potentially life-threatening infection was the basis for marketing approval. A phase IV commitment that included a large simple trial was required. In more than 18,000 subjects, the trial revealed no TdP events (*see* Chapter 13). Additionally, post-marketing experience to date has noted about 15 TdP in close to 20 million patients treated, though most if not all had alternative explanations for the TdP event (e.g., concomitant use with sotalol, etc.).

TERFENADINE APPROVED IN 1985—TAKEN OFF THE MARKET IN 1998, CISAPRIDE APPROVED IN 1993—EFFECTIVELY TAKEN OFF THE MARKET IN 2000

Surprisingly, the debates and endless reviews relating to terfenadine (a nonsedating antihistamine) and cisapride (a prokinetic gastrointestinal drug for reflux disease) were not related so much to whether or not TdP was related to their use (even though the incidence was rare, in the range of <1/10,000 to 100,000 exposures), but initially as to whether there was objective demonstration of prolongation of the QT_C interval duration. After further QT studies with terfenadine a mean change from baseline of about 6 ms on average was demonstrated. Although QT_C prolongation was known and production of TdP was uncontested, terfenadine remained on the market ("appropriately" labeled) until another nonsedating antihistamine that did not have the QT_C effects became available. This represents another example of the loosely interpreted principle that "something better than something else" (in this case nonsedating properties) was "worth" the risk.

At the time of cisapride approval, no ECG trial had been conducted. Retrospectively, the then existing data can be interpreted to show an effect on QTc duration in the same range as terfenadine existed. Cisapride was finally removed from active marketing when the FDA and the sponsor (each, initially unwilling to accept the rare reports as representing a risk) accepted that the increasing risk of voluntary post-marketing reports of TdP was not worth the benefit of some relief of dyspepsia.

MIBEFRADIL APPROVED IN 1997—TAKEN OFF THE MARKET IN 1998

Mibefradil, the first selective T-type calcium channel antagonist was withdrawn from the market primarily because of drug–drug interactions (there were serious events associated with at least 24 other drugs commonly used in cardiovascular medicine). The interactions were produced from mainly CYP3A4 inhibition produced by mibefradil. The withdrawal from the market was neither based on its effects on cardiac repolarization nor the observed cases of TdP.

The QT_C issues associated with mibefradil's original approval illustrate the difficulty in defining what to measure as well as how to interpret whatever one measures. The analysis is recounted here, cursorily, because to my knowledge this was the singular (and only) time that the FDA actually looked at raw ECG data and measured QT intervals from raw ECG recordings. The QT_C data we derived were only corrected by Bazett's formula, which was the standard in the mid to late 1990s.

In the original NDA routine analysis of routine ECGs obtained in the clinical trials (hypertension and angina were the target populations' disease indications) produced data that showed that mibefradil prolonged the QT_C interval and the prolongation was dose-related. Were that accepted as fact, mibefradil would not have been approved. Consequently, a great deal of attention was paid to analysis of the QT_C variable by both the sponsors and FDA, and perhaps because of that attention, the implications of the effects of mibefradil on the CYP3A4 system were largely overlooked.

All ECGs that were declared by the previous routine analysis to have had a prolongation of the QT_C was the material that was to be analyzed, by patient and week in study, by myself from original ECGs, calipers, an EXCEL spreadsheet, and two sponsor representatives. After 31 patients' ECGs were examined (probably in the order of 200 or so ECGs) I decided to stop looking at ECGs, because the same phenomenon was boringly and consistently observed in the first 31 patients. So boring and consistent were they, that I decided it was a waste of time to look at any more.

Basically, one had to be sensitive to minuscule U waves seen in the prerandomization records. Surprisingly, U waves could be detected in over 50% of the patients' ECGs. What was measured was both the QT and QU interval if there was a U wave detected (or suggested) in the prerandomized ECGs. Both intervals were then corrected for heart rate by the Bazett formula. In those patients in whom no U wave was detected at baseline, there was a prolongation in the QT_C because no QU had been able to be measured at baseline. In those individuals in whom a U wave was detectable at baseline, there was no change in QU_C although the QT_C was prolonged.

In each of the patients that had a U wave detectable at baseline, lining up the ECGs as a function of weeks in study (e.g., baseline, wk 1, wk 2, wk 4, wk 8, etc.) showed the U wave growing (as a function of time in study), and becoming indistinguishable from the T. Thus, we concluded and the Cardiac and Renal Drugs Advisory Committee concurred, that there was no effect of mibefradil on ventricular repolarization, although there was an alteration of morphology. We and our panel of advisors did not know how to consider this abnormal form of repolarization, and thus we decided that mibefradil should be approved for both hypertension and angina, and that nothing more than a description of the phenomenon should appear in the package insert.

Our conclusion was based on many factors in addition to the lack of effect on intervals. Included among those factors: mibefradil (after very careful exploration of a wide range of concentrations) did nothing but shorten the action potential duration in an in vitro model; animal models of TdP were not able to demonstrate TdP induction by mibefradil; ECGs that showed similar phenomenology when verapamil was administered at high doses in man; some in-silico work produced by Dr. Denis Noble relating mibefradil's known effects on ion channels to surface ECGs; and finally by the relatively event free database associated with the mibefradil development program (though the one patient with a confounded case of TdP may be considered differently today).

Not long after approval (a few months) there were 14 cases of TdP reported to the voluntary adverse drug reaction system of the FDA. Only one of these reports was not confounded by many factors (such as concomitant cisapride use, concomitant bepridil use, congestive heart failure, etc.) and was not considered by the FDA at the time to be sufficient to substantively establish a causative relationship between use of mibefradil and TdP. Subsequently, a report by Glaser et al. *(5)* established a causal relationship by re-challenge. Thus, some agents may have a negative repolarization interval signal but induce repolarization changes with QTc-U wave complexes that may provide, as in the case of mibefradil, a substrate allowing TdP. Thus, careful consideration must be given to the process of ECG acquisition and exposition, and ECGs must be looked at in addition to any analysis of ECG intervals.

SUMMARY OF ANECDOTES

Although the above is an incomplete list of possible anecdotes, the list provided exemplifies that serious post-marketing actions have been based entirely upon clinical events of TdP, and that pre-marketing decision making is spotty at best and in error at worst. Of particular note is that the anecdotes, and my memory, do not include discussions related to the maximum (i.e., peak effect) on QTc in temporal relationship to dose, nor any form of *safety margin* (related to effects at maximum body burden of parent drug and/or metabolites). Such deficiencies in concept have been currently remedied, at least in the Division of Cardiac and Renal Drug Products.

Perhaps more importantly, despite particular recent emphasis on QT measurements (e.g., the Division of Cardiac and Renal Drug Products had around 50 consults per year in early 2000 related to effects of drugs on QT intervals from other FDA divisions), the imprecise value of the QT interval as a predictor of clinical events seems brutally clear. Most of those consultations resulted in determining that there was no definitive information in the data collected and that repeat measurements needed to be made

MEASUREMENT OF THE QT DURATION AND CORRECTION FOR HEART RATE

This book as well as other numerous publications delineates the rather staggering amount of information that has occurred as a consequence of the focus on QT measurements in the drug developing arena. Among the most important being the recognition that using a fixed exponent (in the form of $QT_c = (QT)/RR^{exp}$) is the poorest way to make the heart rate correction for QT to derive the corrected QT or QTc interval. An article by Browne and co-workers *(6)* analyzed the effects of atropine on the QT interval in patients with pacemakers. The effects of atropine when unpaced and the QT interval was estimated by Bazett correction to increase the QT by an average of 43 msec, whereas the actual effect of atropine in the same patients when they were paced was to decrease the QT interval by 24 ms (a 67 ms error).

It now appears reasonable to conclude that the relationship between QT interval and heart rate interval (RR) varies from individual to individual *(7)*, and that the individual relationship is preserved over long times. Moreover, the exponent that can be obtained by fitting the RR QT data from each individual has wide variations from the single fixed exponent values that are commonly used to calculate the QT_C duration. Many examples exist in the author's experience where an apparent QT_C effect calculated by a fixed exponent Bazett or Fridericia method disappears when the individual correction formula method is used.

DIGITAL ECGS: THE CURRENT RECOMMENDATION

Almost all commercially available ECG machines digitize the analog signal recoded from the limb and precordial leads—the original data is recorded in digital format—and then converts the digitized ECG back to an analog waveform for purposes of writing it to paper (so that the ECG can be viewed in conventional format). Among the more rational recent events was the notion that digital ECGs (not paper) should be submitted in support of an NDA and/or other submissions to the FDA for any purpose. Numerous public meetings have been held where the details of this notion have been discussed. At present, the FDA is requesting raw ECG data in the FDA XML schema routinely for all ECG trials (*see* Chapter 16).

Thus, in November 2002 the FDA Concept Paper *(8)* was generated as an attempt to summarize what has been learned since the mid-1980s about the regulatory impact of drugs that affect the QTc interval. The use of digital rather than paper ECGs that are processed, stored, and available for review, as well as careful consideration of methods for ECG analysis and interpretation and the conduct of a trial dedicated to reveal the ECG changes in the target species (man) are detailed in this FDA publication.

EXPERIMENTAL DESIGN WHEN EVALUATING THE QT

Although terfenadine should have sensitized everyone to the P450 system, and indeed it is very unusual for any drug presented for approval today not to have carefully delineated those effects, as late as 1997 (mibefradil) an important signal was missed while pursuing a misleading analysis. Such oversights may again occur, but not when designing an appropriate QT evaluation according to current concepts. The concept of having maximum body burden of parent drug and metabolites at steady state (perhaps requiring the presence of a metabolic inhibitor) is now a clearly enunciated (and although sometimes not enforced) request of the FDA.

Among the more important developments, other than collecting and preserving raw data in original form, is defining a purpose for evaluation of the QT. The first principle is to make the measurement appropriately, thus avoiding the endless arguments over the prolongation or lack of prolongation of the QT. Although there may be no exact way to interpret the results, there should be no doubt as to the drug's effects on this variable as a function of dose. The next is the principle that appropriate experimental design must incorporate the use of a positive control. In other words, not finding an effect on QT for a new drug depends heavily upon the entire clinical trial and its analysis being such that it could find a prolongation, if it had been present. Not a novel concept, but now finally being applied.

Lastly, is the notion that the 12 lead ECGs should be recorded continuously (for new Holter technology methods, *see* Chapter 8) and analyzed at discrete time after dose. After the first analysis is complete, if one concludes that other time points should have been measured to better define the time course of effect, one has a recording that contains the data; as opposed to having to repeat the trial because paper was not collected at those times.

SUMMARY

Perhaps the next decade or two will evolve a more sensible and defensible overall position. For now, evaluation of the QT (as primitive and as nonpredictive as it is) remains the singular means of dispensing "safety concerns." It is the sponsor's task to show that the drug is "safe," not FDA's task to show that the drug is "unsafe." Real risk of rare events can only be explicitly excluded by controlled clinical trials that involve tens to hundreds of thousands of randomized patients; an unachievable and impractical plan. At least from the perspective of QT effects, such "safety assurance" can be currently offered by suitably measuring the QT_C in a suitably designed trial that includes a positive control (*see* Chapter 11). As that becomes common to development programs, discussion can center around the measurement having suitable predictive value in contrast with current discussions that center around the question of is there an effect on the QT_C. Additionally, and aside from the quantitation of intervals, analysis and display of data must incorporate actually being able to see the intervals superimposed upon the raw data. That is a form of progress. Perhaps more will become available as the phenomenology of TdP is elucidated *(9)* and more systematic approaches to assessing risk are evolved.

Such considerations are especially important for treatments that are intended only for symptomatic relief, or where efficacy can be shown with only a small sample size. Alternatives are for a new chemical entity to convincingly show that it is the only therapy available, it is more effective than therapies currently available, its effect is favorable utilizing a morbid/mortal endpoint (and consequently there is no need to worry about rare serious adverse effects), or to conduct trials of at least 100,000 persons to establish that the new therapy is safe (the latter, although seemingly heroic, can only exclude events occurring at a frequency of less than 1 per 160,000 if no events are detected).

REFERENCES

1. Symposium on the QT Interval Prolongation: Is it harmful or beneficial? Edited by Joel Morganroth MD to be Published by Yorke Medical Publishers—August 26, 1993 as a monograph in the American Journal of Cardiology.
2. Gussak I, Brugada P, Brugada J, Wright RS, Kopecky SL, Chaitman BR, Bjerregaard P. Idiopathic short QT interval: a new clinical syndrome? Cardiology 2000;94:99–102.
3. Brugada R, Hong K, Dumaine R, Cordeiro J, Gaita F, Borggrefe M, et al. Sudden death associated with short-QT syndrome linked to mutations in HERG. Circulation. 2004;109:30–35.
4. Schimpf R, Wolpert C, Bianchi F, Giustetto C, Gaita F, Bauersfeld U, Borggrefe M. Congenital short QT syndrome and implantable cardioverter defibrillator treatment: inherent risk for inappropriate shock delivery. J Cardiovasc Electrophysiol. 2003;14:1278–1279.
5. Glaser S, Steinbach M, Opitz C, Wruck U, Kleber FX. Torsades de pointes caused by Mibefradil. Eur J Heart Fail. 2001;3:627–630.
6. Browne KF, Zipes DP, Heger JJ, Prystowsky EN. Influence of the autonomic nervous system on the Q-T interval in man. Am J Cardiol. 1982;50:1099–1103.
7. Malik M, Farbom P, Batchvarov V, Hnatkova K, Camm AJ. Relation between QT and RR intervals is highly individual among healthy subjects: implication for hear rate correction of the QT interval. Heart 2002;87:220–228
8. Food and Drug Administration and Health Canada. The clinical evaluation of QT/QTc interval prolongation and proarrhythmic potential for non-antiarrhythmic drugs. Preliminary Concept paper, November 15, 2002 http//www.fda.gov/cder/workshop.htm#upcoming
9. Fenichel, RR, Malik, M, Antzelevitch, C, Sanguinetti, M, Roden, DM, Priori, S, et alDrug-induced Torsades de Pointes and implications for drug development. J Cardiovasc Electrophsiol2004;15:1–21.

II   Preclinical and Pharmacogenomic Cardiac Safety Evaluations

2   Molecular Physiology of Ion Channels That Control Cardiac Repolarization

Jeanne M. Nerbonne, PhD
and Robert S. Kass, PhD

CONTENTS

INTRODUCTION

The mammalian heart operates as an electromechanical pump, the proper functioning of which depends critically on the sequential activation of cells throughout the myocardium and the coordinated activation of the ventricles (Fig. 1). Electrical signaling in the heart is mediated through regenerative action potentials that reflect the synchronized activity of multiple ion channels that open, close, and inactivate in response to changes in membrane potential (Fig. 1). The rapid upstroke of the action potential (phase 0) in ventricular and atrial cells, for example, is attributed to inward currents through voltage-gated Na$^+$ (Nav) channels. Phase 0 is followed by a rapid phase of repolarization (phase 2), reflecting Nav channel inactivation and the activation of voltage-gated outward K$^+$ (Kv)

From: *Cardiac Safety of Noncardiac Drugs:*
Practical Guidelines for Clinical Research and Drug Development
Edited by: J. Morganroth and I. Gussak © Humana Press Inc., Totowa, NJ

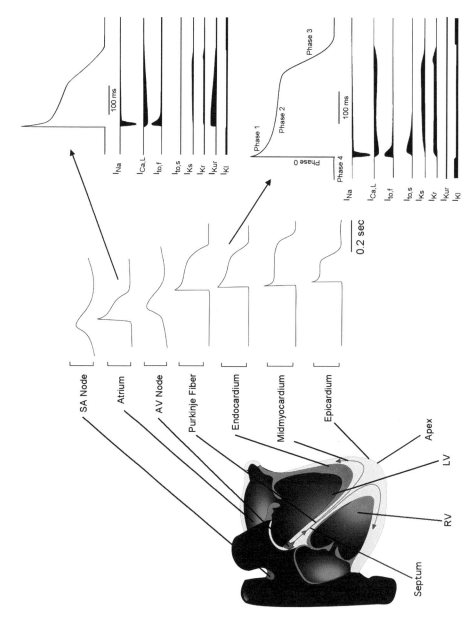

Fig. 1. Regulation of cardiac membrane excitability. Left Panel: schematic of the human heart and the waveforms of the action potentials recorded in different regions of the heart. Right panel: action potentials and underlying ionic currents in adult human atrial (top) and ventricular (bottom) myocytes. The contributions of some K$^+$ currents, such as I$_{Kr}$ and I$_{Kur}$, are distinct in atrial and in ventricular cells.

currents (Fig. 1). In ventricular cells, this transient repolarization or *notch* influences the height and duration of the action potential plateau (phase 2), which depends on the balance of inward (Ca^{2+} and Na^+) currents and outward (K^+) currents. The main contributor of inward current during the plateau phase is Ca^{2+} influx through high threshold, L-type voltage-gated Ca^{2+} (Cav) channels. The (L-type Ca^{2+}) channels undergo Ca^{2+} and voltage-dependent inactivation and, as these channels inactivate, the outward K^+ currents predominate resulting in a second, rapid phase (phase 3) of repolarization back to the resting potential (Fig. 1). The height and duration of the plateau, as well as the time-and voltage-dependent properties of the underlying Na^+, Ca^{2+}, and K^+ channels determine action potential durations in individual cardiac cells. Changes in the properties or the densities of any of these channels, owing to underlying cardiac disease or as a result of the actions of cardiac and noncardiac drugs, therefore, is expected to have dramatic effects on action potential waveforms, refractory periods, and cardiac rhythms.

Electrophysiological studies have detailed the properties of the major voltage-gated inward (Na^+ and Ca^{2+}) and outward (K^+) currents (Table 1) that determine the heights and the durations of cardiac action potentials. In contrast to the Na^+ and Ca^{2+} currents, there are multiple types of myocardial K^+ currents, particularly Kv currents. At least two types of transient outward currents, $I_{to,f}$ and $I_{to,s}$, and several components of delayed rectification, including I_{Kr} ($I_{K(rapid)}$) and I_{Ks} ($I_{K(slow)}$), for example, have been distinguished (Table 1). There are marked regional differences in the expression patterns of these currents, differences that contribute to regional variations in action potential waveforms *(1–3)*. The time- and voltage-dependent properties of the Kv currents in myocytes isolated from different species and/or from different regions of the heart are similar, however, suggesting that the molecular correlates of the underlying channels are also the same. The pore forming (α) and accessory (β, δ, and γ) subunits encoding myocardial Na^+, Ca^{2+}, and K^+ channels have been identified, and considerable progress has been made in defining the relationships between these subunits and functional cardiac Na^+, Ca^{2+}, and K^+ channels.

The densities and the properties of voltage-gated cardiac Na^+, Ca^{2+}, and K^+ currents change during development, reshaping action potential waveforms *(4)* and modifying the sensitivity to cardiac, as well as noncardiac, drugs. Alterations in the densities and properties of voltage-gated Na^+, Ca^{2+}, and K^+ currents also occur in a number of myocardial disease states *(5–12)*. These changes can lead directly or indirectly to arrhythmia generation, as well as influence the sensitivity of individuals to the effects of cardiac and noncardiac drugs that influence the properties and/or the functional expression of these channels. There is, therefore, considerable interest in defining the properties of myocardial ion channels, as well as in delineating molecular mechanisms controlling the regulation, the modulation, and the functional expression of these channels.

INWARD VOLTAGE-GATED NA⁺ CURRENTS IN THE MYOCARDIUM

Voltage-gated Nav channels open rapidly on membrane depolarization and underlie the rising phases of the action potentials in ventricular and atrial myocytes (Fig. 1). The threshold for Nav channel activation is quite negative (-55 mV), and activation is steeply voltage-dependent *(13)*. In addition, Nav channels inactivate rapidly and, during the plateau phase of ventricular action potentials, most of the Nav channels are in an inactivated and nonconducting state *(14–16)*. There is, however, a finite probability (approx 1%) of channel reopening at voltages corresponding to the action potential plateau *(14–17)*. Although the resulting plateau (or "window") Nav current is small in magnitude *(18)*,

Table 1

Cardiac Currents Contributing to Action Potential Repolarization

Channel Type	Current Name	Activation	Inactivation	Recovery	Species	Tissue[1]
NaV	I_{Na}	very fast	fast	fast	cat, dog, ferret, human, mouse, rat	A, P, V, SAN[3], AVN[3]
CaV	$I_{Ca(L)}$	fast	moderat	fast	cat, dog, ferret, human, mouse, rat	A, P, V, SAN, AVN
	$I_{Ca(T)}$	fast	fast	slow	cat, dog, guinea pig, rat	A, P, SAN, AVN
Kv(I_{to})	$I_{to,f}$	fast	fast	fast	cat, dog, ferret, human, mouse, rat	A, P, V
	$I_{to,s}$	fast	moderate	slow	ferret, human, mouse, rat, rabbit	V (A, AVN, SA)[4]
Kv(I_K)	I_{Kr}	moderate	fast	slow	cat, dog, guinea pig, human, mouse, rabbit, rat	A, P, V, SAN, AVN
	I_{Ks}	very slow	no	—	dog, guinea pig, human, rat	A, P, V, SAN
	I_{Kur}	very fast	very slow	slow	dog, human	A
	$I_{K,slow1}$	very fast	slow	slow	mouse	A, V
	I_{Kp}	fast	no	—	guinea pig	V
	$I_{K,slow2}$	fast	very slow	slow	mouse	A, V
	I_K	slow	slow	slow	rat	V
	I_{ss}	slow	no	—		A, V, AVN
Kir	I_{K1}	—	—	—	cat, dog, ferret, human, mouse, rabbit, rat	A, P, V

[1] A = atrial; P = Purkinje; V = ventricular; SAN = sinoatrial node; AVN = atrioventricular node.
[2] Inactivation is Ca^{2+}-, as well as voltage dependent.
[3] Seen in some, but not all, AV and SAN cells.
[4] Seen in atrial and nodal cells only in rabbit.

particularly when compared with the Nav current during phase 0, it does contribute to maintaining the depolarized state, and plays a role in action potential repolarization, particularly in the ventricles.

Although the Nav channel "window" current has been recognized as a determinant of cardiac action potential waveforms for a great many years now *(19,20)*, the identification of inherited mutations in the genes encoding myocardial Nav channels and the delineation of the molecular consequences of these mutations *(14–16)* have clearly demonstrated that plateau Nav currents play a very important role in action potential repolarization. Interestingly, there are regional differences in the expression of the persistent Nav current component *(21)*, differences that may contribute to regional heterogeneities in action potential amplitudes and durations *(1–3)*, as well as impact arrhythmia susceptibility.

INWARD VOLTAGE-GATED MYOCARDIAL CA^{2+} CURRENTS

Two broad classes of voltage-gated Ca^{2+} (Cav) currents/channels, low-voltage-activated (LVA) and high-voltage-activated (HVA), Cav channels, have been distinguished based primarily on differences in the (voltage) threshold of channel activation *(22)*. Similar to Nav channels, the LVA Cav channels activate at relatively hyperpolarized membrane potentials, and these channels activate and inactivate rapidly. HVA Cav channels, in contrast, open on depolarization to membrane potentials more positive than − 20 mV, and these channels inactivate in tens to hundreds of milliseconds. There is considerable variability in the detailed kinetic and pharmacological properties of HVA Ca^{2+} channels expressed in different cell types, and multiple HVA channel types, referred to as L, N, P, Q, or R, have been described *(22,23)*. LVA channels are also often referred to as T (transient) type Ca^{2+} channels *(23)*.

In mammalian cardiac myocytes, L-type HVA Cav currents predominate *(24)*. In response to membrane depolarization, L-type cardiac Cav channels open with a delay relative to the Nav channels, and these channels contribute little to phase 0 (Fig. 1). The Ca^{2+} influx through the L-type Cav channels, however, triggers the release of Ca^{2+} from intracellular Ca^{2+} stores and excitation-contraction coupling *(24)*. At positive potentials, L-type Cav channels undergo rapid voltage- and Ca^{2+}-dependent inactivation, contributing to the termination of action potential plateau and repolarization. It is clear, therefore, that cardiac and noncardiac drugs that modulate the influx of Ca^{2+} through these channels could have profound effects on action potential waveforms and the generation of normal cardiac rhythms.

DIVERSITY OF VOLTAGE-GATED MYOCARDIAL K$^+$ CURRENTS

Voltage-gated K$^+$ (Kv) channel currents influence the amplitudes and durations of cardiac action potentials and, in most cells, two classes of Kv currents have been distinguished: 1. transient outward K$^+$ currents, I$_{to}$, and 2. delayed, outwardly rectifying K$^+$ currents, I$_K$ (Table 1). I$_{to}$ channels activate and inactivate rapidly and underlie the early phase (phase 1) of repolarization, whereas I$_K$ channels determine the latter phase (phase 3) of repolarization (Fig. 1). These are broad classifications, however, and there are multiple Kv currents (Table 1) expressed in cardiac cells. Differences in the expression patterns and the properties of these currents contribute to the observed variations in action potential waveforms recorded in different cardiac cell types (Fig. 1) and in different species *(1–3)*.

The early phase (phase 1) of repolarization is attributed to the activation of Ca^{++}-independent, 4-aminopyridine-sensitive transient outward K^+ currents, variably referred to as I_{to}, I_{to1}, or I_t (25,26). Electrophysiological and pharmacological studies, however, have now clearly demonstrated that there are actually two distinct cardiac transient outward K^+ currents, $I_{to, fast}$ ($I_{to,f}$) and $I_{to,slow}$ ($I_{to,s}$) (27–30). Rapidly activating and inactivating transient outward K^+ currents that are also characterized by rapid recovery from steady-state inactivation are referred to as $I_{to, fast}$ ($I_{to,f}$) (28). The rapidly activating transient outward K^+ currents that recover slowly from inactivation are referred to as $I_{to,slow}$ ($I_{to,s}$) (28). $I_{to,f}$ is a prominent repolarizing current in ventricular and atrial cells in most species (27–37), and is readily distinguished from other Kv currents, including $I_{to,s}$, using the spider K^+ channel toxins, *Heteropoda* toxin-2 or -3 (38). The fact that the properties of $I_{to,f}$ in different species and cell types are similar led to the suggestion that the molecular correlates of the underlying ($I_{to,f}$) channels are the same (25), and considerable experimental evidence in support of this hypothesis has now been provided. Nevertheless, there are differences in the detailed biophysical properties of $I_{to,f}$ channels (39), suggesting that there likely are subtle, albeit important, differences in the molecular compositions of these channels in different cells/species.

In rabbit myocardium, the prominent transient outward K^+ current (I_t) inactivates slowly and recovers from steady-state inactivation very slowly (40–42), and would be classified as $I_{to,s}$. In some species, $I_{to,f}$ and $I_{to,s}$ are co-expressed and differentially distributed (28–30). In all cells isolated from adult mouse right (RV) and left (LV) ventricles, for example, $I_{to,f}$ is expressed, whereas $I_{to,s}$ is undetectable (28–30). In the mouse interventricular septum, in contrast, $I_{to,f}$ and $I_{to,s}$ are co-expressed in approx 80% of the cells, and in $\approx$ 20% of the cells, only $I_{to,s}$ is evident.

Delayed rectifier Kv currents, I_K, have also been characterized extensively in cardiac myocytes and, in most cells, multiple components of I_K (Table 1) are co-expressed. Two prominent components of I_K, I_{Kr} ($I_{K,rapid}$) and I_{Ks} ($I_{K,slow}$), for example, were first distinguished in guinea pig myocytes based on differences in time- and voltage-dependent properties (43–47). I_{Kr} activates rapidly, inactivates very rapidly, displays marked inward rectification and is selectively blocked by several class III antiarrhythmics (44,47). In contrast, no inward rectification is evident for I_{Ks}, and this current is not blocked by the compounds that affect I_{Kr} (44,47). In human (48,49), canine (50), and rabbit (51) ventricular cells, both I_{Kr} and I_{Ks} are expressed and contribute to repolarization. In adult rodent hearts, however, neither I_{Kr} nor I_{Ks} is a prominent repolarizing Kv current, and there are additional components of I_K (Table 1). In rat ventricular myocytes, for example, there are novel delayed rectifier Kv currents, referred to as I_K and I_{ss} (Table 1) (33,52). In mouse ventricular myocytes, three distinct Kv currents, $I_{K,slow1}$, $I_{K,slow2}$, and I_{ss}, are co-expressed (28,53–59). It is clear, therefore, that in efforts focused on evaluating the possibility that there will be unwanted cardiac effects of drugs with clinical potential, it will be important to select the experimental species used in the assays carefully.

In rat (60), canine (61), and human (62,63) atrial myocytes, a novel, rapidly activating and slowly inactivating outward K^+ current, referred to as I_{Kur} ($I_{Kultra rapid}$), is expressed (Table 1). It has been suggested that the expression of I_{Kur}, together with $I_{to,f}$ in atrial myocytes, contributes to the more rapid repolarization evident in atrial, compared with ventricular, myocytes (Fig. 1). However, in guinea pig (64) and mouse (53,57–59) ventricular myoctyes there are voltage-gated outward K^+ currents with biophysical properties similar to atrial I_{Kur}. The rapidly activating μM 4-AP-sensitive component of mouse ventricular $I_{K,slow}$, $I_{K,slow1}$ (57,59) should probably be renamed I_{Kur} (Table 1). Importantly, I_{Kur} is not expressed in human ventricular myocytes or in Purkinje fibers, suggesting that I_{Kur} channels might represent a therapeutic target for the treatment of atrial arrhythmias without complicating effects on ventricular function or performance. The potential of this pharmacological strategy, however, will have to be determined by the atrial specificity/selectivity of the reagents to be developed.

REGIONAL AND DEVELOPMENTAL DIFFERENCES IN ACTION POTENTIAL WAVEFORMS AND IONIC CURRENTS

There are marked regional differences in action potential waveforms in the myocardium (Fig. 1), and these contribute to the normal propagation of activity through the heart and the generation of normal cardiac rhythms. An important determinant of the observed regional differences in action potential waveforms is heterogeneity in Kv current expression *(1–3)*. There are, for example, large variations in ventricular $I_{to,f}$ densities *(27–29,31,32,35,36,65–67)*. In (canine) LV, $I_{to,f}$ density is five- to sixfold higher in epicardial and midmyocardial, than in endocardial, cells *(65)*. The density of $I_{to,s}$ is quite variable *(27–30)*, being detected only in endocardial *(27)* and septum *(28,29)* cells. There are also regional differences in I_{Ks} and I_{Kr} densities. In (canine) LV, for example I_{Ks} density is higher in epicardial and endocardial cells than in M cells *(49)*. In cells isolated from the (guinea pig) LV free wall, I_{Kr} density is higher in subepicardial, than in midmyocardial or subendocardial, myocytes *(68)*. At the base of the LV, in contrast, I_{Kr} and I_{Ks} densities are significantly lower in endocardial than in midmyocardial or epicardial cells *(69)*. These differences contribute to the variations in action potential waveforms recorded in different regions (right vs left; apex vs base) and layers (epicardial, midmyocardial, and endocardial) of the ventricles. In addition, these electrophysiological differences clearly suggest that there will be regional differences in the physiological effects of drugs that affect the properties and/or the functional expression of cardiac Kv channels, differences that could increase the propensity to develop life-threatening arrhythmias.

During postnatal development, myocardial action potentials shorten markedly *(4)*. In ventricular myocardium, for example, phase 1 repolarization becomes more pronounced with age, and functional $I_{to,f}$ density is increased *(52,70–77)*. In addition, action potentials in neonatal cells are insensitive to 4-AP, and voltage-clamp recordings reveal that $I_{to,f}$ is undetectable, whereas, in cells from 60 d postnatal animals, $I_{to,f}$ is present and phase 1 repolarization is clearly evident *(71)*. $I_{to,f}$ density is also low in neonatal mouse *(75)* and rat *(52,70,72,74,76)* ventricular myocytes, and increases several fold during early postnatal development. In rat, the properties of the currents in 1–2 d ventricular myocytes *(76)* are also distinct from those of $I_{to,f}$ in postnatal d 5 to adult cells *(52)* in that inactivation and recovery from inactivation are slower. Indeed, the properties of the transient outward currents in postnatal d 1–2 rat ventricular cells *(76)* more closely resemble $I_{to,s}$ than $I_{to,f}$. In rabbit ventricular myocytes, transient outward K^+ current density increases and the kinetic properties of the currents also change during postnatal development *(73)*. In this case, however, the rate of recovery of the currents is ten times faster in neonatal (mean recovery time ~ 100 ms) than in adult (mean recovery time ~ 1300 ms) cells *(73)*. The slow recovery of the transient outward currents underlies the marked broadening of action potentials at high stimulation frequencies in adult (but not in neonatal) rabbit ventricular myocytes *(73)*. These observations suggest that $I_{to,f}$ is prominent in neonatal rabbit cells and that $I_{to,s}$ dominates repolarization in adult cells. In addition, these observations again reveal species differences in the ionic currents shaping action potential waveforms, again demonstrating the importance of the selection of species in efforts focused on determining drug effects in the myocardium.

Delayed rectifier K^+ current expression also changes during postnatal development. For example, both I_{Kr} and I_{Ks} are readily detected in neonatal mouse ventricular myocytes (77), whereas these currents are not detected in adult cells (28,29). Because I_{Kr} and I_{Ks} are prominent repolarizing K^+ currents in adult human cardiac cells, developmental changes in the expression and/or the properties of these currents will lead to marked changes in action potential waveforms and altered sensitivity to drugs that affect the properties and the functioning of these channels.

INWARDLY RECTIFYING K^+ CHANNELS CONTRIBUTE TO ACTION POTENTIAL REPOLARIZATION

In addition to Kv currents, the inwardly rectifying K^+ (Kir) current (I_{K1}) plays a role in myocardial action potential repolarization (Table 1), and there are marked regional differences in I_{K1} expression in atria, ventricles and conducting tissues (78,79). In atrial and ventricular myocytes and in cardiac Purkinje cells, I_{K1} plays a role in establishing the resting membrane potential, the plateau potential and contributes to phase 3 repolarization (Fig. 1). The strong inward rectification evident in these channels is attributed to block by intracellular Mg^{2+} (80) and by polyamines (81,82). The fact that channel conductance is high at negative membrane potentials underlies the contribution of I_{K1} to resting membrane potentials (79). The voltage dependent properties of I_{K1} channels, however, are such that the conductance is very low at potentials positive to approx –40 mV (78). Nevertheless, because the driving force on K^+ is high at depolarized potentials, I_{K1} channels do contribute outward K^+ current during the plateau phase of the action potential, as well as during phase 3 repolarization (Fig. 1), particularly in ventricular cells. Cardiac and noncardiac drugs that affect the properties or the functioning of I_{K1} channels, therefore, could have rather profound effects on myocardial action potential waveforms, propagation, and rhythmicity and these effects are expected to be region specific, owing to the differential expression of these channels.

MOLECULAR CORRELATES OF VOLTAGE-GATED CARDIAC NA+ (NAV) CHANNELS

Functional cardiac Nav channels reflect the coassembly of Nav pore-forming (α) subunits and accessory (β) subunits. The Nav channel α subunits (Fig. 2A) belong to the "S4" superfamily of voltage-gated ion channel genes. Although a number of Nav α subunits have been identified, Nav1.5 (*SCN5A*) is the one predominantly expressed in the myocardium, and Nav1.5 is the locus of mutations linked to one form of inherited long QT syndrome, LQT3 (Fig. 2A), as well as Brugada syndrome and conduction defects (14–17). Each Nav α subunit has four homologous domains (I to IV), and each domain contains six α-helical transmembrane repeats (S1–S6) (Fig. 2A). The cytoplasmic linker between domains III and IV is a pivotal component of Nav channel inactivation, and a critical isoleucine, phenylalanine, and methionine (IFM) motif in this linker has been identified as the inactivation gate (84–86).

During the plateau phase of ventricular action potentials, approx 99% of the Nav channels are in an inactivated, nonconducting state in which the inactivation gate is

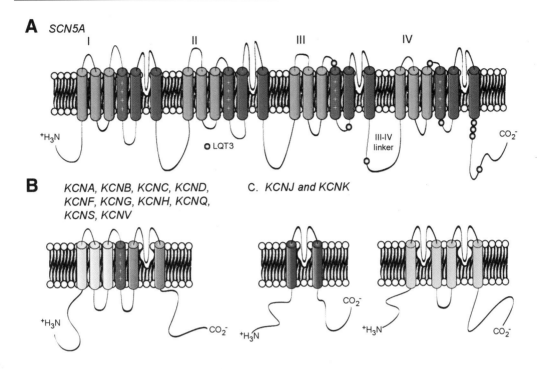

Fig. 2. Pore-forming (α) subunits of cardiac ion channels. Membrane topologies of the α subunits encoding Nav (A), Kv (B), and Kir channels (C) are illustrated. A four transmembrane, two-pore domain K+ (K2P) channel α subunit is also illustrated in C.

thought to occlude the inner mouth of the pore through specific interactions with sites on S6 *(87)* or the S4-S5 loop *(88)* in domain IV. Inherited LQT3 mutations (i.e., ΔKPQ) in the domain III–IV linker in Nav1.5 disrupt inactivation *(89)*. This (ΔKPQ) and other LQT3 mutations result in sustained (bursting) Nav current activity *(89)*, resulting in action potential prolongation in theoretical models *(90)* and in mice genetically engineered with LQT3 mutant Nav channels *(91)*. Analysis of other *SCN5A* mutations, linked both to LQT3 and the Brugada syndrome, however, has revealed that this is not the only mechanism by which altered Nav channel function can prolong cardiac action potentials. A critical role for the carboxy (C)-terminal tail of Nav1.5 channel in the control of channel inactivation, for example, has now been defined *(92–94)*. Point mutations in the C-terminus shift the voltage-dependence of inactivation, promote sustained Na+ channel activity, change the kinetics of both the onset of and recovery from inactivation, and alter drug-channel interactions *(95–98)*. Single channel studies reveal that the C-terminus has pronounced effects on repetitive channel openings *(99)*. Modeling studies suggest that this (C-terminal) domain can adopt a predominantly α-helical structure and that only the proximal region of the C-terminus, which contains this helical domain, appears to measurably affect channel inactivation. Interactions likely occur, therefore, between the structured region of the C-terminus and other components of the channel protein, and these interactions appear to function to stabilize the channel in an inactivated state at depolarized membrane potentials. Drugs that affect these interactions, therefore, will alter Nav channel inactivation, influence action potential waveforms, and affect rhythmicity.

Modeling studies *(100,101)* have also provided insights into the mechanistic basis of the pathophysiology of other LQT3 mutations. The I1768V mutation, for example, does not cause channel bursting, but rather speeds recovery (from inactivation) at hyperpolarized potentials. Computational analysis predicts that this mutation will have a significant effect during action potential repolarization, a prediction that was verified experimentally *(102)*. Similarly, subtle changes in Nav channel gating are caused by a commonly occurring *SCN5A* variant (S1102Y) which is associated with an elevated arrhythmia risk in African Americans *(103)*. This variant causes subtle changes in channel activation and inactivation that are not likely to alter myocyte functioning in mutation carriers, unless these carriers are treated with drugs that block cardiac K^+ channels (103). In this case, computational analysis, in combination with the experimental data, suggests a novel mechanism underlying susceptibility to drug-induced QT prolongation *(103)*.

Functional Nav channels (Fig. 3) are thought to reflect the coassembly of Nav α subunits with accessory Nav β subunits *(104)*, and three different Nav β subunit genes, *SCN1b (105,106)*, *SCN2b (107,108)*, and *SCN3b (109)* have been identified. Co-expression of either *SCN1b* or *SCN3b* with *SCN5A* affects Nav channel kinetics and current densities *(110)*, and *SCN2b (111)* co-expression affects the Ca^{2+} permeability of functional Nav channels *(112)*. The fact that Navβ subunits interact with ankyrin B *(113)*, a cytoskeletal adaptor protein *(114)*, suggests that an important function of these subunits may be to regulate Nav channel function through the cytoskeleton. Consistent with this hypothesis, electrophysiological recordings from myocytes isolated from ankyrin $B^+/-$ hearts reveal increased Nav channel bursting *(115)*. Interestingly, molecular genetic studies have revealed that a loss-of-function mutation in ankyrin B (E1425G) underlies LQT4 *(116)*.

MOLECULAR CORRELATES OF VOLTAGE-GATED CARDIAC CA^{2+} (CAV) CHANNELS

Similar to Nav channels, Cav channel pore-forming (α) subunits belong to the "S4" superfamily of voltage-gated ion channel genes, and these subunits combine with auxiliary β and $\alpha_2\delta$ subunits to form functional Cav channels (Fig. 3). Four distinct subfamilies of Cav α_1 subunits, Cav1, Cav2, Cav3, and Cav4 *(117)*, have been identified, each with many subfamily members. Expression studies reveal that these genes encode Cav channels with distinct time- and voltage-dependent properties and pharmacological sensitivities. Functional expression of any of the Cav1 α subunits, Cav1.1, Cav1.2, Cav1.3, or Cav1.4, for example, reveals L-type HVA Ca^{2+} channel currents, which activate at approx −20 mV and are selectively blocked by dihydropyridine Ca^{2+} channel antagonists. One member of this Cav1 subfamily, Cav1.2, is composed of 44 invariant and six alternative exons *(118)*. Cav1.2 encodes the α_{1C} ($\alpha_1$1.2) protein, and three different isoforms of the α_{1C} protein, $\alpha_1$1.2a, $\alpha_1$1.2b, and $\alpha_1$1.2c *(119,120)*, have been identified. Although nearly identical (>95 %) in amino acid sequences, these isoforms are differentially expressed, and the cardiac specific isoform is $\alpha_1$1.2a *(119)*.

There are two distinct types of Cav accessory subunits, Cavβ and Cav$\alpha_2\delta$ subunits. The β subunits are cytosolic proteins that are believed to form part of each functional L-type Cav channel protein complex (Fig. 3). Four different Cavβ subunits, Cavβ_1 *(121,122)*, Cavβ_2 *(123,124)*, Cavβ_3 *(123–125)*, and Cavβ_4 *(125,126)* have been identified. Each Cavβ subunit has three variable regions (the carboxyl terminus, the amino terminus, and small region in the center of the linear protein sequence) flanking two highly conserved domains. The conserved domains mediate the interaction(s) with Cavα_1 subunits, and the variable domains determine the functional effects of Cavβ subunit

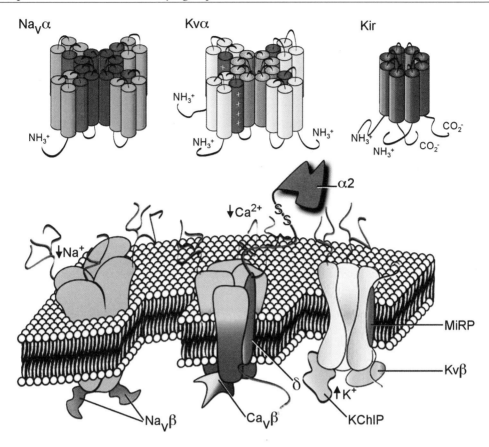

Fig. 3. Molecular compositions of functional cardiac Nav, Cav, and Kv channels. Upper panel: the four domains of Nav (and Cav) α subunit form monomeric Nav (and Cav) channels, whereas four Kv or Kir α subunits combine to form tetrameric Kv and Kir channels. Lower panel: schematic illustrating functional cardiac Nav, Cav, and Kv channels, composed of the pore-forming α subunits and a variety of accessory subunits.

co-expression *(127)*. In co-expression studies, all four Cavβ subunits associate with Cavα₁ subunits and modify the amplitudes, as well as the time- and voltage-dependent properties, of the currents *(128–133)*.

In addition to Cavβ subunits, a disulfide-linked, transmembrane accessory subunit, Cavα₂δ, is also found in the complex of functional Cav channels (Fig. 3). The first Cavα₂δ subunit was cloned from skeletal muscle *(134)*, and there are several members of the Cavα₂δ–1 subfamily, as well as two homologous, Cavα₂δ–2 and Cavα₂δ–3, subfamilies *(135)*. The Cavα₂δ subunits are heavily glycosylated proteins that are cleaved posttranslationally to yield disulfide-linked α₂ and δ proteins. The Cavα₂ domain is extracellular and the Cavδ domain has a large hydrophobic region, which inserts into the membrane (Fig. 3) and anchors the Cavα₂δ complex *(136–138)*. The functional roles of Cavα₂δ are somewhat variable and seem to depend on the identities of the co-expressed Cavα₁ and Cavβ subunits and the expression environment. In general, co-expression of Cavα₂δ–1 alters channel gating and increases current amplitudes, compared with the currents produced on expression of Cavα₁ and Cavβ subunits alone *(135,136,138–140)*. The increase in current density reflects improved targeting of Cavα₁ subunits to the membrane, an effect attributed to the α₂ subunit domain *(141)*.

MOLECULAR CORRELATES OF VOLTAGE-GATED
CARDIAC K⁺ (Kv) CHANNELS

Kv channel pore-forming (α) subunits are six transmembrane spanning domain proteins with an "S4" domain and a K⁺-selective pore (Fig. 2), and functional Kv channels reflect the tetrameric assembly of four α subunits (Fig. 3). Ten homologous Kv α subunit subfamilies, *KCNA, KCNB, KCNC, KCND, KCNF, KCNG, KCNH, KCNQ, KCNS,* and *KCNV*, have been identified (Fig. 2) and in most subfamilies, there are several members *(2)*. In addition to the multiplicity of Kv α subunits, further functional Kv channel diversity can arise through alternative splicing of transcripts and through the formation of heteromultimeric channels *(2)*.

The *KCNH2* subunit, which encodes the ether-a-go-go-related *(143)* or ERG1 protein *(144)*, is the locus of mutations (Fig. 2B) underlie familial long QT syndrome, LQT2 *(145)*. Expression of ERG1 in Xenopus oocytes reveals inwardly rectifying voltage-gated, K⁺-selective currents *(146,147)* with properties similar to cardiac I_{Kr}. There are additional members of the *KCNH* subfamily *(2)*, although none of these appear to be expressed in the heart. Another Kvα subunit, KvLQT1 *(KCNQ1)*, has also been linked to inherited arrhythmias, and mutations in *KCNQ1* (Fig. 2C) underlie LQT1 *(147)*. Although heterologous expression of *KCNQ1* alone reveals rapidly activating and noninactivating K⁺ currents, co-expression with minK produces slowly activating K⁺ currents that resemble the slow component of cardiac delayed rectification, I_{Ks} *(149,150)*. There are additional *KCNQ* subfamily members, *KCNQ2* and *KCNQ3*, although these are not expressed in the heart *(151–153)*. Interestingly, however, *KCNQ2* and *KCNQ3* have been identified as loci of mutations leading to benign familial neonatal convulsions *(151,153)*.

Similar to cardiac Nav and Cav channels, accessory subunits also contribute to the generation of functional cardiac Kv channels. The first identified Kv accessory subunit, minK *(KCNE1)*, is a small (130 amino acids) protein with a single membrane spanning domain *(154–156)* that appears to co-assemble with KvLQT1 to form functional I_{Ks} channels *(149,150)*. Additional minK homologues, MiRP1 *(KCNE2)*, MiRP2 *(KCNE3)*, and MiRP3 *(KCNE4)* have also been identified, and it has been suggested that MiRP1 functions as an accessory subunit of ERG1 in the generation of I_{Kr} *(157,158)*. Although it is unclear whether minK, MiRP1 or other *KCNE* subfamily members contribute to the formation of cardiac Kv channels in addition to I_{Ks} and I_{Kr}, it has been reported that MiRP2 assembles with Kv3.4 in mammalian skeletal muscle *(159)* and with Kv4.x α subunits in heterologous expression systems *(160)*. These observations suggest the interesting possibility that *KCNE* subunits can assemble with different Kv α subunits and contribute to the formation of multiple types of myocardial Kv channels.

The accessory Kvβ subunits are low molecular weight (~ 45 kD) cytosolic proteins, first identified in the brain *(161,162)*. There are four homologous Kv β subunits, Kv β1, Kv β2, Kv β3, and Kv β4, and both Kv β1 and Kv β2 are expressed in the heart *(163–168)*. The presence of Kvβ subunits affects the properties and the cell surface expression of Kv α subunit-encoded K⁺ channels *(163–167)*. Heterologous expression studies suggest that the effects of the Kv β subunits are subfamily specific, i.e., Kv β1, Kv β2, and Kv β3 interact with the Kv 1 subfamily of α subunits *(169,170)*, whereas Kv β4 is specific for the Kv2 subfamily *(171)*. It is not known, however, which Kv α subunit(s) the Kv β1 and Kv β2 subunits associate with in the myocardium.

A distinct Kv channel accessory protein, referred to as KChAP (K⁺ channel accessory protein), was identified in a yeast two hybrid screen *(172)*. Co-expression of KChAP with

Kv2.1 (or Kv2.2) increases functional Kv2.x-induced current densities without measurably affecting the time-dependent and/or the voltage-dependent properties of the currents, suggesting that KChAP functions as a chaperon protein *(172)*. Interestingly, KChAP can also interact with the N-termini of Kv1.x α subunits and with the C-termini of Kvβ1.x subunits *(172)*, suggesting that KChAP may be a multifunctional protein contributing to the generation of several cardiac Kv channels.

A yeast two hybrid screen also lead to the identification of the KChIPs (Kv channel interacting proteins) *(173)*. Of these, only KChIP2 appears to be expressed in the heart (173,174), although there are several splice variants of KChIP2 *(174–176)*. The KChIPs contain multiple EF-hand domains and belong to the recovering family of neuronal Ca^{2+}-sensing (NCS) proteins *(177)*. When co-expressed with Kv4 α subunits, the KChIPs increase current densities, slow current inactivation, speed recovery from inactivation and shift the voltage-dependence of activation *(173)*. However, KChIP co-expression reportedly does not affect the properties or the densities of Kv1.4- or Kv2.1-encoded K^+ currents, suggesting that the modulatory effects of the KChIP proteins are specific for α subunits of the Kv4 subfamily *(173)*. In addition, although the binding of the KChIP proteins to Kv4 α subunits is not Ca^{2+}-dependent, mutations in EF hand domains 2, 3, and 4 eliminate the modulatory effects of KChIP1 on heterologously expressed Kv4.2-encoded K^+ channels *(173)*. It has also been shown that KChIP2 co-immunoprecipitates with Kv4.2 and Kv4.3 α subunits from adult mouse ventricles, consistent with a role for this subunit in the generation of Kv4-encoded cardiac $I_{to,f}$ channels *(178)*. Interestingly, a gradient in KChIP2 message expression is observed through the thickness of the ventricular wall in canine and human heart, suggesting that KChIP2 underlies the observed differences in $I_{to,f}$ densities in the epicardium and endocardium in human and canine ventricles *(174,179)*. However, in rat and mouse there is no gradient in KChIP2 expression, and it appears that differences in Kv4.2 underlie the regional variations in $I_{to,f}$ densities in rodents *(178,180)*.

Although the link is less clear than for Nav channels *(113–115)*, there is evidence to suggest that myocardial Kv channels are also regulated through interactions with the actin cytoskeleton. Using a yeast two-hybrid screen, for example, it has been shown that Kv1α subunits, Kv1.5 and Kv1.4, bind to α-actinin-2 *(181,182)*. In addition, when heterologously expressed, Kv1.5 and α-actinin-2 co-immunoprecipitate, and treatment of cells with cytochalasin B or D reduces the functional cell surface expression of Kv1.5-encoded K^+ channels *(181,182)*. It has also been reported that α subunits of the Kv4 subfamily interact directly with another actin-binding protein, filamin *(183)*, and that disruption of the cytoskeleton increases the density of heterologously expressed Kv4-encoded K^+ currents *(184)*. Although the role of cytoskeletal-channel interactions in the myocardium and the molecular mechanisms involved in mediating these interactions remain to be defined, it seems reasonable to suggest that cardiac Kv (and other) channels function as components of macromolecular complexes. Clearly, drugs that interact with any of the complex components or that affect interactions between complex components could, in principle, affect channel properties and myocardial function.

RELATIONS BETWEEN KV SUBUNITS AND FUNCTIONAL CARDIAC KV CURRENTS

Considerable experimental evidence has accumulated documenting a role for Kv α subunits of the Kv4 subfamily in the generation of cardiac $I_{to,f}$ channels *(185–188)*. In ventricular myocytes isolated from transgenic mice expressing a dominant negative pore mutant of Kv4.2 (Kv4.2W362F), Kv4.2DN in the myocardium, for example, $I_{to,f}$ is eliminated *(187)*. In addition, biochemical and electrophysiological studies suggest that Kv4.2 and Kv4.3 are associated in adult mouse ventricles and that functional mouse ventricular $I_{to,f}$ are heteromeric *(178)*. However, in large mammals, including humans, it appears that $I_{to,f}$ channels are Kv4.3 homomultimers because Kv4.2 is not expressed *(189)*. The fact that the properties of $I_{to,s}$ are different from $I_{to,f}$ (Table 1), suggested that the molecular correlates of $I_{to,s}$ and $I_{to,f}$ channels are also distinct. Direct experimental support for this hypothesis was provided with the demonstration that $I_{to,s}$ is eliminated *(29)* in ventricular myocytes isolated from mice with a targeted deletion in the Kv1.4 gene *(190)*. Given the similarities in current properties, it seems reasonable to suggest that Kv1.4 also encodes $I_{to,s}$ in other species, including humans.

As noted earlier, *KCNH2* is the locus of mutations in LQT2 and has been shown to encode I_{Kr} *(145–147)*, and *KCNQ1*, the locus of mutations leading in LQT1 *(148)*, encodes cardiac I_{Ks} *(149,140)*. The fact that mutations in the transmembrane domain of minK alter the properties of heterologously expressed *KCNQ1* and minK Kv channels suggests that the transmembrane segment of minK also contributes to the I_{Ks} channel pore *(191–194)*. Alternative experimental strategies, primarily in mice, have been exploited to define the molecular correlates of several other myocardial Kv currents. A role for Kv2 α subunits in the generation of mouse ventricular $I_{K,slow2}$, for example, was revealed with the demonstration that $I_{K,slow2}$ is selectively attenuated in ventricular myocytes isolated from transgenic mice expressing a truncated Kv2.1 α subunit that functions as a dominant negative *(55)*. Subsequently, it was also shown that $I_{K,slow1}$ is eliminated in ventricular myocytes isolated from mice with targeted deletion of Kv1.5 (57), revealing that Kv1.5 encodes mouse ventricular $I_{K,slow1}$ *(57,59)*. These findings, together with the previous results obtained on cells isolated from Kv1.4 null animals, in which $I_{to,s}$ is eliminated *(29)*, suggest that, in contrast to the Kv 4 α subunits *(178)*, myocardial Kv 1 α subunits, Kv1.4 and Kv1.5, do not associate in situ. Rather, functional cardiac Kv1 α subunit-encoded K+ channels are homomeric, composed of Kv1.4 α subunits ($I_{to,s}$) or Kv1.5 α subunits ($I_{K,slow1}$, I_{Kur}).

MOLECULAR CORRELATES OF OTHER CARDIAC K+ CURRENTS

In cardiac and other cells, the inwardly rectifying K+ (Kir) channels are encoded by a large and diverse subfamily of Kir channel α subunit genes, each of which encodes a protein with two transmembrane domains (Fig. 2C). Similar to Kv channels, Kir subunits assemble as tetramers to form K+ selective pores (Fig. 3). Based on the properties of the currents produced in heterologous expression systems, it has been suggested that Kir2 α subunits encode cardiac I_{K1} channels *(195)*, and several members of the Kir 2 subfamily are expressed in the myocardium *(196)*. Direct support for a role for Kir 2 α subunits in the generation of I_{K1} channels was provided in studies completed on myocytes isolated from mice with a targeted deletion of Kir2.1 (Kir2.1–/–) or Kir 2.2 (Kir2.2–/–) *(197,198)*. Although the Kir2.1–/– mice have cleft palate and die shortly after birth *(197)*, voltage-clamp recordings from newborn Kir2.1–/– ventricular myocytes revealed that I_{K1} is absent *(198)*. A small, slowly activating inward rectifier current, distinct from I_{K1}, however, is evident in Kir2.1–/– myocytes. Voltage-clamp recordings from adult Kir2.2–/– ventricular myocytes reveal that I_{K1} is reduced *(198)*. Taken together, these results suggest that both Kir2.1 and Kir2.2 contribute to functional cardiac I_{K1} channels. The observation that Kir2.2 does not generate I_{K1} channels in the absence of Kir2.1, however, further suggests that functional cardiac I_{K1} channels are heteromeric.

A novel type of K$^+$ channel α subunit with four transmembrane spanning regions and two pore domains (Fig. 2C) was identified with the cloning of TWIK-1 *(199)*. Both pore domains are functional and TWIK subunits assemble as dimers, rather than tetramers *(200)*. There are a great many four transmembrane and two pore domain K$^+$ (K2P) channel α subunit *(KCNK)* genes, and expression studies suggest that the members of various K2P subunit subfamilies give rise to currents that display distinct current-voltage-relations and differential sensitivities to a variety of modulators, including pH and fatty acids *(200)*. Nevertheless, the physiological roles of these subunits/channels in the myocardium, as well as in other cell types, remain to be determined. The K2P subunits TREK-1 and TASK-1, for example, are both expressed in the heart and heterologous expression of either of these subunits gives rise to instantaneous, noninactivating K$^+$ currents that display little or no voltage-dependence *(200)*. These properties have led to suggestions that these subunits contribute to "background" or "leak" currents *(201)*, and interestingly, expressed TREK-1 or TASK-1 currents are similar to the current referred to as I_{Kp} in guinea pig ventricular myocytes *(64,202)*.

SUMMARY AND CONCLUSIONS

Electrophysiological studies have clearly identified multiple types of voltage-gated inward and outward currents that contribute to action potential repolarization in the mammalian myocardium (Table 1). Interestingly, the outward currents are more numerous and more diverse than the inward currents, and cardiac myocytes express a repertoire of Kv channels/currents that contribute importantly to shaping the waveforms of action potentials, as well as influencing automaticity and refractoriness. Changes in the properties or the functioning of cardiac Kv channels during development, owing to underlying cardiac disease or resulting from the actions of cardiac or non-cardiac drugs, can, therefore, have rather dramatic effects on myocardial action potential waveforms and the generation of normal cardiac rhythms.

In addition to the demonstrated importance of repolarizing Kv currents in the myocardium, however, it is also quite clear that Cav channel currents and the Nav channel "window" current also contribute importantly to action potential repolarization. This has been very elegantly demonstrated for Nav channels with the characterization of inherited mutations in the cardiac Nav *SCN5A* gene, mutations that underlie Long QT3, Brugada syndrome, and conduction defects. Functional characterization of these mutants and computer simulations of cellular electrical activity together have provided new insights into the effects of altered channel functioning on action potential waveforms and rhythmicity *(100,101,117,138,139,203)*. These studies demonstrate that small changes in Nav channel currents can have profound effects on repolarization because the plateau phase of the action potential is maintained by the delicate balance of small (inward and outward) currents. It is very clear, therefore, that cardiac or noncardiac drugs that affect Nav channel currents will influence action potential durations. Because cardiac Cav channels also control the plateau phase of cardiac action potentials and action potential repolarization, changes in Cav channel currents will also have functional consequences. Indeed, it seems reasonable to suggest that drugs that affect the functional expression and/or the properties of any of the (inward or outward current) channels that contribute to shaping action potentials would have been expected to impact the propagation of activity and the generation of cardiac rhythms. When considering screening of noncardiac (as well as cardiac) drugs, therefore, effects on all of the various cardiac ion channels that contribute to repolarization must be considered.

In addition to the diversity of voltage-gated ion channel pore-forming α subunits, molecular and biochemical studies have now demonstrated that there are multiple accessory subunits that contribute to the formation of the various cardiac inward and outward current channels. Recent studies also suggest that channel subunit interactions with the actin cytoskeleton are important in determining functional cardiac (Nav and Kv) channel expression. Although it seems quite clear that the relationships between channel subunits and regulatory molecules are important in determining channel expression and/or properties, very little is presently known about the molecular interactions involved and/or the role(s) of these interactions in determining the properties and/or the functioning of the various cardiac ion channels involved in mediating repolarization. Nevertheless, these channel subunit-subunit and channel subunit-regulatory protein interactions are also potential sites of action of cardiac and noncardiac drugs. It seems reasonable to suggest, therefore, that defining the molecular correlates/compositions of the channels controlling cardiac action potential waveforms in detail will facilitate future efforts focused on delineating the mechanisms controlling the properties and the functional expression of these channels in the developing, aging, damaged, or diseased myocardium. In addition, however, this information will provide fresh new insights into the repertoire of proteins that play roles in regulating the properties and the expression of myocardial ion channels and into the detailed molecular mechanisms involved in mediating these effects. Probing these molecular mechanisms in detail is requisite to understanding the factors controlling channel expression and properties during normal cardiac development, as well as in the aged, damaged, and/or diseased myocardium. Also, because any step in the regulatory pathway could potentially be affected by cardiac and/or noncardiac drugs, it will become increasingly important to understand these pathways in detail, as well as how the various drugs might affect one or more steps in channel regulatory pathways, to minimize potentially dangerous, life-threatening drug effects. Clearly, a major focus of future research will be on defining the molecular mechanisms controlling the properties and the functioning of myocardial ion channels in great detail.

REFERENCES

1. Antzelevitch C, Dumaine R. Electrical heterogeneity in the heart: physiological, pharmacological and clinical implications. In Handbook of Physiology. Vol. 1. Solaro RJ, ed.. New York: Oxford, 2002:654–692.
2. Nerbonne JM. Molecular analysis of voltage-gated K⁺ channel diversity and functioning in the mammalian heart. In Handbook of Physiology. Vol. 1. Solaro RJ, ed. New York: Oxford, 2002:568–594.
3. Nerbonne JM, Guo W. Heterogeneous expression of voltage-gated potassium channels in the heart: Roles in normal excitation and arrhythmias. J Cardiovasc Electrophysiol 2002;13:406–409.
4. Wetzel GT, Klitzner TS. Developmental cardiac electrophysiology recent advances in cellular physiology. Cardiovasc Res 1996; 31 Spec No:E52–E60.
5. Beuckelmann DJ, Näbauer M, Erdmann E. Alterations of K⁺ currents in isolated human ventricular myocytes from patients with terminal heart failure. Circ Res 1993; 73:379–385.
6. Näbauer M, Beuckelmann DJ, Erdmann E. Characteristics of transient outward current in human ventricular myocytes from patients with terminal heart failure. Circ Res 1993; 73:386–394.
7. Boyden PA, Jeck CD. Ion channel function in disease. Cardiovasc Res 1995; 29:312–318.
8. Bailly P, Benitah JP, Mouchoniere M, Vassort G, Lorente P. Regional alteration of the transient outward current in human left ventricular septum during compensated hypertrophy. Circulation 1997; 96:1266–1274.

9. Näbauer M, Kääb S. Potassium channel down-regulation in heart failure. Cardiovasc Res 1998; 37: 324–334.

10. Bolli R, Marbán E. Molecular and cellular mechanisms of myocardial stunning. Physiol Rev 1999; 79:609–634.

11. Tomaselli GF, Marbán E. Electrophysiological remodeling in hypertrophy and heart failure. Cardiovasc Res 1999; 42:270–283.

12. Van Wagoner D. Electrophysiological remodeling in human atrial fibrillation. Pacing and Clin Electrophysiol 2003; 26:1572–1575.

13. Catterall WA. From ionic currents to molecular mechanisms: the structure and function of voltage-gated sodium channels. Neuron 2000; 26:13–25.

14. Bennett PB. Long QT syndrome: biophysical and pharmacologic mechanisms in LQT3. J Cardiovasc Electrophysiol 2000; 11:819–822.

15. Keating MT, Sanguinetti MC. Molecular and cellular mechanisms of cardiac arrhythmias. Cell 2001; 104:569–580.

16. Balser JR. Inherited sodium channelopathies: models for acquired arrhythmias? Am J Physiol 2002; 282:H1175-H1180.

17. Clancy CE, Kass RS. Defective cardiac ion channels: from mutations to clinical syndromes. J Clin Invest 2002; 110:1075–1077.

18. Attwell D, Cohen I, Eisner D, Ohba M, Ojeda C. The steady state TTX-sensitive ("window") sodium current in cardiac Purkinje fibres. Pflugers Arch 1979; 379:137–142.

19. Weidmann S. Effect of current flow on the membrane potential of cardiac muscle. J Physiol 1951; 115:227–236.

20. Salata JJ, Wasserstrom JA. Effects of quinidine on action potentials and ionic currents in isolated canine ventricular myocytes. Circ Res 1988; 62:324–337.

21. Sakmann BF, Spindler AJ, Bryant SM, Linz KW, Noble D. Distribution of a persistent sodium current across the ventricular wall in guinea pigs. Circ Res 2000; 87:910–914.

22. Bean BP. Classes of calcium channels in vertebrate cells. Ann Rev Physiol 1989; 51:367–384.

23. Perez-Reyes E. T type Ca channels. Physiol Rev 2003; 83:117–161.

24. Bers D, Perez-Reyes E. Ca channels in cardiac myocytes: Structure function in Ca influx and intracellular Ca release. Cardiovasc Res 1999; 42:339–360.

25. Barry DM, Nerbonne JM. Myocardial potassium channels: electrophysiological and molecular diversity. Annu Rev Physiol 1996; 58:363–394.

26. Campbell DL, Rasmusson RL, Qu Y, Strauss HC. The calcium-independent transient outward potassium current in isolated ferret right ventricular myocytes. I. Basic characterization and kinetic analysis. J Gen Physiol 1993; 101:571–601.

27. Brahmajothi MV, Campbell DL, Rasmusson RL, Morales MJ, Trimmer JS, Nerbonne JM, Strauss HC. Distinct transient outward potassium current (Ito) phenotypes and distribution of fast-inactivating potassium channel alpha subunits in ferret left ventricular myocytes. J Gen Physiol 1999; 113:581–600.

28. Xu H, Guo W, Nerbonne JM. Four kinetically distinct depolarization-activated K^+ currents in adult mouse ventricular myocytes. J Gen Physiol 1999; 113:661–678.

29. Guo W, Xu H, London B, Nerbonne JM. Molecular basis of transient outward K^+ current diversity in mouse ventricular myocytes. J Physiol 1999; 521 Pt 3:587–599.

30. Guo W, Li H, London B, Nerbonne JM. Functional consequences of elimination of $I_{(to,f)}$ and $I_{(to,s)}$: early afterdepolarizations, atrioventricular block, and ventricular arrhythmias in mice lacking Kv1.4 and expressing a dominant-negative Kv4 alpha subunit. Circ Res 2000; 87:73–79.

31. Furukawa T, Myerburg RJ, Furukawa N, Bassett AL, Kimura S. Differences in transient outward currents of feline endocardial and epicardial myocytes. Circ Res 1990; 67:1287–1291.

32. Litovsky SH, Antzelevitch C. Transient outward current prominent in canine ventricular epicardium but not endocardium. Circ Res 1988; 62:116–126.

33. Apkon M, Nerbonne JM. Characterization of two distinct depolarization-activated K+ currents in isolated adult rat ventricular myocytes. J Gen Physiol 1991; 97:973–1011.

34. Wettwer E, Amos G, Gath J, Zerkowski HR, Reidemeister JC, Ravens U. Transient outward current in human and rat ventricular myocytes. Cardiovasc Res 1993; 27:1662–1669.

35. Wettwer E, Amos GJ, Posival H, Ravens U. Transient outward current in human ventricular myocytes of subepicardial and subendocardial origin. Circ Res 1994; 75:473–482.

36. Konarzewska H, Peeters GA, Sanguinetti MC. Repolarizing K^+ currents in nonfailing human hearts. Similarities between right septal subendocardial and left subepicardial ventricular myocytes. Circulation 1995; 92:1179–1187.

37. Yue L, Feng J, Li GR, Nattel S. Transient outward and delayed rectifier currents in canine atrium: properties and role of isolation methods. Am J Physiol 1996; 270:H2157—H2168.

38. Sanguinetti MC, Johnson JH, Hammerland LG, et al. Heteropodatoxins: peptides isolated from spider venom that block Kv4.2 potassium channels. Mol Pharmacol 1997; 51:491–498.

39. Akar FG, Wu RC, Deschenes I, Armoundas AA, Piacentino V, Houser SR, Tomaselli GF. Phenotypic differences in transient outward K^+ current of human and canine ventricular myocytes: insights into molecular composition of ventricular I_{to}. Am J Physiol 2004; 286:H602–H609.

40. Giles WR, Imaizumi Y. Comparison of potassium currents in rabbit atrial and ventricular cells. J Physiol 1988; 405:123–145.

41. Fedida D, Giles WR. Regional variations in action potentials and transient outward current in myocytes isolated from rabbit left ventricle. J Physiol 1991; 442:191–209.

42. Wang Z, Feng J, Shi H, Pond A, Nerbonne JM, Nattel S. Potential molecular basis of different physiological properties of the transient outward K^+ current in rabbit and human atrial myocytes. Circ Res 1999; 84:551–561.

43. Horie M, Hayashi S, Kawai C. Two types of delayed rectifying K^+ channels in atrial cells of guinea pig heart. Jpn J Physiol 1990; 40:479–490.

44. Sanguinetti MC, Jurkiewicz NK. Delayed rectifier outward K^+ current is composed of two currents in guinea pig atrial cells. Am J Physiol 1991; 260:H393–H399.

45. Walsh KB, Arena JP, Kwok WM, Freeman L, Kass RS. Delayed-rectifier potassium channel activity in isolated membrane patches of guinea pig ventricular myocytes. Am J Physiol 1991; 260: H1390–H1393.

46. Anumonwo JM, Freeman LC, Kwok WM, Kass RS. Delayed rectification in single cells isolated from guinea pig sinoatrial node. Am J Physiol 1992; 262:H921– H925.

47. Follmer CH, Colatsky TJ. Block of delayed rectifier potassium current, IK, by flecainide and E-4031 in cat ventricular myocytes. Circulation 1990; 82:289–293.

48. Wang Z, Fermini B, Nattel S. Rapid and slow components of delayed rectifier current in human atrial myocytes. Cardiovasc Res 1994; 28:1540–1546.

49. Li GR, Feng J, Yue L, Carrier M, Nattel S. Evidence for two components of delayed rectifier K^+ current in human ventricular myocytes. Circ Res 1996; 78:689–696.

50. Liu DW, Antzelevitch C. Characteristics of the delayed rectifier current (I_{Kr} and I_{Ks}) in canine ventricular epicardial, midmyocardial, and endocardial myocytes. A weaker I_{Ks} contributes to the longer action potential of the M cell. Circ Res 1995; 76:351–365.

51. Veldkamp MW, van Ginneken AC, Bouman LN. Single delayed rectifier channels in the membrane of rabbit ventricular myocytes. Circ Res 1993; 72:865–878.

52. Xu H, Dixon JE, Barry DM, Trimmer JS, Merlie JP, McKinnon D, Nerbonne JM. Developmental analysis reveals mismatches in the expression of K^+ channel alpha subunits and voltage-gated K^+ channel currents in rat ventricular myocytes. J Gen Physiol 1996; 108:405–419.

53. Fiset C, Clark RB, Larsen TS, Giles WR. A rapidly activating sustained K^+ current modulates repolarization and excitation-contraction coupling in adult mouse ventricle. J Physiol 1997; 504(Pt 3):557–563.

54. Zhou J, Jeron A, London B, Han X, Koren G. Characterization of a slowly inactivating outward current in adult mouse ventricular myocytes. Circ Res 1998; 83:806–814.

55. Xu H, Barry DM, Li H, Brunet S, Guo W, Nerbonne JM. Attenuation of the slow component of delayed rectification, action potential prolongation, and triggered activity in mice expressing a dominant-negative Kv2 alpha subunit. Circ Res 1999; 85:623–633.

56. London B, Jeron A, Zhou J, Buckett P, Han X, Mitchell GF, Koren G. Long QT and ventricular arrhythmias in transgenic mice expressing the N terminus and first transmembrane segment of a voltage-gated potassium channel. Proc Natl Acad Sci USA 1998; 95:2926–2931.

57. London B, Guo W, Pan XH, Lee JS, Shusterman V, Logothetis DA, Nerbonne JM, Hill JA. Targeted replacement of Kv1.5 in the mouse leads to loss of the 4 amino pyridine-sensitive component of $I_{K,slow}$ and resistance to drug-induced QT prolongation. Circ Res 2001; 88:940–946.

58. Zhou J, Kodirov S, Murata M, Buckett PD, Nerbonne JM, Koren G. Regional upregulation of Kv2.1-encoded current, $I_{K,slow1}$, in Kv1 DN mice is abolished by crossbreeding with Kv2 DN mice. Am J Physiol 2003; 284:H491–H500.

59. Li H, Guo W, Yamada KA, Nerbonne JM. Selective elimination of one component of delayed rectification, $I_{K,slow1}$, in mouse ventricular myocytes expressing a dominant negative $Kv1.5\alpha$ subunit. Am J Physiol 2004; 286:H319–H328.

60. Boyle WA, Nerbonne JM. Two functionally distinct 4-aminopyridine-sensitive outward K^+ currents in rat atrial myocytes. J Gen Physiol 1992; 100:1041–1067.

61. Yue L, Feng J, Li GR, Nattel S. Characterization of an ultra rapid delayed rectifier potassium channel involved in canine atrial repolarizzation. J Physiol 1996;496:647–662.

62. Wang Z, Fermini B, Nattel S. Sustained depolarization-induced outward current in human atrial myocytes. Evidence for a novel delayed rectifier K⁺ current similar to Kv1.5 cloned channel currents. Circ Res 1993; 73:1061–1076.

63. Wang Z, Fermini B, Nattel S. Delayed rectifier outward current and repolarization in human atrial myocytes. Circ Res 1993; 73:276–285.

64. Yue D, Marbán E. A novel potassium channel that is active and conductive at depolarized potentials. Pflügers Arch 1988;413:127–133.

65. Liu DW, Gintant GA, Antzelevitch C. Ionic basis for electrophysiological distinctions among epicardial, midmyocardial, and endocardial myocytes from the free wall of the canine left ventricle. Circ Res 1993; 72:671–687.

66. Clark RB, Bouchard RA, Salinas-Stefanon E, Sanchez-Chapula J, Giles WR. Heterogeneity of action potential waveforms and potassium currents in rat ventricle. Cardiovasc Res 1993; 27:1795–1799.

67. Furukawa T, Kimura S, Furukawa N, Bassett AL, Myerburg RJ. Potassium rectifier currents differ in myocytes of endocardial and epicardial origin. Circ Res 1992; 70:91–103.

68. Main MC, Bryant SM, Hart G. Regional differences in action potential characteristics and membrane currents of guinea-pig left ventricular myocytes. Exp Physiol 1998; 83:747–761.

69. Bryant SM, Wan X, Shipsey SJ, Hart G. Regional differences in the delayed rectifier current (I_{Kr} and I_{Ks}) contribute to the differences in action potential duration in basal left ventricular myocytes in guinea-pig. Cardiovasc Res 1998; 40:322–331.

70. Kilborn MJ, Fedida D. A study of the developmental changes in outward currents of rat ventricular myocytes. J Physiol 1990; 430:37–60.

71. Jeck CD, Boyden PA. Age-related appearance of outward currents may contribute to developmental differences in ventricular repolarization. Circ Res 1992; 71:1390–1403.

72. Wahler GM, Dollinger SJ, Smith JM, Flemal KL. Time course of postnatal changes in rat heart action potential and in transient outward current is different. Am J Physiol 1994; 267:H1157—H1166.

73. Sanchez-Chapula J, Elizalde A, Navarro-Polanco R, Barajas H. Differences in outward currents between neonatal and adult rabbit ventricular cells. Am J Physiol 1994; 266:H1184—H1194.

74. Shimoni Y, Fiset C, Clark RB, Dixon JE, McKinnon D, Giles WR. Thyroid hormone regulates postnatal expression of transient K⁺ channel isoforms in rat ventricle. J Physiol 1997; 500 (Pt 1):65–73.

75. Wang L, Duff HJ. Developmental changes in transient outward current in mouse ventricle. Circ Res 1997; 81:120–127.

76. Wickenden AD, Kaprielian R, Parker TG, Jones OT, Backx PH. Effects of development and thyroid hormone on K⁺ currents and K+ channel gene expression in rat ventricle. J Physiol 1997; 504(Pt 2):271–286.

77. Wang L, Feng Z, Kondo C, Sheldon RS, Duff HJ. Developmental changes in the delayed rectifier K+ channels in mouse heart. Circ Res 1996; 79:79–85.

78. Nichols CG, Lopatin AN. Inward rectifier potassium channels. Annu Rev Physiol 1997; 59:171–191.

79. Lopatin AN, Nichols CG. Inward rectifiers in the heart: an update on I_{K1}. J Mol Cell Cardiol 2001; 33:625–638.

80. Vandenberg CA. Inward rectification of a potassium channel in cardiac ventricular cells depends on internal magnesium ions. Proc Natl Acad Sci USA 1987; 84:2560–2564.

81. Ficker E, Taglialatela M, Wible BA, Henley CM, Brown AM. Spermine and spermidine as gating molecules for inward rectifier K⁺ channels. Science 1994; 266:1068–1072.

82. Lopatin AN, Makhina EN, Nichols CG. Potassium channel block by cytoplasmic polyamines as the mechanism of intrinsic rectification. Nature 1994; 372:366–369.

83. Patton DE, West JW, Catterall WA, Goldin AL. Amino acid residues required for fast Na⁺-channel inactivation: charge neutralizations and deletions in the III-IV linker. PNAS, USA 1992; 89: 10905–10909.

84. Vassilev PM, Scheuer T, Catterall WA. Identification of an intracellular peptide segment involved in sodium channel inactivation. Science 1988; 241:1658–1661.

85. Vassilev P, Scheuer T, Catterall WA. Inhibition of inactivation of single sodium channels by a site-directed antibody. Proc Natl Acad Sci USA 1989; 86:8147–8151.

86. West JW, Patton DE, Scheuer T, Wang Y, Goldin AL, Catterall WA. A cluster of hydrophobic amino acid residues required for fast Na⁺-channel inactivation. Proc Natl Acad Sci USA 1992; 89:10910–10914.

87. McPhee JC, Ragsdale DS, Scheuer T, Catterall WA. A critical role for transmembrane segment IVS6 of the sodium channel alpha subunit in fast inactivation. Journal of Biological Chemistry 1995; 270: 12025–12034.

88. McPhee JC, Ragsdale DS, Scheuer T, Catterall WA. A critical role for the S4-S5 intracellular loop in domain IV of the sodium channel alpha-subunit in fast inactivation. Journal of Biological Chemistry 1998; 273:1121–1129.

89. Bennett PB, Yazawa K, Makita N, George AL. Molecular mechanism for an inherited cardiac arrhythmia. Nature 1995; 376:683–685.

90. Clancy CE, Rudy Y. Linking a genetic defect to its cellular phenotype in a cardiac arrhythmia. Nature 1999; 400:566–569.

91. Nuyens D, Stengl M, Dugarmaa S, Rossenbacker T, Compernolle V, Rudy Y, Smits JF, Flameng W, Clancy CE, Moons L, Vos MA, Dewerchin M, Benndorf K, Collen D, Carmeliet E, Carmeliet P. Abrupt rate accelerations or premature beats cause life-threatening arrhythmias in mice with long-QT3 syndrome. Nat Med 2001; 7:1021–1027.

92. Bennett PB. Long QT syndrome: biophysical and pharmacologic mechanisms in LQT3. J Cardiovasc Electrophysiol 2000; 11:819–822.

93. Kambouris NG, Nuss HB, Johns DC, Marban E, Tomaselli G, Balser JR. A revised view of cardiac sodium channel "blockade" in the long-QT syndrome. J Clin Invest 2000; 105:1133–1140.

94. Viswanathan PC, Bezzina CR, George AL, Jr, Roden DM, Wilde AA, Balser JR. Gating-dependent mechanisms for flecainide action in SCN5A-linked arrhythmia syndromes. Circulation 2001; 104:1200–1205.

95. Abriel H, Wehrens XH, Benhorin J, Kerem B, Kass RS. Molecular pharmacology of the sodium channel mutation D1790G linked to the long-QT syndrome. Circulation 2000; 102:921–925.

96. Benhorin J, Taub R, Goldmit M, Kerem B, Kass RS, Windman I, Medina A. Effects of flecainide in patients with new SCN5A mutation: mutation-specific therapy for long-QT syndrome? Circulation 2000; 101:1698–1706.

97. Liu H, Tateyama M, Clancy CE, Abriel H, Kass RS. Channel openings are necessary but not sufficient for use-dependent block of cardiac Na+ channels by flecainide: Evidence from the analysis of disease-linked mutations. J Gen Physiol 2002; 120:39–51.

98. Keating MT, Atkinson D, Dunn C, Timothy K, Vincent GM, Leppert M. Evidence of genetic heterogeneity in the long QT syndrome. Science 1993; 260:1960–1961.

99. Cormier JW, Rivolta I, Tateyama M, Yang AS, Kass RS. Secondary structure of the human cardiac Na+ channel C terminus. Evidence for a role of helical structures in modulation of channel inactivation. J Biol Chem 2002; 277:9233–9241.

100. Luo CH, Rudy Y. A dynamic model of the cardiac ventricular action potential. I. Simulations of ionic currents and concentration changes. Circ Res 1994; 74:1071–1096.

101. Luo CH, Rudy Y. A dynamic model of the cardiac ventricular action potential. II. After depolarizations, triggered activity, and potentiation. Circ Res 1994; 74:1097–1113.

102. Clancy CE, Tateyama M, Liu H, Wehrens HHT, Kass RS. Non-equilibrium gating in cardiac Na+ channels: An original mechanism of arrhythmia. Circulation 2003; 107:2233–2237.

103. Splawski I, Timothy KW, Tateyama M, Clancy CE, Malhotra A, Beggs AH, Cappuccio FP, Sagnella GA, Kass RS, Keating MT. Variant of SCN5A sodium channel implicated in risk of cardiac arrhythmia. Science 2002; 297:1333–1336.

104. Isom LL, De Jongh KS, Catterall WA. Auxiliary subunits of voltage-gated ion channels. Neuron 1994; 12:1183–1194.

105. Isom LL, De Jongh KS, Patton DE, Reber BF, Offord J, Charbonneau H, Walsh K, Goldin AL, Catterall WA. Primary structure and functional expression of the beta 1 subunit of the rat brain sodium channel. Science 1992; 256:839–842.

106. Makita N, Sloan-Brown K, Weghuis DO, Ropers HH, George AL, Jr. Genomic organization and chromosomal assignment of the human voltage-gated Na+ channel beta 1 subunit gene (SCN1B). Genomics 1994; 23:628–634.

107. Isom LL, Ragsdale DS, De Jongh KS, Westenbroek RE, Reber BF, Scheuer T, Catterall WA. Structure and function of the beta 2 subunit of brain sodium channels, a transmembrane glycoprotein with a CAM motif. Cell 1995; 83:433–442.

108. Jones JM, Meisler MH, Isom LL. Scn2b, a voltage-gated sodium channel beta2 gene on mouse chromosome 9. Genomics 1996; 34:258–259.

109. Morgan K, Stevens EB, Shah B, Cox PJ, Dixon AK, Lee K, Pinnock RD, Hughes J, Richardson PJ, Mizuguchi K, Jackson AP. beta 3: an additional auxiliary subunit of the voltage-sensitive sodium channel that modulates channel gating with distinct kinetics. Proc Natl Acad Sci USA 2000; 97: 2308–2313.

110. Fahmi AI, Patel M, Stevens EB, Fowden AL, John JE 3rd, Lee K, Pinnock R, Morgan K, Jackson AP, Vandenberg JI. The sodium channel beta-subunit SCN3b modulates the kinetics of SCN5a and is expressed heterogeneously in sheep heart. J Physiol 2001; 537:693–700.

111. Dhar Malhotra J, Chen C, Rivolta I, Abriel H, Malhotra R, Mattei LN, Brosius FC, Kass RS, Isom LL. Characterization of sodium channel alpha- and beta-subunits in rat and mouse cardiac myocytes. Circulation 2001; 103:1303–1310.

112. Santana LF, Gomez AM, Lederer WJ. Ca^{2+} flux through promiscuous cardiac Na^+ channels: slip-mode conductance. Science 1998; 279:1027–1033.

113. Malhotra JD, Koopmann MC, Kazen-Gillespie KA, Feltman N, Hortsch M, Isom LL. Structural requirements for interaction of sodium channel $\beta 1$ subunits with ankyrin. J Biol Chem 2002; 277:26681–26688.

114. Chauhan VS, Tuvia S, Buhusi M, Bennett V, Grant AO. Abnormal cardiac Na^+ channel properties and QT heart rate adaptation in neonatal ankyrin B knockout mice. Circ Res 2000; 86:441–447.

115. Bennett PB. Anchors aweigh! Ion channels, cytoskeletal proteins and cellular excitability. Circ Res 2000; 86:367–368.

116. Mohler PJ, Schott J-J, Gramolini AO, Dilly KW, Guatimosim S, duBell WH, Song L-S, Haurogné K, Kyndt F, Ali ME, Rogers TB, Lederer WJ, Escande D, LeMarec H, Bennett V. Ankyrin B mutation causes type 4 long-QT cardiac arrhythmia and sudden cardiac death. Nature 2003; 421:634–637.

117. Ertel EA, Campbell KP, Harpold MM, et al. Nomenclature of voltage-gated calcium channels. Neuron 2000; 25:533–535.

118. Soldatov NM. Genomic structure of human L-type Ca^{2+} channel. Genomics 1994; 22:77–87.

119. Mikami A, Imoto K, Tanabe T, Niidome T, Mori Y, Takeshima H, Narumiya S, Numa S. Primary structure and functional expression of the cardiac dihydropyridine-sensitive calcium channel. Nature 1989; 340:230–233.

120. Biel M, Ruth P, Bosse E, Hullin R, Stuhmer W, Flockerzi V, Hofmann F. Primary structure and functional expression of a high voltage activated calcium channel from rabbit lung. FEBS Lett 1990; 269:409–412.

121. Ruth P, Rohrkasten A, Biel M, Bosse E, Regulla S, Meyer HE, Flockerzi V, Hofmann F. Primary structure of the beta subunit of the DHP-sensitive calcium channel from skeletal muscle. Science 1989; 245:1115–1118.

122. Pragnell M, Sakamoto J, Jay SD, Campbell KP. Cloning and tissue-specific expression of the brain calcium channel beta-subunit. FEBS Lett 1991; 291:253–258.

123. Perez-Reyes E, Castellano A, Kim HS, Bertrand P, Baggstrom E, Lacerda AE, Wei XY, Birnbaumer L. Cloning and expression of a cardiac/brain beta subunit of the L-type calcium channel. J Biol Chem 1992; 267:1792–1797.

124. Hullin R, Singer-Lahat D, Freichel M, Biel M, Dascal N, Hofmann F, Flockerzi V. Calcium channel beta subunit heterogeneity: functional expression of cloned cDNA from heart, aorta and brain. Embo J 1992; 11:885–890.

125. Castellano A, Wei X, Birnbaumer L, Perez-Reyes E. Cloning and expression of a neuronal calcium channel beta subunit. J Biol Chem 1993; 268:12359–12366.

126. Vance CL, Begg CM, Lee WL, Haase H, Copeland TD, McEnery MW. Differential expression and association of calcium channel alpha1B and beta subunits during rat brain ontogeny. J Biol Chem 1998; 273:14495–14502.

127. Pragnell M, De Waard M, Mori Y, Tanabe T, Snutch TP, Campbell KP. Calcium channel beta-subunit binds to a conserved motif in the I-II cytoplasmic linker of the alpha 1-subunit. Nature 1994; 368:67–70.

128. Gregg RG, Messing A, Strube C, Beurg M, Moss R, Behan M, Sukhareva M, Haynes S, Powell JA, Coronado R, Powers PA. Absence of the beta subunit (cchb1) of the skeletal muscle dihydropyridine receptor alters expression of the alpha 1 subunit and eliminates excitation-contraction coupling. Proc Natl Acad Sci USA 1996; 93:13961–13966.

129. Yamaguchi H, Hara M, Strobeck M, Fukasawa K, Schwartz A, Varadi G. Multiple modulation pathways of calcium channel activity by a beta subunit. Direct evidence of beta subunit participation in membrane trafficking of the alpha1C subunit. J Biol Chem 1998; 273:19348–19356.

130. Beurg M, Sukhareva M, Strube C, Powers PA, Gregg RG, Coronado R. Recovery of Ca^{2+} current, charge movements, and Ca^{2+} transients in myotubes deficient in dihydropyridine receptor beta 1 subunit transfected with beta 1 cDNA. Biophys J 1997; 73:807–818.

131. Wei SK, Colecraft HM, DeMaria CD, Peterson BZ, Zhang R, Kohout TA, Rogers TB, Yue DT. Ca^{2+} channel modulation by recombinant auxiliary beta subunits expressed in young adult heart cells. Circ Res 2000; 86:175–184.

132. Chien AJ, Zhao X, Shirokov RE, Puri TS, Chang CF, Sun D, Rios E, Hosey MM. Roles of a membrane-localized beta subunit in the formation and targeting of functional L-type Ca^{2+} channels. J Biol Chem 1995; 270:30036–30044.

133. Chien AJ, Gao T, Perez-Reyes E, Hosey MM. Membrane targeting of L-type calcium channels. Role of palmitoylation in the subcellular localization of the beta2a subunit. J Biol Chem 1998; 273: 23590–23597.

134. Ellis SB, Williams ME, Ways NR, Brenner R, Sharp AH, Leung AT, Campbell KP, McKenna E, Koch WJ, Hui A, Schwartz A, Harpold MM. Sequence and expression of mRNAs encoding the alpha 1 and alpha 2 subunits of a DHP-sensitive calcium channel. Science 1988; 241:1661–1664.

135. Klugbauer N, Marais E, Lacinova L, Hofmann F. A T-type calcium channel from mouse brain. Pflugers Arch 1999; 437:710–715.

136. Gurnett CA, De Waard M, Campbell KP. Dual function of the voltage-dependent Ca^{2+} channel alpha 2 delta subunit in current stimulation and subunit interaction. Neuron 1996; 16:431–440.

137. Gurnett CA, Felix R, Campbell KP. Extracellular interaction of the voltage-dependent Ca^{2+} channel alpha2delta and alpha1 subunits. J Biol Chem 1997; 272:18508–18512.

138. Wiser O, Trus M, Tobi D, Halevi S, Giladi E, Atlas D. The alpha 2/delta subunit of voltage sensitive Ca^{2+} channels is a single transmembrane extracellular protein which is involved in regulated secretion. FEBS Lett 1996; 379:15–20.

139. Bangalore R, Mehrke G, Gingrich K, Hofmann F, Kass RS. Influence of L-type Ca channel alpha 2/delta-subunit on ionic and gating current in transiently transfected HEK 293 cells. Am J Physiol 1996; 270:H1521–1528.

140. Felix R, Gurnett CA, De Waard M, Campbell KP. Dissection of functional domains of the voltage-dependent Ca^{2+} channel alpha2delta subunit. J Neurosci 1997; 17:6884–6891.

141. Shistik E, Ivanina T, Puri T, Hosey M, Dascal N. Ca^{2+} current enhancement by alpha 2/delta and beta subunits in Xenopus oocytes: contribution of changes in channel gating and alpha 1 protein level. J Physiol 1995; 489 (Pt 1):55–62.

142. Pongs O. Molecular biology of voltage-dependent potassium channels. Physiol Rev 1992; 72:S69–S88.

143. Warmke JW, Ganetzky B. A family of potassium channel genes related to eag in Drosophila and mammals. Proc Natl Acad Sci USA 1994; 91:3438–34342.

144. Pond AL, Scheve BK, Benedict AT, Petrecca K, Van Wagoner DR, Shrier A, Nerbonne JM. Expression of distinct ERG proteins in rat, mouse, and human heart. Relation to functional I_{Kr} channels. J Biol Chem 2000; 275:5997–6006.

145. Curran ME, Splawski I, Timothy KW, Vincent GM, Green ED, Keating MT. A molecular basis for cardiac arrhythmia: HERG mutations cause long QT syndrome. Cell 1995; 80:795–803.

146. Sanguinetti MC, Jiang C, Curran ME, Keating MT. A mechanistic link between an inherited and an acquired cardiac arrhythmia: HERG encodes the I_{Kr} potassium channel. Cell 1995; 81:299–307.

147. Trudeau MC, Warmke JW, Ganetzky B, Robertson GA. HERG, a human inward rectifier in the voltage-gated potassium channel family. Science 1995; 269:92–95.

148. Wang Q, Curran ME, Splawski I, et al. Positional cloning of a novel potassium channel gene: KVLQT1 mutations cause cardiac arrhythmias. Nat Genet 1996; 12:17–23.

149. Barhanin J, Lesage F, Guillemare E, Fink M, Lazdunski M, Romey G. K(V)LQT1 and lsK (minK) proteins associate to form the $I_{(Ks)}$ cardiac potassium current. Nature 1996; 384:78–80.

150. Sanguinetti MC, Curran ME, Zou A, et al. Coassembly of KvLQT1 and minK (IsK) proteins to form cardiac $I_{(Ks)}$ potassium channel. Nature 1996; 384:80–83.

151. Biervert C, Schroeder BC, Kubisch C, Berkovic SF, Propping P, Jentsch TJ, Steinlein OK. A potassium channel mutation in neonatal human epilepsy. Science 1998; 279:403–406.

152. Wang Z, Yue L, White M, Pelletier G, Nattel S. Differential distribution of inward rectifier potassium channel transcripts in human atrium versus ventricle. Circulation 1998; 98:2422–2428.

153. Schroeder BC, Kubisch C, Stein V, Jentsch TJ. Moderate loss of function of cyclic-AMP-modulated KCNQ2/KCNQ3 K^+ channels causes epilepsy. Nature 1998; 396:687–690.

154. Murai T, Kakizuka A, Takumi T, Ohkubo H, Nakanishi S. Molecular cloning and sequence analysis of human genomic DNA encoding a novel membrane protein which exhibits a slowly activating potassium channel activity. Biochem Biophys Res Commun 1989; 161:176–181.

155. Folander K, Smith JS, Antanavage J, Bennett C, Stein RB, Swanson R. Cloning and expression of the delayed-rectifier IsK channel from neonatal rat heart and diethylstilbestrol-primed rat uterus. Proc Natl Acad Sci USA 1990; 87:2975–2979.

156. Lesage F, Attali B, Lazdunski M, Barhanin J. IsK, a slowly activating voltage-sensitive K^+ channel. Characterization of multiple cDNAs and gene organization in the mouse. FEBS Lett 1992; 301:168–172.

157. Abbott GW, Goldstein SA. A superfamily of small potassium channel subunits: form and function of the minK-related peptides (MiRPs). Q Rev Biophys 1998; 31:357–398.

158. Abbott GW, Sesti F, Splawski I, Buck ME, Lehmann MH, Timothy KW, Keating MT, Goldstein SA. MiRP1 forms I_{Kr} potassium channels with HERG and is associated with cardiac arrhythmia. Cell 1999; 97:175–187.

159. Abbott GW, Butler MH, Bendahhou S, Dalakas MC, Ptacek LJ, Goldstein SA. MiRP2 forms potassium channels in skeletal muscle with Kv3.4 and is associated with periodic paralysis. Cell 2001; 104:217–231.

160. Zhang M, Jiang M, Tseng GN. minK-related peptide 1 associates with Kv4.2 and modulates its gating function: potential role as beta subunit of cardiac transient outward channel? Circ Res 2001; 88:1012–1019.

161. Muniz ZM, Parcej DN, Dolly JO. Characterization of monoclonal antibodies against voltage-dependent K+ channels raised using alpha-dendrotoxin acceptors purified from bovine brain. Biochemistry 1992; 31:12297–12303.

162. Rettig J, Heinemann SH, Wunder F, Lorra C, Parcej DN, Dolly JO, Pongs O. Inactivation properties of voltage-gated K+ channels altered by presence of beta-subunit. Nature 1994; 369:289–294.

163. Castellino RC, Morales MJ, Strauss HC, Rasmusson RL. Time- and voltage-dependent modulation of a Kv1.4 channel by a beta-subunit (Kv beta 3) cloned from ferret ventricle. Am J Physiol 1995; 269:H385—H391.

164. England SK, Uebele VN, Kodali J, Bennett PB, Tamkun MM. A novel K+ channel beta-subunit (hKv beta 1.3) is produced via alternative mRNA splicing. J Biol Chem 1995; 270:28531–28534.

165. England SK, Uebele VN, Shear H, Kodali J, Bennett PB, Tamkun MM. Characterization of a voltage-gated K+ channel beta subunit expressed in human heart. Proc Natl Acad Sci USA 1995; 92:6309–6313.

166. Majumder K, De Biasi M, Wang Z, Wible BA. Molecular cloning and functional expression of a novel potassium channel beta-subunit from human atrium. FEBS Lett 1995; 361:13–16.

167. Morales MJ, Castellino RC, Crews AL, Rasmusson RL, Strauss HC. A novel beta subunit increases rate of inactivation of specific voltage-gated potassium channel alpha subunits. J Biol Chem 1995; 270:6272–6277.

168. Deal KK, England SK, Tamkun MM. Molecular physiology of cardiac potassium channels. Physiol Rev 1996; 76:49–67.

169. Nakahira K, Shi G, Rhodes KJ, Trimmer JS. Selective interaction of voltage-gated K+ channel beta-subunits with alpha-subunits. J Biol Chem 1996; 271:7084–7089.

170. Sewing S, Roeper J, Pongs O. Kv beta 1 subunit binding specific for shaker-related potassium channel alpha subunits. Neuron 1996; 16:455–463.

171. Fink M, Duprat F, Lesage F, Heurteaux C, Romey G, Barhanin J, Lazdunski M. A new K+ channel beta subunit to specifically enhance Kv2.2 (CDRK) expression. J Biol Chem 1996; 271:26341–26348.

172. Wible BA, Yang Q, Kuryshev YA, Accili EA, Brown AM. Cloning and expression of a novel K+ channel regulatory protein, KChAP. J Biol Chem 1998; 273:11745–11751.

173. An WF, Bowlby MR, Betty M, Cao J, Ling HP, Mendoza G, Hinson JW, Mattsson KI, Strassle BW, Trimmer JS, Rhodes KJ. Modulation of A-type potassium channels by a family of calcium sensors. Nature 2000; 403:553–556.

174. Rosati B, Pan Z, Lypen S, Wang HS, Cohen I, Dixon JE, McKinnon D. Regulation of KChIP2 potassium channel beta subunit gene expression underlies the gradient of transient outward current in canine and human ventricle. J Physiol 2001; 533:119–125.

175. Bahring R, Dannenberg J, Peters HC, Leicher T, Pongs O, Isbrandt D. Conserved Kv4 N-terminal domain critical for effects of Kv channel-interacting protein 2.2 on channel expression and gating. J Biol Chem 2001; 276:23888–23894.

176. Decher N, Uyguner O, Scherer CR, Karaman B, Yuksel-Apak M, Busch AE, Steinmeyer K, Wollnik B. hKChIP2 is a functional modifier of hKv4.3 potassium channels: cloning and expression of a short hKChIP2 splice variant. Cardiovasc Res 2001; 52:255–264.

177. Burgoyne RD, Weiss JL. The neuronal calcium sensor family of Ca^{2+}-binding proteins. Biochem J 2001; 353:1–12.

178. Guo W, Li H, Aimond F, Johns DC, Rhodes KJ, Trimmer JS, Nerbonne J. Role of heteromultimers in the generation of myocardial transient outward K+ currents. Circ Res 2002; 90:586–593.

179. Rosati B, Grau F, Rodriguez S, Li H, Nerbonne JM, McKinnon D. Co-ordinate patterns of KChIP2 mRNA, protein and transient outward current expression throughout canine ventricle. J Physiol, London 2003;548:815–822.

180. Dixon JE, McKinnon D. Quantitative analysis of potassium channel mRNA expression in atrial and ventricular muscle of rats. Circ Res 1994; 75:252–260.

181. Maruoka ND, Steele DF, Au BP, Dan P, Zhang X, Moore ED, Fedida D. alpha-actinin-2 couples to cardiac Kv1.5 channels, regulating current density and channel localization in HEK cells. FEBS Lett 2000;473:188–194.

182. Cukovic D, Lu GW, Wible B, Steele DF, Fedida D. A discrete amino terminal domain of Kv1.5 and Kv1.4 potassium channels interacts with the spectrin repeats of alpha-actinin-2. FEBS Lett 2001;498:87–92.

183. Petrecca K, Miller DM, Shrier A. Localization and enhanced current density of the Kv4.2 potassium channel by interaction with the actin binding protein filamin. J Neurosci 2000; 20:8736–8744.

184. Wang Z, Eldstrom JR, Jantzi J, Moore ED, Fedida D. Increased focal Kv4.2 channel expression at the plasma membrane is the result of actin depolymerization. Am J Physiol 2004; 286:H749–H759.

185. Fiset C, Clark RB, Shimoni Y, Giles WR. Shal-type channels contribute to the Ca^{2+}-independent transient outward K^+ current in rat ventricle. J Physiol 1997; 500 (Pt 1):51–64.

186. Johns DC, Nuss HB, Marban E. Suppression of neuronal and cardiac transient outward currents by viral gene transfer of dominant-negative Kv4.2 constructs. J Biol Chem 1997; 272:31598–31603.

187. Barry DM, Xu H, Schuessler RB, Nerbonne JM. Functional knockout of the transient outward current, long-QT syndrome, and cardiac remodeling in mice expressing a dominant-negative Kv4 alpha subunit. Circ Res 1998; 83:560–567.

188. Wickenden AD, Lee P, Sah R, Huang Q, Fishman GI, Backx PH. Targeted expression of a dominant-negative K(v)4.2 K(+) channel subunit in the mouse heart. Circ Res 2002;90:497–499.

189. Dixon JE, Shi W, Wang HS, McDonald C, Yu H, Wymore RS, Cohen IS, McKinnon D. Role of the Kv4.3 K^+ channel in ventricular muscle. A molecular correlate for the transient outward current. Circ Res 1996; 79:659–668.

190. London B, Wang DW, Hill JA, Bennett PB. The transient outward current in mice lacking the potassium channel gene Kv1.4. J Physiol 1998; 509 (Pt 1):171–182.

191. Goldstein SA, Miller C. Site-specific mutations in a minimal voltage-dependent K^+ channel alter ion selectivity and open-channel block. Neuron 1991; 7:403–408.

192. Takumi T, Ohkubo H, Nakanishi S. Cloning of a membrane protein that induces a slow voltage-gated potassium current. Science 1988; 242:1042–1045.

193. Wang KW, Tai KK, Goldstein SA. MinK residues line a potassium channel pore. Neuron 1996; 16:571–577.

194. Tai KK, Goldstein SA. The conduction pore of a cardiac potassium channel. Nature 1998; 391: 605–608.

195. Takahashi N, Morishige K, Jahangir A, Findlay I, Koyama H, Kurachi Y. Molecular cloning and functional expression of cDNA encoding a second class of inward rectifier potassium channels in the mouse brain. J Biol Chem 1994; 269:23274–23279.

196. Liu GX, Derst C, Schlichthorl G, Heinen S, Seebohm G, Bruggemann A, Kummer W, Veh RW, Daut J, Preisig-Muller R. Comparison of cloned Kir2 channels with native inward rectifier K^+ channels from guinea-pig cardiomyocytes. J Physiol 2001; 532:115–126.

197. Zaritsky JJ, Eckman DM, Wellman GC, Nelson MT, Schwarz TL. Targeted disruption of Kir2.1 and Kir2.2 genes reveals the essential role of the inwardly rectifying K^+ current in K^+-mediated vasodilation. Circ Res 2000; 87:160–166.

198. Zaritsky JJ, Redell JB, Tempel BL, Schwarz TL. The consequences of disrupting cardiac inwardly rectifying K^+ current (I_{K1}) as revealed by the targeted deletion of the murine Kir2.1 and Kir2.2 genes. J Physiol 2001; 533:697–710.

199. Lesage F, Guillemare E, Fink M, Duprat F, Lazdunski M, Romey G, Barhanin J. TWIK-1, a ubiquitous human weakly inward rectifying K^+ channel with a novel structure. Embo J 1996; 15:1004–1011.

200. Lesage F, Lazdunski M. Potassium channels with two P domains. In: Jan LY, ed. Current topics in membranes. Vol. 46. San Diego: Academic Press, 1999:199–222.

201. Goldstein SA, Bockenhauer D, O'Kelly I, Zilberberg N. Potassium leak channels and the KCNK family of two-P-domain subunits. Nat Rev Neurosci 2001; 2:175–184.

202. Backx PH, Marban E. Background potassium current active during the plateau of the action potential in guinea pig ventricular myocytes. Circ Res 1993; 72:890–900.

203. Clancy CE, Rudy Y. Na^+ channel mutation that causes both Brugada and long-QT syndrome phenotypes: a simulation study of mechanism. Circulation 2002; 105:1208–1213.

3

Cellular, Molecular, and Pharmacologic Mechanisms Underlying Drug-Induced Cardiac Arrhythmogenesis

Charles Antzelevitch, PhD

CONTENTS

INTRODUCTION

Pharmacologic agents can contribute to cardiac arrhythmogenesis by altering conduction, repolarization, or automaticity, and by inducing triggered activity in the form of early or delayed afterdepolarizations. Modulation of ion channel activity by drugs contributes to the development of both passive and active cardiac arrhythmias. The mechanisms responsible for active cardiac arrhythmias are generally divided into two major categories: (1) enhanced or abnormal impulse formation, and (2) re-entry (Fig. 1). Re-entry occurs when a propagating impulse fails to die out after normal activation of the heart and persists to re-excite the heart after expiration of the refractory period. Evidence implicating re-entry as a mechanism of cardiac arrhythmias stems back to the turn of the twentieth century *(1–16)*. The mechanisms responsible for abnormal impulse

From: *Cardiac Safety of Noncardiac Drugs:*
Practical Guidelines for Clinical Research and Drug Development
Edited by: J. Morganroth and I. Gussak © Humana Press Inc., Totowa, NJ

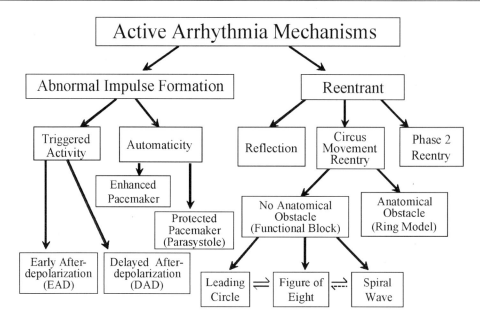

Fig. 1. Classification of active cardiac arrhythmias.

formation include enhanced automaticity and triggered activity. Automaticity can be further subdivided into normal and abnormal and triggered activity, consisting of early afterdepolarizations (EADs) and delayed afterdepolarizations (DADs).

Inhibition of inward currents by sodium and calcium channel blockers generally slows conduction, reduces excitability, and leads to the development of bradyarrhythmias secondary to sinoatrial and atrioventricular block, all examples of passive arrhythmias. Inward current inhibition can also lead to active arrhythmias by creating the substrate for re-entry in the form of unidirectional block and slow conduction, or by causing loss of the action potential dome and marked abbreviation of the action potential in epicardium. In the latter case, sodium and calcium channel block can give rise to transmural as well as epicardial dispersion of repolarization, leading to the development of phase 2 re-entry-mediated extrasystoles, ST segment elevation, and polymorphic ventricular tachycardia (VT), all electrophysiologic features of the Brugada syndrome *(17,18)*. Augmentation of late inward currents or inhibition of outward repolarizing current generally gives rise to an increase in action potential duration (APD), as well as EAD-induced triggered activity. Because APD prolongation is often inhomogeneous, drugs that inhibit outward repolarizing currents or augment late inward depolarizing currents commonly amplify transmural dispersion of repolarization, thus providing the substrate for the development of torsade de pointes (TdP) arrhythmias, characteristic of the long QT syndrome (LQTS) *(19)*. Our focus in this chapter will be on drugs that contribute to the development of the acquired long QT syndrome, the most frequently encountered form of drug-induced channelopathy.

ROLE OF ELECTRICAL HETEROGENEITY IN ACQUIRED LONG QT SYNDROME

Prolongation of the QT interval in the electrocardiogram (ECG) occurs when the action potential of a significant proportion of cells in the ventricular myocardium are prolonged, as a result of a reduction in one or more repolarizing currents and/or an augmentation of inward currents. The effect of a drug on APD is determined by the balance between its action to alter inward and outward currents. A prolonged APD can be caused by drug effects on a single, or on many ion channels, pumps or exchangers. Inhibition of the rapidly activating delayed rectifier potassium channels (I_{Kr}) is the most common cause of drug-induced QT prolongation *(20)*. Many drugs that block I_{Kr}, including agents like quinidine, amiodarone, azimilide, also inhibit the slowly activating delayed rectifier (I_{Ks}). Some drugs and toxins, including DPI 201–106, anthopleurin-A, and ATX-II *(21–23)*, prolong the QT interval by augmenting late I_{Na}. As discussed later, many drugs block multiple cardiac ion channels, thus causing a more complex alteration of action potential morphology.

I_{Kr} block and QT prolongation have attracted considerable attention in recent years as a result of their association with life-threatening cardiac arrhythmias, such as TdP *(24–28)*. Nine drugs have been withdrawn from the market worldwide over the past decade because of this problem: terodiline, lidoflazine, terfenadine, astemizole, grepafloxicin, droperidol, sertindole, levomethadyl, and cisapride. In the United States, more drugs have been withdrawn from the market over the past decade because of their propensity to cause life-threatening polymorphic ventricular tachycardia or TdP, than for any other reason *(24)*. Another agent, recently withdrawn from the U.S. market, namely mibefradil, is suspected but not proven to possess this problem.

Antiarrhythmic drugs with Class III action capable of prolonging cardiac repolarization by blocking potassium channels were among the first to be linked to this arrhythmogenic syndrome. Syncope arising following the initiation of quinidine therapy has been recognized for over 80 yr *(29)*. The incidence of TdP in patients treated with quinidine is estimated to range between 2.0 and 8.8% *(29–31)*. DL-sotalol has been associated with an incidence ranging from 1.8 to 4.8 % *(32–34)*. A similar incidence has been described for newer class III agents, such as dofetilide *(35)* and ibutilide. An ever-increasing number and variety of noncardiovascular agents, most acting via inhibition of I_{kr}, have also been shown to aggravate and/or precipitate TdP *(24,25)*. Over 50 commercially available or investigational noncardiovascular and 20 cardiovascular nonantiarrhythmic drugs have been implicated.

The principal substrate for the development of TdP is thought to arise as a consequence of an increase in dispersion of repolarization secondary to amplification of electrical heterogeneities intrinsic to ventricular myocardium *(26,37–44)*. Studies conducted over the past 15 yr have highlighted regional differences in electrical properties of ventricular cells as well as differences in the response of the different cell types to pharmacological agents and pathophysiological states *(39,41)*. Among the heterogeneities uncovered are electrical and pharmacologic distinctions between endocardium and epicardium of the canine, feline, rabbit, rat, mouse, and human heart, as well as differences in the electrophysiologic characteristics and pharmacologic responsiveness of M cells located in the deep structures of the ventricular myocardium. The hallmark of the M cell is the ability of its action potential to prolong more than that of epicardial and endocardial cells in response to a slowing of rate and/or upon exposure to drugs with QT-prolonging actions *(45)*. The ionic basis for the prolonged APD of M cells includes a smaller I_{Ks} and a larger late I_{Na} *(46,47)* and sodium-calcium exchange current (I_{Na-Ca}) *(48)* compared to epicardial and endocardial cells. Other currents, including the rapidly activating delayed rectifier (I_{Kr}) and inward rectifier (I_{K1}) currents are similar in the three cell types in the canine heart *(47)*.

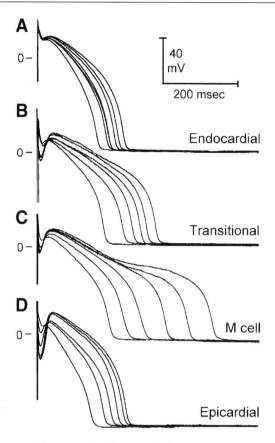

Fig. 2. Transmembrane activity recorded from cells isolated from the epicardial (Epi), M and endocardial (Endo) regions of the canine left ventricle at basic cycle lengths (BCL) of 300 to 5000 ms (steady-state conditions). The M and transitional cells were enzymatically dissociated from the midmyocardial region. Deceleration-induced prolongation of APD in M cells is much greater than in epicardial and endocardial cells. The spike and dome morphology is also more accentuated in the epicardial cell. At slow rates, the transmural dispersion of action potential duration exceeds 200 ms.

The net result is a decrease in repolarizing current during phases 2 and 3 of the M cell action potential. These ionic distinctions also sensitize the M cells to a variety of pharmacological agents *(49)*.

INSCRIPTION OF THE T WAVE

Figure 2 shows action potentials recorded from cardiac myocytes isolated from the different regions of the left ventricular wall and stimulated over a wide range of basic cycle lengths. At slow rates of stimulation, the transmural differences in repolarization time exceed 200 ms. What type of differences can we expect when these cells are in the intact wall of the ventricle and electrotonically interacting with each other, and how do these distinctions in repolarization time contribute to the inscription of the T wave? The arterially-perfused wedge preparation was developed to address these issues. In the example illustrated in Fig. 3, transmural dispersion of repolarization in the left ventricular wedge preparation is 57 ms under control conditions. The intrinsic differences in repo-

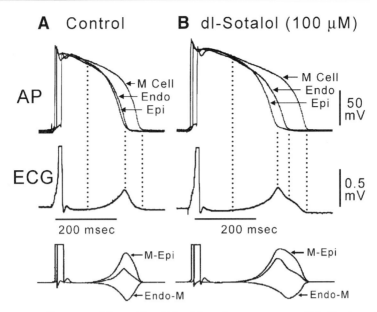

Fig. 3. Voltage gradients on either side of the M region are responsible for inscription of the electrocardiographic T wave. Top: Action potentials simultaneously recorded from endocardial, epicardial and M region sites of an arterially-perfused canine left ventricular wedge preparation. Middle: ECG recorded across the wedge. Bottom: Computed voltage differences between the epicardium and M region action potentials (ΔV_{M-Epi}) and between the M region and endocardium responses (ΔV_{Endo-M}). If these traces are representative of the opposing voltage gradients on either side of the M region, responsible for inscription of the T wave, then the weighted sum of the two traces should yield a trace (middle trace in bottom grouping) resembling the ECG, which it does. The voltage gradients are weighted to account for differences in tissue resistivity between M and Epi and Endo and M regions, thus yielding the opposing currents flowing on either side of the M region. A: Under control conditions the T wave begins when the plateau of epicardial action potential separates from that of the M cell. As epicardium repolarizes, the voltage gradient between epicardium and the M region continues to grow giving rise to the ascending limb of the T wave. The voltage gradient between the M region and epicardium (ΔV_{M-Epi}) reaches a peak when the epicardium is fully repolarized—this marks the peak of the T wave. On the other end of the ventricular wall, the endocardial plateau deviates from that of the M cell, generating an opposing voltage gradient (ΔV_{Endo-M}) and corresponding current that limits the amplitude of the T wave and contributes to the initial part of the descending limb of the T wave. The voltage gradient between the endocardium and the M region reaches a peak when the endocardium is fully repolarized. The gradient continues to decline as the M cells repolarize. All gradients are extinguished when the longest M cells are fully repolarized. B: DL-sotalol (100 µ*M*) prolongs the action potential of the M cell more than those of the epicardial and endocardial cells, thus widening the T wave and prolonging the QT interval. The greater separation of epicardial and endocardial repolarization times also gives rise to a notch in the descending limb of the T wave. Once again, the T wave begins when the plateau of epicardial action potential diverges from that of the M cell. The same relationships as described for panel A are observed during the remainder of the T wave. The sotalol-induced increase in dispersion of repolarization across the wall is accompanied by a corresponding increase in the Tpeak-Tend interval in the pseudo-ECG. (Modified from ref. *50* with permission.)

larization time are thus reduced from over 200 to 57 ms as a result of electrotonic interaction among the different cell types. In the presence of DL-sotalol, the M cell action potential is prolonged more than epicardium and endocardium, leading to an increase of TDR to 94 ms.

Studies involving the arterially perfused wedge have provided significant insight into the cellular basis of the T wave showing that currents flowing down voltage gradients on either side of the M region are in large part responsible for the T wave (Fig. 3) *(50)*. The interplay between these opposing forces establishes the height and width of the T wave and the degree to which either the ascending or descending limb of the T wave is interrupted, leading to a bifurcated or notched appearance of the T wave. The voltage gradients result from a more positive plateau potential in the M region than in epicardium or endocardium and from differences in the time-course of phase 3 of the action potential of the three predominant ventricular cell types.

Apico-basal repolarization gradients measured along the epicardial surface have been suggested to play a role in the registration of the T wave *(51)*. More recent studies involving the perfused wedge suggest little or no contribution, owing to the fact that the ECG recorded along the apico-basal axis fails to display a T wave (Fig. 4) *(50)*. These findings suggest that in this part of the canine left ventricular wall (anterior, mid-apico-basal) the inscription of the T wave is largely the result of voltage gradients along the transmural axis.

U WAVE VS T2 WAVE

A number of theories have been proposed to explain the origin of the U wave since the initial description of this wave by Einthoven *(52)*. These include delayed repolarization of the ventricular septum *(53)*, papillary muscles *(54)*, negative afterpotentials *(55,56)*, Purkinje system *(57,58)*, early or delayed afterdepolarizations *(56)*, or "mechano-electrical feedback" *(59,60)*.

One popular hypothesis ascribes the U wave to delayed repolarization of the His-Purkinje system *(57,58)*. The small mass of the specialized conduction system is difficult to reconcile with the sometimes very large U wave deflections reported in the literature, especially in cases of acquired and congenital long QT syndrome. In 1996, we suggested that the M cells, more abundant in mass and possessing delayed repolarization characteristics similar to those of Purkinje fibers, may be responsible for the inscription of the pathophysiologic U wave *(61)*. More recent findings discussed earlier clearly indicate that what many clinicians refer to as an accentuated or inverted U wave is not a U wave, but rather a component of the T wave whose descending or ascending limb (especially during hypokalemia) is interrupted (Fig. 5) *(50,62)*. A transient reversal in current flow across the ventricular wall caused by shifting voltage gradients between epicardium and the M region and endocardium and the M region underlies this phenomena. The data suggest that the *pathophysiologic U wave* that develops under conditions of acquired or congenital LQTS is part of the T wave and that the various hump morphologies represent different levels of interruption of the ascending limb of the T wave, arguing for use of the term T2 in place of U to describe these events, as previously suggested by Lehmann et al. *(50,63)*.

Delayed repolarization of the M cells, although it contributes to the inscription of T2 (pathophysiologic U wave), is unlikely to be responsible for the normal U wave, the very small distinct deflection following the T wave. The repolarization of the His–Purkinje system as previously suggested by Hoffman et al. *(57)* and by Watanabe and co-workers *(58)* remains a plausible hypothesis. Repolarization of the Purkinje system is temporally aligned with the expected appearance of the U wave in the perfused wedge preparation *(50)*. A test of this hypothesis awaits the availability of an experimental model displaying a prominent U wave (most animal species do not manifest a U wave).

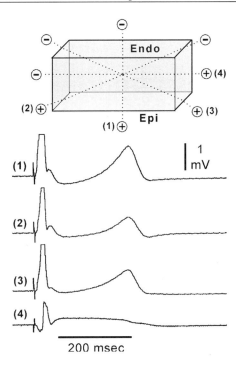

Fig. 4. Contribution of transmural vs. apico-basal and anterior-posterior gradients to the registration of the T wave. The four ECG traces were simultaneously recorded at 0°, 45°, –45°, and 90° (apico-basal) angles relative to the transmural axis of an arterially perfused left ventricular wedge preparation. Inscription of the T wave is largely the result of voltage gradients along the transmural axis. (Modified from ref. *50* with permission.)

A second very plausible hypothesis that also lacks direct experimental and clinical evidence is that the normal U wave is associated with the mechanical activity of the heart (mechano-electrical feedback). Initially proposed by Lepeshkin *(56)* and more recently advocated by Surawicz *(64)*, this hypothesis emphasizes the coincidence between the start of the U wave and the second heart sound, suggesting that mechanical mechanisms associated with the opening of the AV valves generate afterpotentials that are responsible for the appearance of the normal U wave.

The distinction between a T2 and U wave is critically important from the standpoint of identifying potential risk of agents that prolong the QT interval. A continuous spectrum of TU transitions can make distinction of the two difficult at times. Such a distinction, however, becomes paramount when studying the effects of agents with Class III antiarrhythmic actions. QTc may be grossly underestimated if a T2 is judged to be a U wave and excluded from the measurement of the QT interval. Figure 6 shows a clinical example in a patient receiving amiodarone, illustrating how such confusion can arise. The prominent apparent U waves are actually T2 waves. If excluded from the measurement of QT, a value of 400 ms would be obtained, far shorter than the actual QT interval of 600 msec.

To discern between T2 and U waves, it is sometimes helpful to compare the U wave in leads V2-3 where the U wave is generally largest with leads aVL, I, II and V5 where the U wave is less prominent. Leads aVL and I usually lack a visible U wave.

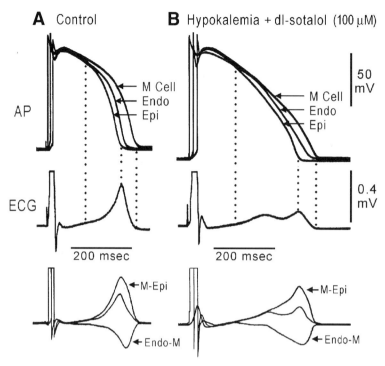

Fig. 5. Transient shift of voltage gradients on either side of the M region results in T wave bifurcation. The format is the same as in Fig. 3. All traces were simultaneously recorded from an arterially perfused left ventricular wedge preparation. A: Control. B: In the presence of hypo-kalemia ($[K^+]_o$ = 1.5 mM), the IKr blocker dl-sotalol (100 μM) prolongs the QT interval and produces a bifurcation of the T wave, a morphology some authors refer to as T-U complex. The rate of repolarization of phase 3 of the action potential is slowed giving rise to smaller opposing transmural currents that cross-over producing a low amplitude bifid T wave. Initially the voltage gradient between the epicardium and M regions (M-Epi) is greater than that between endocardium and M region (Endo-M). When endocardium pulls away from the M cell, the opposing gradient (Endo-M) increases, interrupting the ascending limb of the T wave. Predominance of the M-Epi gradient is restored as the epicardial response continues to repolarize and the Epi-M gradients increases, thus resuming the ascending limb of the T wave. Full repolarization of epicardium marks the peak of the T wave. Repolarization of both endocardium and the M region contribute importantly to the descending limb. BCL = 1000 ms. (Modified from ref. *50* with permission.)

EXPERIMENTAL MODELS OF LONG QT SYNDROME

Differences in the time course of repolarization of the three ventricular myocardial cell types generates voltage gradients that not only inscribe the T wave in the ECG, but also have the potential to create a vulnerable window for the development of re-entrant arrhythmias. This substrate develops when the heterogeneities intrinsic to ventricular myocardium are amplified. Preferential prolongation of the M cell action potential is one mechanism by which transmural dispersion of repolarization can be amplified to yield an arrhythmogenic substrate under long QT conditions. Studies employing the arterially-perfused wedge preparation have provided insight into the mechanisms that underlie congenital and acquired LQTS (Fig. 7). The wedge model is capable of developing and sustaining a variety of arrhythmias, including TdP.

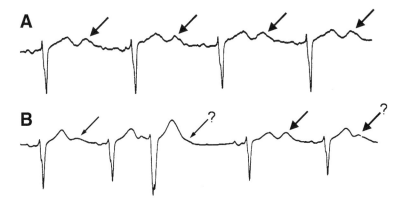

Fig. 6. Spectrum of T-U transitions recorded in the 71-yr-old male on amiodarone (for atrial fibrillation). Lead II. (**A**) The U wave (thick arrows) is completely separated from the T wave and may be erroneously excluded in measurement of the QT interval. The QTc (without the U) is 400 ms, too short for a patient on amiodarone, whereas the QTc (with the U) is 600 ms, very long even for a patient on amiodarone. In this case, the U wave is pathologic (T2) and the QT is abnormally prolonged. (**B**) ECG recorded the next day in the same patient The U waves are greatly diminished (thin arrows) but appear to become much more prominent (thick arrows) following a post-extrasystolic compensatory pause. The post-pause T2 augmentation suggests that, regardless of their origin, these pathophysiologic waves reflect early afterdepolarizations (EADs), increased dispersion of repolarization or both. Question marks indicate intermediate T-U configurations that are very difficult to classify as either T2 or U. (Courtesy of Dr. Sami Viskin.)

The example illustrated in Figure 7A shows that I_{Ks} block alone produces a homogeneous prolongation of repolarization across the ventricular wall, but does not induce arrhythmias. The addition of isoproterenol leads to abbreviation of epicardial and endocardial APD with little or no change in the APD of the M cell, resulting in a marked augmentation of transmural dispersion of repolarization (TDR) and the development of spontaneous and stimulation-induced TdP (65). Generally, these cellular changes give rise to a broad-based T wave and a long QT interval characteristic of LQT1, similar to that observed clinically in patients with the LQT1 form of LQTS (Fig. 7G). The development of TdP in this model (Fig. 8A) is exquisitely sensitive to β adrenergic stimulation consistent with the high sensitivity of congenital LQTS, LQT1 in particular, to sympathetic stimulation (66).

I_{Kr} block with D-sotalol also causes a greater prolongation of the M cell action potential as well as a slowing of phase 3 of the action potential of all three cell types, resulting in low amplitude T waves, prolonged QT interval, large transmural dispersion of repolarization, and the development of spontaneous as well as stimulation-induced TdP (Fig. 7B). The addition of hypokalemia further accentuates the reduction in the amplitude of the T wave, giving rise to a deeply notched or bifurcated appearance, similar to that commonly seen in patients with the LQT2 syndrome (Fig. 7H) (50,62).

Augmentation of late I_{Na} with ATX-II (62) markedly prolongs the QT interval, delays the onset of the T wave, in some cases also widening it, and causes a sharp rise in transmural dispersion of repolarization as a result of a greater prolongation of the APD of the M cell (Fig. 7C). A relatively large effect of ATX-II to prolong the APD of epicardium and endocardium leads to a relatively long delay in the onset of the T wave, consistent with the late-appearing T wave pattern and prolonged isoelectric ST segment commonly observed in patients with the LQT3 form of the long QT syndrome (Fig. 7I).

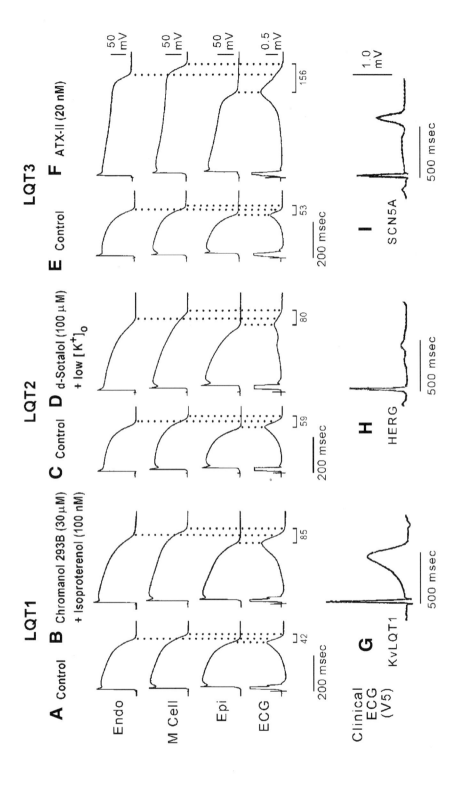

In all three cases described previously, the pharmacological interventions significantly prolong the QT interval as a consequence of the prolongation of APD, but because the action potential of the M cell is preferentially prolonged, QT prolongation is accompanied by a very substantial increase in TDR, creating the substrate for reentry. When TDR approached 90 ms TdP may develop (Fig. 8).

The tachyarrhythmia most commonly encountered in congenital and acquired LQTS is TdP, an atypical polymorphic ventricular tachycardia. TdP most commonly develops in patients receiving an I_{Kr} blocker, especially in the presence of hypokalemia and slow heart rates or long pauses, conditions similar to those under which I_{Kr} blockers induce early afterdepolarizations (EAD) and triggered activity in isolated Purkinje fibers and M cells. An EAD-induced extrasystole is believed to be responsible for the premature beat that initiates TdP, but the maintenance of the arrhythmia is generally thought to be a result of circus movement re-entry *(19,26)*. In the wedge model, TdP can occur spontaneously or be induced with programmed electrical stimulation. Figure 8 illustrates examples of TdP induced by exposure of the wedge preparation to I_{Kr} and I_{Ks} blockers or agents that augment late I_{Na}, mimicking the LQT1, LQT2, and LQT3 forms of LQTS. The extrasystoles that precipitate spontaneous TdP are presumably caused by EADs arising from either Purkinje fibers or deep subendocardial M cells.

Figure 9 illustrates another example of TdP. With coronary perfusate adjusted to temperatures approaching physiological levels, spontaneous TdP was observed. EADs are known to be exquisitely temperature-sensitive and are readily suppressed as temperature is reduced. When the perfusate was cooled all focal extrasystolic activity was suppressed and spontaneous TdP was no longer observed, but the arrhythmia could be readily induced with a single premature beat applied to the epicardium, the site of briefest refractoriness. The action potential recordings demonstrate the persistence of a substrate

---

Fig. 7. Transmembrane action potentials and transmural electrocardiograms (ECG) in the LQT1 (**A** and **B**), LQT2 (**C** and **D**), and LQT3 (**E** and **F**) models (arterially perfused canine left ventricular wedge preparations), and clinical ECG lead V5 of patients with LQT1 (*KvLQT1* defect) (**G**), LQT2 (*HERG* defect) (**H**) and LQT3 (*SCN5A* defect) (**I**) syndromes. Isoproterenol + chromanol 293B— an IKs blocker, D-sotalol + low [K^+]$_o$, and ATX-II - an agent that slows inactivation of late I_{Na} are used to mimic the LQT1, LQT2 and LQT3 syndromes, respectively. Panels A–F depict action potentials simultaneously recorded from endocardial (Endo), M and epicardial (Epi) sites together with a transmural ECG. BCL = 2000 ms. In all cases, the peak of the T wave in the ECG is coincident with the repolarization of the epicardial action potential, whereas the end of the T wave is coincident with the repolarization of the M cell action potential. Repolarization of the endocardial cell is intermediate between that of the M cell and epicardial cell. Transmural dispersion of repolarization across the ventricular wall, defined as the difference in the repolarization time between M and epicardial cells, is denoted below the ECG traces. B: Isoproterenol (100 n*M*) in the presence of chromanol 293B (30 μ*M*) produced a preferential prolongation of the APD of the M, resulting in an accentuated transmural dispersion of repolarization and broad-based T waves as commonly seen in LQT1 patients (G). D: D-Sotalol (100 μ*M*) in the presence of low potassium (2 mM) gives rise to low-amplitude T waves with a notched or bifurcated appearance as a result of a very significant slowing of repolarization as commonly seen in LQT2 patients (H). F: ATX-II (20 n*M*) markedly prolongs the QT interval, widens the T wave, and causes a sharp rise in the dispersion of repolarization. ATX-II also produces a marked delay in onset of the T wave as a result of relatively large effects of the drug on the APD of epicardium and endocardium, consistent with the late-appearing T wave pattern observed in LQT3 patients (I). (Modified from refs.*62,65* with permission.)

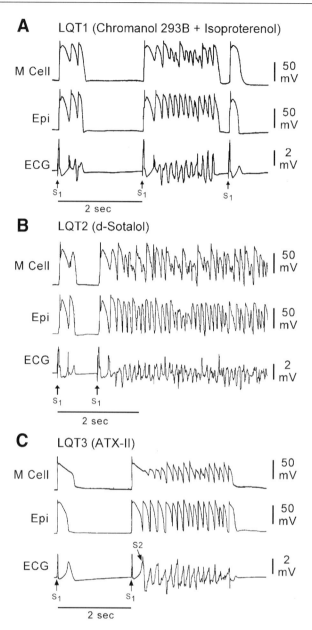

Fig. 8. Polymorphic ventricular tachycardia displaying features of TdP in the LQT1 (**A**), LQT2 (**B**), and LQT3 (**C**) models (arterially perfused canine left ventricular wedge preparations). Isoproterenol + chromanol 293B, D-sotalol, and ATX-II are used to mimic the 3 LQTS syndromes, respectively. Each trace shows action potentials simultaneously recorded from M and epicardial (Epi) cells together with a transmural ECG. The preparation was paced from the endocardial surface at a BCL of 2000 ms (S1). (A and B) Spontaneous TdP induced in the LQT1 and LQT2 models, respectively. In both models, the first groupings show spontaneous ventricular premature beat (or couplets) that fail to induce TdP, and a second grouping that show spontaneous premature beats that succeed. The premature response appears to originate in the deep subendocardium (M or Purkinje). (C) Programmed electrical stimulation induces TdP in the LQT3 model. ATX-II produced very significant dispersion of repolarization (first grouping). A single extrastimulus (S2) applied to the epicardial surface at an S1–S2 interval of 320 ms initiates TdP (second grouping). (Modified from refs. *62,65* with permission.)

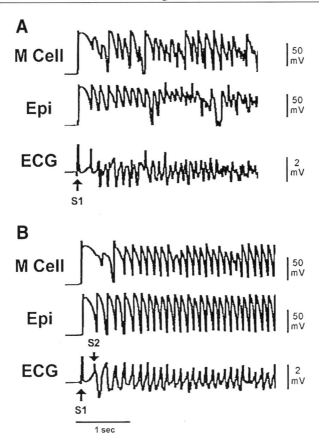

Fig. 9. Spontaneous and stimulation-induced polymorphic ventricular tachycardia with features of TdP occurring in a canine arterially-perfused left ventricular wedge preparation. **(A)** Spontaneous TdP in a preparation pretreated with chromanol (30 umol/L) + isoproterenol (100 nmol/L). A spontaneous premature beat with a coupling interval of 285 ms, likely originating from subendocardial Purkinje system, initiates an episode of TdT. **(B)** The perfusate temperature was cooler (36°C) and extrasystolic activity was absent, presumably as a result of the absence of early afterdepolarization-induced triggered activity. The presence of a reentrant substrate in the form of a transmural dispersion of repolarization is evidenced by the ability to induce TdP with a single extrasystole applied to epicardium (site of briefest refractoriness). S1–S1 = 2000 ms. (Modified from ref. *19* with permission.)

for re-entry in the form of a transmural dispersion of repolarization. Taken together these observations provide strong evidence in support of re-entry as the basis for TdP. This conclusion is shared by most, but not all investigators in the field *(26)*.

Whereas polymorphic ventricular tachycardia can arise as a consequence of both focal and re-entrant mechanisms, in the presence and absence of a prolonged QT interval, the available data point to the following hypothesis as the basis for most LQTS-related TdP (Fig. 10). The hypothesis presumes the presence of electrical heterogeneity in the form of transmural dispersion of repolarization under baseline conditions. This intrinsic heterogeneity is amplified by agents that reduce net repolarizing current via a reduction in I_{Kr} or I_{Ks} or augmentation of late I_{Ca} or late I_{Na}. Conditions leading to a reduction in I_{Kr} or augmentation of late I_{Na} produce a preferential prolongation of the M cell action potential. As a consequence, the QT interval prolongs and is accompanied by a dramatic

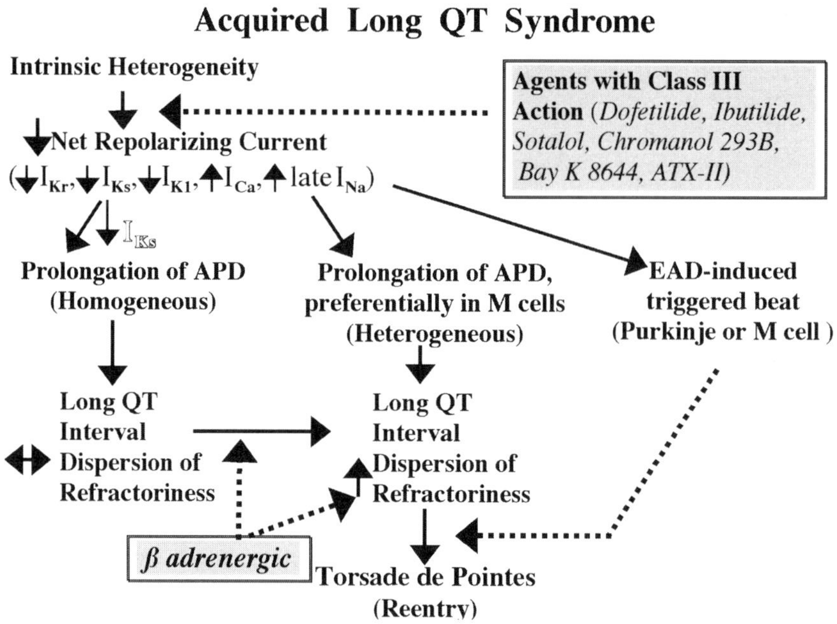

Acquired Long QT Syndrome

Fig. 10. Proposed cellular and ionic mechanisms for the long QT syndrome.

increase in transmural dispersion of repolarization that creates a vulnerable window for the development of re-entry. The reduction in net repolarizing current also predisposes to the development of EAD-induced triggered activity in M and Purkinje cells that provide the extrasystole that triggers TdP when it falls within the vulnerable period. β adrenergic agonists further amplify transmural heterogeneity (transiently) in the case of I_{Kr} block, but reduce it in the case of I_{Na} promoters *(67,68)*. In contrast, conditions leading to a reduction in I_{Ks} cause a *homogeneous* prolongation of APD throughout the ventricular wall, leading to a prolongation of the QT interval, but with no increase in transmural dispersion of repolarization. TdP does not occur spontaneously nor can it be induced by programmed stimulation under these conditions until a β-adrenergic agonist is introduced. Isoproterenol dramatically increases transmural dispersion of repolarization and refractoriness under these conditions by abbreviating the APD of epicardium and endocardium, thus creating a vulnerable window that an EAD-induced triggered response can invade to generate TdP.

MULTI-ION CHANNEL INHIBITORS

Drugs affecting two or more ion channels, such as quinidine, cisapride, pentobarbital, amiodarone, ranolazine, and azimilide produce a more complex response. In the case of quinidine, relatively low therapeutic levels of the drug (3–5 μ*M*), produce a marked prolongation of the M cell APD but not of epicardium and endocardium, consistent with a predominant effect of the drug to block I_{Kr} at this concentration. Higher concentrations of quinidine produce a further prolongation of the epicardial and endocardial action potential, consistent with an effect of the drug to block I_{Ks}, but *abbreviation* of the APD of the M cell, caused by its action to suppress late I_{Na} *(69)*. Thus, at low concentrations, quinidine prolongs QT and transmural dispersion of repolarization (TDR), whereas at

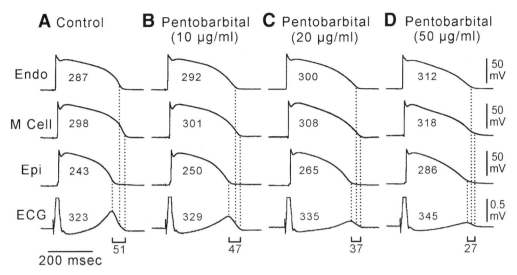

Fig. 11. Dose-dependent effect of sodium pentobarbital (10, 20, 50 µg/mL) on transmembrane and ECG activity in an arterially perfused canine left ventricular wedge preparation. All traces show action potentials simultaneously recorded from endocardial (Endo), M and epicardial (Epi) sites together with a transmural ECG. BCL = 2000 ms. Pentobarbital prolongs the QT interval and increases APD of the endocardial and epicardial cells more than that of the M cell, thus reducing transmural dispersion of repolarization and flattening the T wave in a dose-dependent manner. Numbers associated with each action potential indicate the APD_{90} value. Numbers associated with the ECG denote the QT interval, and those beneath the ECG represent the transmural dispersion of repolarization. (From ref. *71* with permission.)

higher concentrations the prolongation of QT is not accompanied by an increase in TDR. This may be the reason why quinidine produces TdP at low therapeutic concentrations, but not at high therapeutic or toxic concentrations *(41,70)*.

Pentobarbital is an example of an agent that prolongs the QT interval but reduces transmural dispersion of repolarization (Fig. 11) *(71)*. Like high concentrations of quinidine, pentobarbital does this by inhibiting I_{Kr}, I_{Ks}, and I_{Na} most prominently *(72)*. This multichannel inhibition leads to a greater prolongation of APD in epicardial and endocardial cells than in M cells, causing a significant reduction in TDR. The effect of the drug on late I_{Na} (and I_{Ca}) also suppresses D-sotalol-induced EAD activity in M cells. Thus, despite its actions to prolong QT, pentobarbital does not induce TdP *(71)* As a result of its actions to reduce transmural dispersion and inhibit EAD-induced triggered activity, the anesthetic is effective in *suppressing* D-sotalol-induced TdP *(40)*.

Another agent that acts to prolong the QT interval, but which generally produces either a decrease or a relatively small increase of TDR is amiodarone. Amiodarone is a potent antiarrhythmic drug used in the management of both atrial and ventricular arrhythmias, which induces TdP only rarely. In addition to its β-blocking properties, amiodarone is known to block the sodium, potassium, and calcium channels in the heart. Its antiarrhythmic efficacy and low incidence of proarrhythmia relative to other agents with class III actions are attributed to its complex pharmacology. When administered chronically (30–40 mg/kg/d orally for 30–45 d), amiodarone produces a greater prolongation of APD in epicardium and endocardium of the dog heart, but less of an increase, or even a decrease at slow rates, in the M region, thereby reducing transmural dispersion of repolarization *(73)* Like pentobarbital, chronic amiodarone therapy can suppress the ability of the I_{Kr}

blocker, D-sotalol, to induce a marked dispersion of repolarization or early afterdepolarization activity. Amiodarone is the only class III antiarrhythmic agent that has thus far failed to produce TdP in the chronic AV block (CAVB) dog (74)

Ranolazine, a novel anti-anginal agent, has been shown to possess ionic and cellular actions similar to those of amiodarone (75). Ranolazine blocks I_{Kr} (IC_{50} = 12), late I_{Na}, late I_{Ca}, peak I_{Ca}, I_{Na-Ca} (IC_{50} = 5.9, 50, 296, and 91 μM, respectively) and I_{Ks} (17% at 30 μM). In left ventricular (LV) tissue and wedge preparations, ranolazine produces a concentration-dependent prolongation of APD in epicardium, but abbreviation of APD of M cells, leading to either no change or a reduction in TDR. The result is a modest prolongation of the QT interval. Prolongation of APD and QT by ranolazine is fundamentally different from that of other drugs that block I_{Kr} and induce TdP, in that APD prolongation is rate-independent (i.e., does not display reverse rate-dependent prolongation of APD), and is not associated with EADs, triggered activity, increased spatial dispersion of repolarization, or polymorphic VT. TdP arrhythmias were not observed spontaneously nor could they be induced in the perfused wedge preparation with programmed electrical stimulation. Indeed, ranolazine was found to possess significant antiarrhythmic activity, acting to suppress the arrhythmogenic effects of other QT-prolonging drugs. Thus, ranolazine produces ion channel effects similar to those observed following pentobarbital or chronic exposure to amiodarone (reduced I_{Kr}, I_{Ks}, late I_{Na}, and I_{Ca}). Ranolazine's actions to reduce TDR and suppress EADs suggest that, in addition to its anti-anginal actions, the drug possesses antiarrhythmic activity (76). These results highlight the fact that I_{Kr} block does not in and of itself predict the arrhythmogenic potential of pharmacological agents.

This conclusion is supported by a recent study contrasting I_{Kr} block potency of a wide variety of drugs with clinical risk of TdP (77). The results indicate that not all drugs that cause TdP are potent I_{Kr} blockers and that I_{Kr} block is not necessarily associated with TdP, suggesting that other properties of the drugs contribute to their propensity to cause TdP. Antiarrhythmic drugs that prolong QT without inducing TdP have in common the ability to inhibit I_{Ks}, I_{Kr}, and I_{Na} (and/or I_{Ca}) and thus to prolong refractoriness without increasing transmural dispersion of repolarization. Indeed, in some cases transmural dispersion may be reduced.

Another pharmacological agent capable of prolonging the QT interval without increasing TDR is I_{Ks} block. Chromanol 293B, a relatively selective I_{Ks} blocker produces a homogeneous prolongation of APD across the ventricular wall (Fig. 12) (65). Despite a prominent prolongation of QT, chromanol 293B never produces TdP in experimental models, either spontaneously or in response to programmed stimulation. The addition of a β adrenergic agent leads to a marked abbreviation of APD of epicardium and endocardium, but not of the M cell resulting in the development of a marked dispersion of repolarization that is accompanied by the development of TdP, both spontaneous and stimulation-induced. These observations provide support for the hypothesis that the principal problem with LQTS is not long QT intervals, but rather the dispersion of repolarization that often accompanies prolongation of the QT interval. The spatial dispersion of repolarization creates a vulnerable window that can be captured by an extrasystole arising as consequence of the development of an EAD, thus precipitating re-entry, the mechanism thought to be responsible for most cases of TdP (Fig. 10). In support of this hypothesis is the observation that most drugs that induce TdP in the clinic cause an increase in spatial dispersion of repolarization and EADs. Spatial dispersion refers to dispersion of ventricular repolarization across the LV wall (transmural) between the left and right ventricle (interventricular), or between the base and apex of the heart. Drugs that block I_{Kr} /I_{Ks} and prolong the QT interval, but which do not increase spatial

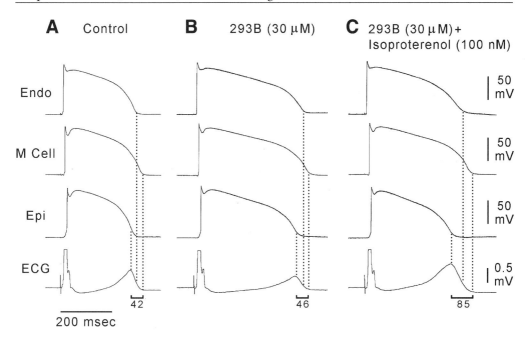

Fig. 12. I_{Ks} block alone prolongs QT interval without increasing transmural dispersion of repolarization. Ation potentials and transmural ECG under control conditions (**A**) after addition of chromanol 293B (30 µmol/L) (**B**), and after further addition of isoproterenol (100 nmol/L) (**C**). All traces depict action potentials simultaneously recorded from endocardial (Endo), M and epicardial (Epi) sites together with a transmural ECG. BCL = 2000 ms. (A) Control (B) I_{Ks} block with chromanol 293B prolongs the action potentials of the three cell types and the QT interval, but does not increase TDR (42 to 46 ms) or widen the T wave. (C) Isoproterenol in the continued presence of chromanol 293B abbreviated the action potential of epicardial and endocardial cells, but not that of the M cell, resulting in an accentuated TDR (85 ms) and broad-based T waves as commonly seen in LQT1 patients.

dispersion of repolarization or induce EADs, do not induce TdP either in the clinic or in experimental models (Table 1).

Whereas no single cell-based assay, in vitro heart preparation, or in vivo animal model can predict which drugs will induce TdP in humans with absolute accuracy *(19,24–26,43)*, studies conducted in M cell and epicardial tissues and arterially perfused wedge preparations isolated from the canine heart have yielded promising results with a sensitivity of 90% and a specificity of 100% in detecting agents that predispose to TdP (Table 2). Agents that increased TDR correlated well with their ability to induce TdP in the clinic. Conversely, drugs for which TdP has not been reported failed to produce an increase in TDR in these experimental models. Thus, among in vitro models canine isolated tissues and wedge preparations appear to be highly predictive in the identification of drugs with the potential to cause TdP.

In vivo models have also proved useful in the identification of drugs associated with a risk for TdP. A model initially developed by Carlsson et al. *(78)* consists of α-chloralose-anesthetized rabbits pretreated with methoxamine, an α_1 agonist. This model has a very high sensitivity to QT prolonging drugs, especially pure I_{Kr} blockers. Experience with drugs other than relatively pure I_{Kr} blockers is limited. The sensitivity and specificity of the rabbit model is therefore not well defined. Increasing concentrations of terfenadine and quinidine failed to induce TdP in the model *(79)*.

Table 1

Drugs That Block I_{Kr} and/or I_{Ks}, Prolong the QT Interval or Induce Torsade de Pointes and Their Ability to Induce EADs and Increase Dispersion of Ventricular Repolarization*

Drug[a]	Blocks I_{Kr}/I_{Ks}	QT_c interval	Prolongs TdP reported	Induces EADs	Increases dispersion of repolarization[b]	References
Antiarrhythmics						
Almokalant	+	+	+	+	+	98–100,101–103
Amiodarone	+	+	+	–	+/–	74,77,104–109
Azimilide	+	+	+	+	+	110–114
Dofetilide	+	+	+	+	+	77,79,113,115–118
Ibutilide	+	+	+	+	+	36,77,117,119–121
Quinidine	+	+	+	+	+	30,41,77,79,116,122–125
Sotalol	+	+	+	+	+	33,40,112,117,126–131
Antihistamines						
Astemizole	+	+	+	+	+	132–137
Terfenadine	+	+	+	+	+	79,132–134,138–141
Antibiotics						
Erythromycin	+	+	+	+	+	142–148
Calcium channel antagonists						
Diltiazem	+	+/–	–	–	–	149–152
Verapamil	+	+/–	–	–	–	77,149,153–157
Mibefradil	+	+	+	+	–	158–160
Bepridil	+	+	+	+	+	153,161–165

54

Psychotherapeutic					
Sertindole	+	+	+	−	128,166–169
Droperidol	+	+	+	?	170–174
Miscellaneous					
Cisapride	+	+	+	+	175–180
Sodium pentobarbital	+	−	−	+	71,72
Ketanserin	+	+	+	+	181–183
Ranolazine	+	−	−	−	76,184

*Includes drugs known to inhibit I_{Kr} and I_{Ks}, prolong QT or induce TdP, for which data are available relative to their actions to cause EADs or increase dispersion of ventricular repolarization.

+, response to drug noted; −, lack of response to drug noted; +/−, response noted in some studies but not others; ?, data not found.

[a]Based on a review of the literature of QT-prolonging drugs reported to inhibit I_{Kr} and/or I_{Ks}. Data are derived from humans, nonclinical models, or both. Nonclinical models include anesthetized animals, isolated hearts, multicellular and single cardiac-cell preparations.

[b]Dispersion of repolarization includes both QT dispersion (i.e., interlead variability of QT interval in humans) and/or transmural and inter-ventricular dispersion of repolarization (i.e., differences in action potential duration) in non-clinical models.

Modified from (26).

Table 2
Association of Increased Transmural Dispersion of Repolarization
and Early Afterdepolarization Activity in Canine Left Ventricular
Myocardium With the Occurrence of Torsade de Pointes in Humans

Drug/condition (ref.)	Canine LV tissues studied				Effect in canine LV		Effect in humans	
	M*	Epi*	PF*	Wedge	EADs	⇑TDR	⇑QT	TdP
Amiodarone (73)	✓	✓			−	−	+	±
Azimilide (185)	✓	✓			+	+	+	+
Cisapride (178)	✓	✓	✓	✓	+	+	+	+
Erythromycin (144)	✓	✓	✓		+	+	+	+
⇓$_{Ks}$ with β stim (68)	✓	✓	✓	✓	−	+	+	+
⇓$_{Ks}$ with β block (68)	✓	✓	✓	✓	−	−	+	−
Sodium Pentobarbital (71)	✓	✓	✓		−	−	+	−
Quinidine, low conc (186)	✓	✓	✓		+	+	+	+
Quinidine, high conc (186)	✓	✓	✓		−	−	+	−
Sotalol (62,68,187)	✓	✓	✓	✓	+	+	+	+
Terfenadine*	✓	✓	✓		+	+	+	+
Verapamil*	✓	✓	✓	✓	−	−	±	−
Ranolazine (76,184)	✓	✓	✓	✓	−	−	+	−

Epi, epicardial cells; ⇓$_{Ks}$, LQT1 (I$_{Ks}$ defect) in humans, drug-induced I$_{Ks}$ blockade in dogs; β block, β adrenergic blockade; β stim, β adrenergic stimulation; M, M cells; PF, Purkinje fibers. *unpublished observation.

The chronic AV block dog is an in vivo model closer to humans in its response to QT-prolonging drugs. In this model, dogs undergo ablation of the atrioventricular node, either by injection of formaldehyde via thoracotomy or by application of radiofrequency energy. Bradycardia-induced volume overload leads to biventricular hypertrophy and significant electrical remodeling over a period of 2–4 mo (80,81). In one version of this model, susceptibility to TdP is further increased with use of furosemide to produce hypokalemia (82).

The reported experience is also limited with this model, but drugs known to produce TdP in humans have generally produced TdP in the chronic AV block dogs (Table 3). Quinidine has been a borderline exception; sotalol induced TdP in five of six dogs studied by Weissenburger (83), but quinidine in the same animals induced only less distinctive ventricular tachyarrhythmias.

ALTERNATIVE ELECTROCARDIOGRAM MARKERS OF THE POTENTIAL FOR TORSADE DE POINTES

If QT prolongation and I$_{Kr}$ blocking potency are not reliable indices for predicting the proclivity of a drug to induce TdP, are there better surrogates? From our earlier discussion, transmural dispersion of repolarization might be a more reliable index, but how can we quantitate this parameter from the surface ECG ? Studies involving the arterially-perfused ventricular wedge preparations suggest that the interval between the peak and end of the T wave (Tpeak-Tend) may provide a reasonable index of transmural dispersion of repolarization. When the T wave is upright, the epicardial response is the earliest to

Table 3
TdP in the Chronic AV Block Dog

Drug	N	Incidence of TdP (%)
Almokalant (103)	14	64
Amiodarone (113)	7	0
Azimilide (113)	9	56
Dofetilide (113)	9	67
Dronedarone (113)	8	38
D-sotalol (188)	20	5
D-sotalol (103)	14	0
Ibutilide (25)	12	67

repolarize and the M cell action potential is the latest. Full repolarization of the epicardial action potential coincides with the peak of the T wave and repolarization of the M cells is coincident with the end of the T wave. It therefore follows that the duration of the M cell action potential determines the QT interval, whereas the duration of the epicardial action potential determines the QT peak interval. Another interesting finding stemming from these studies is that the T_{peak}–T_{end} interval may provide an index of transmural dispersion of repolarization (41,50).

The available data suggest that Tpeak-Tend measurements should be limited to precordial leads because these leads may more accurately reflect *transmural* dispersion of repolarization. Recent studies have also provide guidelines for the estimation of transmural dispersion of repolarization in the case of more complex T waves including negative, biphasic, and triphasic T waves (84). In these cases, the interval from the nadir of the first component of the T wave to the end of the T wave provides an accurate electrocardiographic approximation of transmural dispersion of repolarization.

The clinical applicability of these concepts remains to be fully validated. An important step towards validation of the Tpeak-Tend interval as an index of transmural dispersion was provided in a report by Lubinski et al. (85), which showed an increase of this interval in patients with congenital LQTS. Recent studies suggest that the Tpeak-Tend interval may be a useful index of transmural dispersion, and thus may be prognostic of arrhythmic risk under a variety of conditions (86–88).

Direct evidence in support of Tpeak-Tend as a valuable index to predict TdP in patients with LQTS was provided by Yamaguchi and co-workers (89). These authors concluded that Tpeak-Tend is more valuable than QTc and QT dispersion as a predictor of TdP in a patients with acquired LQTS. Further studies are needed to assess the value of these noninvasive indices of electrical heterogeneity and their prognostic value in the assignment of arrhythmic risk.

More recent investigations involving the arterially perfused wedge preparations suggest that the area between the peak and end of the T wave may provide an index of TDR over a wider set of conditions (unpublished observation, Tsuboi and Antzelevitch). It is noteworthy that van Opstal and co-workers (90) recently reported that in the chronic AV block dog, the JT area (area of the entire T wave) correlates well with interventricular dispersion of repolarization, another index of risk for the development of TdP.

Transmural dispersion of repolarization should not be confused with QT dispersion of repolarization, another proposed risk factor that remains somewhat controversial.

INFLUENCE OF GENETICS ON DRUG-INDUCED
LONG QT SYNDROME

The clinical manifestation of drug-induced channelopathies has in recent years been shown to be modulated by genetic factors. Available data suggest that up to 10% of individuals who develop TdP following exposure to QT-prolonging drugs possess mutations associated with LQT syndromes, and may be considered to have a subclinical form of the congenital syndrome *(91–93)*.

Abbot et al. *(94)* were among the first to show that a polymorphism (i.e., a genetic variation that is present in greater than 1% of the population) in an ion channel gene is associated with a predisposition to drug-induced TdP. They identified a polymorphism (T8A) of the *KCNE2* gene encoding for MiRP, a beta subunit of the I_{Kr} channel, that is present in 1.6% of the population and is associated with TdP related to quinidine and to sulfamethoxazole/trimethoprim administration. This finding suggests that common genetic variations may increase the risk for development of drug-related arrhythmias. More recently, Yang et al. *(93)* showed that DNA variants in the coding regions of congenital long-QT disease genes predisposing to acquired LQTS can be identified in approx 10 to 15% of affected subjects, predominantly in genes encoding ancillary subunits, providing further support for the hypothesis that subclinical mutations and polymorphisms may predispose to drug-induced TdP. Splawski et al. *(95)* further advanced this concept. In a population of individuals with drug-induced arrhythmias, they identified a heterozygous polymorphism involving substitution of serine with tyrosine (S1102Y) in the sodium channel gene *SCN5A* among Africans and African-Americans that increased the risk for acquired TdP. The polymorphism was present in 57% of 23 patients with pro-arrhythmic episodes, but in only 13% of controls. These findings suggest that carriers of such polymorphisms can be identified and excluded from treatment with drugs that are associated with a risk of proarrhythmia. It is conceivable that such testing could be applied widely because accurate results could be made available rapidly at relatively low cost.

Genetic variations can also modulate drug-induced channelopathies by influencing the metabolism of drugs. In the case of relatively pure I_{Kr} blockers, there is a clear relationship between plasma levels of drug and the incidence of TdP. Genetic variants of the genes encoding for enzymes responsible for drug metabolism could alter pharmacokinetics so as to cause wide fluctuations in plasma levels, thus exerting a significant proarrhythmic influence *(96,97)* For example, in the case of cytochrome CYP2D6, which is involved in the metabolism of some QT-prolonging drugs (terodiline, thioridazine), multiple polymorphisms have been reported that reduce or eliminate its function; 5–10% of Caucasians and African-Americans lack a functional CYP2D6. Numerous proteins, including drug transport molecules and other drug metabolizing enzymes, are involved in drug absorption, distribution, and elimination. Genetic variants of each of these have the potential to modulate drug concentrations and effects. Multiple substrates and inhibitors of the cytochrome P450 enzymes have been identified. A comprehensive database can be found at http://medicine.iupui.edu/flockhart/.

ACKNOWLEDGMENTS

Supported by grants from the National Institutes of Health (HL 47678), the American Heart Association, Northeast Affiliate, and the Masons of New York State and Florida.

REFERENCES

1. Mayer AG. Rhythmical pulsations is scyphomedusae. Publication 47 of the Carnegie Institute 1906;1–62.
2. Mayer AG. Rhythmical pulsations in scyphomedusae. II. Publication 102 of the Carnegie Institute 1908;115–131.
3. Mines GR. On dynamic equilibrium in the heart. J Physiol 1913; 46:349–382.
4. Mines GR. On circulating excitations in heart muscles and their possible relation to tachycardia and fibrillation. Trans R Soc Can 1914; 8:43–52.
5. Lewis T. The broad features and time-relations of the normal electrocardiogram. Principles of interpretation. The mechanism and graphic registration of the heart beat. London: Shaw & sons, Ltd., 1925: 44–77.
6. Moe GK. Evidence for reentry as a mechanism for cardiac arrhythmias. Rev Physiol Biochem Pharmacol 1975; 72:55–81.
7. Kulbertus HE. In Reentrant Arrhythmias, Mechanisms and Treatment. Kulbertus HE, ed. Baltimore: University Park Press, 1977.
8. Wit AL, Cranefield PF. Re-entrant excitation as a cause of cardiac arrhythmias. Am J Physiol 1978; 235:H1–H17.
9. Wit AL, Allessie MA, Fenoglic JJ, Jr., Bonke FIM, Lammers W, Smeets J. Significance of the endocardial and epicardial border zones in the genesis of myocardial infarction arrhythmias. In Cardiac Arrhythmias: A Decade of Progress. Harrison D, ed. Boston: GK Hall, 1982: 39–68.
10. Spear JF, Moore EN. Mechanisms of cardiac arrhythmias. Annu Rev Physiol 1982; 44:485–497.
11. Janse MJ. Reentry rhythms. In The Heart and Cardiovascular System. Fozzard HA, Haber E, Jennings RB, Katz AM, Morgan HE, eds. New York: Raven Press, 1986: 1203–1238.
12. Hoffman BF, Dangman KH. Mechanisms for cardiac arrhythmias. Experientia 1987; 43:1049–1056.
13. Antzelevitch C. Reflection as a mechanism of reentrant cardiac arrhythmias. Prog Cardiol 1988; 1:3–16.
14. El-Sherif N. Reentry revisited. PACE 1988; 11:1358–1368.
15. Lazzara R, Scherlag BJ. Generation of arrhythmias in myocardial ischemia and infarction. Am J Cardiol 1988; 61:20A–26A.
16. Rosen MR. The links between basic and clinical cardiac electrophysiology. Circulation 1988; 77: 251–263.
17. Antzelevitch C, Brugada P, Brugada J, Brugada R, Towbin JA, Nademanee K. Brugada syndrome: 1992–2002. A historical perspective. J Am Coll Cardiol 2003; 41(10):1665–1671.
18. Antzelevitch C, Brugada P, Brugada J, Brugada R, Shimizu W, Gussak I et al. Brugada Syndrome. A Decade of Progress. Circ Res 2002; 91(12):1114–1119.
19. Antzelevitch C, Shimizu W. Cellular mechanisms underlying the Long QT syndrome. Curr Opin Cardiol 2002; 17(1):43–51.
20. Bednar MM, Harrigan EP, Anziano RJ, Camm AJ, Ruskin JN. The QT interval. Prog Cardiovasc Dis 2001; 43(5 Pt 2):1–45.
21. Gwathmey JK, Slawsky MT, Briggs GM, Morgan JP. Role of intracellular sodium in the regulation of intracellular calcium and contractility. Effects of DPI 201–106 on excitation- contraction coupling in human ventricular myocardium. J Clin Invest 1988; 82:1592–1605.
22. Li CZ, Wang HW, Liu JL, Liu K, Yang ZF, Liu YM. [Effect of ATXII on opening modes of myocyte sodium channel, action potential and QT intervals of ECG]. Sheng Li Xue Bao 2001; 53(2):111–116.
23. Hanck DA, Sheets MF. Modification of inactivation in cardiac sodium channels: Ionic current studies with anthopleurin-A toxin. J Gen Physiol 1995; 106:601–616.
24. Roden DM. Drug-induced prolongation of the QT interval. N Engl J Med 2004; 350(10):1013–1022.
25. Fenichel RR, Malik M, Antzelevitch C, Sanguinetti MC, Roden DM, Priori SG et al. Drug-induced Torsade de Pointes and implications for drug development. J Cardiovasc Electrophysiol 2004; 15:1–21.
26. Belardinelli L, Antzelevitch C, Vos MA. Assessing Predictors of drug-induced Torsade de Pointes. Trends Pharmacol Sci 2003; 24:619–625.
27. Antzelevitch C, el Sherif N, Rosenbaum D, Vos M. Cellular mechanisms underlying the long QT syndrome. J Cardiovasc Electrophysiol 2003; 14(1):114–115.
28. Haverkamp W, Breithardt G, Camm AJ, Janse MJ, Rosen MR, Antzelevitch C et al. The potential for QT prolongation and pro-arrhythmia by non-anti- arrhythmic drugs: Clinical and regulatory implications. Report on a Policy Conference of the European Society of Cardiology. Cardiovasc Res 2000; 47(2):219–233.
29. Selzer A, Wray HW. Quinidine syncope. Paroxysmal ventricular fibrillation occurring during treatment of chronic atrial arrhythmias. Circulation 1964; 30:17–26.

30. Roden DM, Woosley RL, Primm RK. Incidence and clinical features of the quinidine-associated long-QT syndrome: Implications for patient care. Am Heart J 1986; 111:1088–1093.

31. Kay GN, Plumb VJ, Arciniegas JG, Henthorn RW, Waldo AL. Torsade de Pointes: The long-short initiating sequence and other clinical features: observations in 32 patients. J Am Coll Cardiol 1983; 2:806–817.

32. Haverkamp W, Martinez-Rubio A, Hief C, Lammers A, Mühlenkamp S, Wichter T et al. Efficacy and safety of d,l-sotalol in patients with ventricular tachycardia and in survivors of cardiac arrest. J Am Coll Cardiol 1997; 30:487–495.

33. Lehmann MH, Hardy S, Archibald D, Quart B, Macneil DJ. Sex difference in risk of torsade de pointes with d,l-sotalol. Circulation 1996; 94:2535–2541.

34. Hohnloser SH. Proarrhythmia with class III antiarrhythmic drugs: types, risks, and management. Am J Cardiol 1997; 80(8A):82G–89G.

35. Kober L, Bloch Thomsen PE, Moller M, Torp-Pedersen C, Carlsen J, Sandoe E et al. Effect of dofetilide in patients with recent myocardial infarction and left-ventricular dysfunction: a randomised trial. Lancet 2000; 356(9247):2052–2058.

36. Stambler BS, Wood MA, Ellenbogen KA, Perry KT, Wakefield LK, VanderLugt JT. Efficacy and safety of repeated intravenous doses of ibutilide for rapid conversion of atrial flutter or fibrillation. Ibutilide Repeat Dose Study Investigators. Circulation 1996; 94(7):1613–1621.

37. Antzelevitch C. Heterogeneity of cellular repolarization in LQTS: the role of M cells. Eur Heart J 2001; Supplements 3:K-2–K-16.

38. Antzelevitch C, Nesterenko VV, Muzikant AL, Rice JJ, Chen G, Colatsky TJ. Influence of transmural repolarization gradients on the electrophysiology and pharmacology of ventricular myocardium. Cellular basis for the Brugada and long-QT syndromes. Philos Trans R Soc Lond [Biol] 2001; 359:1201–1216.

39. Antzelevitch C, Dumaine R. Electrical heterogeneity in the heart: Physiological, pharmacological and clinical implications. In: Handbook of Physiology. Section 2 The Cardiovascular System. Page E, Fozzard HA, Solaro RJ, eds. New York: Oxford University Press, 2001: 654–692.

40. Weissenburger J, Nesterenko VV, Antzelevitch C. Transmural heterogeneity of ventricular repolarization under baseline and long QT conditions in the canine heart *in vivo*: Torsades de Pointes develops with halothane but not pentobarbital anesthesia. J Cardiovasc Electrophysiol 2000; 11:290–304.

41. Antzelevitch C, Shimizu W, Yan GX, Sicouri S, Weissenburger J, Nesterenko VV et al. The M cell: Its contribution to the ECG and to normal and abnormal electrical function of the heart. J Cardiovasc Electrophysiol 1999; 10(8):1124–1152.

42. Kozhevnikov DO, Yamamoto K, Robotis D, Restivo M, El-Sherif N. Electrophysiological mechanism of enhanced susceptibility of hypertrophied heart to acquired torsade de pointes arrhythmias: tridimensional mapping of activation and recovery patterns. Circulation 2002; 105(9):1128–1134.

43. Vos MA, van Opstal JM, Leunissen JD, Verduyn SC. Electrophysiologic parameters and predisposing factors in the generation of drug-induced Torsade de Pointes arrhythmias. Pharmacol Ther 2001; 92(2-3):109–122.

44. Akar FG, Yan GX, Antzelevitch C, Rosenbaum DS. Unique topographical distribution of M cells underlies reentrant mechanism of torsade de pointes in the long-QT syndrome. Circulation 2002; 105(10):1247–1253.

45. Sicouri S, Antzelevitch C. A subpopulation of cells with unique electrophysiological properties in the deep subepicardium of the canine ventricle. The M cell. Circ Res 1991; 68:1729–1741.

46. Zygmunt AC, Eddlestone GT, Thomas GP, Nesterenko VV, Antzelevitch C. Larger late sodium conductance in M cells contributes to electrical heterogeneity in canine ventricle. Am J Physiol 2001; 281:H689–H697.

47. Liu DW, Antzelevitch C. Characteristics of the delayed rectifier current (IKr and IKs) in canine ventricular epicardial, midmyocardial, and endocardial myocytes. Circ Res 1995; 76:351–365.

48. Zygmunt AC, Goodrow RJ, Antzelevitch C. I_{Na-Ca} contributes to electrical heterogeneity within the canine ventricle. Am J Physiol 2000; 278:H1671–H1678.

49. Antzelevitch C, Zygmunt AC, Dumaine R. Electrophysiology and pharmacology of ventricular repolarization. In Cardiac Repolarization. Bridging Basic and Clinical Sciences. Gussak I, Antzelevitch C, eds. Totowa: Humana Press, NJ, 2003: 63–90.

50. Yan GX, Antzelevitch C. Cellular basis for the normal T wave and the electrocardiographic manifestations of the long QT syndrome. Circulation 1998; 98:1928–1936.

51. Cohen IS, Giles WR, Noble D. Cellular basis for the T wave of the electrocardiogram. Nature 1976; 262:657–661.

52. Einthoven W. Uber die Deutung des Electrokardiogramms. Pflugers Arch 1912; 149:65–86.

53. Zuckerman R, Cabrera-Cosio E. La ondu U. Arch Inst Cardiol Mex 1947; 17:521–532.

54. Furbetta D, Bufalari A, Santucci F, Solinas P. Abnormality of the U wave and the T-U segment of the electrocardiogram: The syndrome of the papillary muscles. Circulation 1956; 14:1129–1137.

55. Nahum LH, Hoff HE. The interpretation of the U wave of the electrocardiogram. Am Heart J 1939; 17:585–598.

56. Lepeschkin E. Genesis of the U wave. Circulation 1957; 15:77–81.

57. Hoffman BF, Cranefield PF. Electrophysiology of the heart. New York: McGraw-Hill, 1960.

58. Watanabe Y. Purkinje repolarization as a possible cause of the U wave in the electrocardiogram. Circulation 1975; 51:1030–1037.

59. Lab MJ. Contraction-excitation feedback in myocardium: Physiologic basis and clinical revelance. Circ Res 1982; 50:757–766.

60. Choo MH, Gibson DG. U waves in ventricular hypertrophy: possible demonstration of mechano-electrical feedback. Br Heart J 1986; 55:428–433.

61. Antzelevitch C, Nesterenko VV, Yan GX. Role of M cells in acquired long QT syndrome, U waves, and torsade de pointes. J Electrocardiol 1996; 28(suppl.):131–138.

62. Shimizu W, Antzelevitch C. Sodium channel block with mexiletine is effective in reducing dispersion of repolarization and preventing Torsade de Pointes in LQT2 and LQT3 models of the long-QT syndrome. Circulation 1997; 96:2038–2047.

63. Lehmann MH, Suzuki F, Fromm BS, Frankovich D, Elko P, Steinman RT et al. T-wave "humps" as a potential electrocardiographic marker of the long QT syndrome. J Am Coll Cardiol 1994; 24:746–754.

64. Surawicz B. U wave: facts, hypotheses, misconceptions, and misnomers. J Cardiovasc Electrophysiol 1998; 9(10):1117–1128.

65. Shimizu W, Antzelevitch C. Cellular basis for the ECG features of the LQT1 form of the long QT syndrome: Effects of b-adrenergic agonists and antagonists and sodium channel blockers on transmural dispersion of repolarization and Torsade de Pointes. Circulation 1998; 98:2314–2322.

66. Schwartz PJ, Priori SG, Spazzolini C, Moss AJ, Vincent GM, Napolitano C et al. Genotype-phenotype correlation in the long-QT syndrome: gene-specific triggers for life-threatening arrhythmias. Circulation 2001; 103(1):89–95.

67. Li GR, Feng J, Yue L, Carrier M. Transmural heterogeneity of action potentials and Ito1 in myocytes isolated from the human right ventricle. Am J Physiol 1998; 275:H369–H377.

68. Shimizu W, Antzelevitch C. Differential effects of beta-adrenergic agonists and antagonists in LQT1, LQT2 and LQT3 models of the long QT syndrome. J Am Coll Cardiol 2000; 35:778–786.

69. Balser JR, Bennett PB, Hondeghem LM, Roden DM. Suppression of time-dependent outward current in guinea-pig ventricular myocytes. Actions of quinidine and amiodarone. Circ Res 1991; 69:519–529.

70. Anyukhovsky EP, Sosunov EA, Feinmark SJ, Rosen MR. Effects of quinidine on repolarization in canine epicardium, midmyocardium, and endocardium. II. In vivo study. Circulation 1997; 96:4019–4026.

71. Shimizu W, McMahon B, Antzelevitch C. Sodium pentobarbital reduces transmural dispersion of repolarization and prevents torsade de pointes in models of acquired and congenital long QT syndrome. J Cardiovasc Electrophysiol 1999; 10:156–164.

72. Sun ZQ, Eddlestone GT, Antzelevitch C. Ionic mechanisms underlying the effects of sodium pentobarbital to diminish transmural dispersion of repolarization. Pacing and Clinical Electrophysiology 20, 11–1116. 1997. Abstract

73. Sicouri S, Moro S, Litovsky SH, Elizari MV, Antzelevitch C. Chronic amiodarone reduces transmural dispersion of repolarization in the canine heart. J Cardiovasc Electrophysiol 1997; 8:1269–1279.

74. van Opstal JM, Schoenmakers M, Verduyn SC, De Groot SH, Leunissen JD, Der Hulst FF et al. Chronic Amiodarone evokes no Torsade de Pointes arrhythmias despite QT lengthening in an animal model of acquired Long-QT Syndrome. Circulation 2001; 104(22):2722–2727.

75. Zygmunt AC, Thomas GP, Belardinelli L, Blackburn B, Antzelevitch C. Ranolazine produces ion channel effects similar to those observed with chronic amiodarone in canine cardiac ventricular myocytes. Pacing Clin.Electrophysiol 25, II–626. 2002. Abstract

76. Antzelevitch C, Belardinelli L, Wu L, Fraser H, Zygmunt AC, Burashnikov A et al. Electrophysiologic Properties of Ranolazine: A Novel Anti-Anginal Agent. J Cardiovasc Pharmacol Therapeut. In press.

77. Yang T, Snyders D, Roden DM. Drug block of I(kr): model systems and relevance to human arrhythmias. J Cardiovasc Pharmacol 2001; 38(5):737–744.

78. Carlsson L, Almgren O, Duker GD. Qtu-Prolongation and Torsades-de-Pointes Induced by Putative Class-III Antiarrhythmic Agents in the Rabbit - Etiology and Interventions. J Cardiovasc Pharmacol 1990; 16:276–285.

79. Lu HR, Remeysen P, De Clerck F. Nonselective I(Kr)-blockers do not induce torsades de pointes in the anesthetized rabbit during alpha1-adrenoceptor stimulation. J Cardiovasc Pharmacol 2000; 36(6):728–736.

80. Vos MA, De Groot SH, Verduyn SC, van der ZJ, Leunissen HD, Cleutjens JP et al. Enhanced susceptibility for acquired torsade de pointes arrhythmias in the dog with chronic, complete AV block is related to cardiac hypertrophy and electrical remodeling. Circulation 1998; 98(11):1125–1135.

81. Sugiyama A, Satoh Y, Shiina H, Takeda S, Hashimoto K. Torsadegenic action of the antipsychotic drug sulpiride assessed using in vivo canine models. J Cardiovasc Pharmacol 2002; 40(2):235–245.

82. Weissenburger J, Chezalviel F, Davy JM, Lainee P, Guhennec C, Penin E et al. Methods and limitations of an experimental model of long QT syndrome. J Pharm Methods 1991; 26:23–42.

83. Weissenburger J, Davy JM, Chezalviel F, Ertzbischoff O, Poirier JM, Engel F et al. Arrhythmogenic activities of antiarrhythmic drugs in conscious hypokalemic dogs with atrioventricular block: comparison between quinidine, lidocaine, flecainide, propranolol and sotalol. J Pharmacol Exp Ther 1991; 259:871–883.

84. Emori T, Antzelevitch C. Cellular basis for complex T waves and arrhythmic activity following combined I(Kr) and I(Ks) block. J Cardiovasc Electrophysiol 2001; 12(12):1369–1378.

85. Lubinski A, Lewicka-Nowak E, Kempa M, Baczynska AM, Romanowska I, Swiatecka G. New insight into repolarization abnormalities in patients with congenital long QT syndrome: the increased transmural dispersion of repolarization. PACE 1998; 21:172–175.

86. Wolk R, Stec S, Kulakowski P. Extrasystolic beats affect transmural electrical dispersion during programmed electrical stimulation. Eur J Clinical Invest 2001;31:293–301.

87. Tanabe Y, Inagaki M, Kurita T, Nagaya N, Taguchi A, Suyama K et al. Sympathetic stimulation produces a greater increase in both transmural and spatial dispersion of repolarization in LQT1 than LQT2 forms of congenital long QT syndrome. J Am Coll Cardiol 2001; 37:911–919.

88. Frederiks J, Swenne CA, Kors JA, van Herpen G, Maan AC, Levert JV et al. Within-subject electrocardiographic differences at equal heart rates: role of the autonomic nervous system. Pflugers Arch 2001; 441(5):717–724.

89. Yamaguchi M, Shimizu M, Ino H, Terai H, Uchiyama K, Oe K et al. T wave peak-to-end interval and QT dispersion in acquired long QT syndrome: a new index for arrhythmogenicity. Clin Sci (Lond) 2003; 105:671–676.

90. van Opstal JM, Verduyn SC, Winckels SK, Leerssen HM, Leunissen JD, Wellens HJ et al. The JT-area indicates dispersion of repolarization in dogs with atrioventricular block. J Interv Card Electrophysiol 2002; 6(2):113–120.

91. Donger C, Denjoy I, Berthet M, Neyroud N, Cruaud C, Bennaceur M et al. KVLQT1 C-terminal missense mutation causes a forme fruste long-QT syndrome. Circulation 1997; 96(9):2778–2781.

92. Napolitano C, Schwartz PJ, Brown AM, Ronchetti E, Bianchi L, Pinnavaia A et al. Evidence for a cardiac ion channel mutation underlying drug-induced QT prolongation and life-threatening arrhythmias [In Process Citation]. J Cardiovasc Electrophysiol 2000; 11(6):691–696.

93. Yang P, Kanki H, Drolet B, Yang T, Wei J, Viswanathan PC et al. Allelic variants in long-QT disease genes in patients with drug-associated torsades de pointes. Circulation 2002; 105(16):1943–1948.

94. Abbott GW, Sesti F, Splawski I, Buck ME, Lehmann MH, Timothy KW et al. MiRP1 forms IKr potassium channels with HERG and is associated with cardiac arrhythmia. Cell 1999; 97:175–187.

95. Splawski I, Timothy KW, Tateyama M, Clancy CE, Malhotra A, Beggs AH et al. Variant of SCN5A sodium channel implicated in risk of cardiac arrhythmia. Science 2002; 297(5585):1333–1336.

96. Ford GA, Wood SM, Daly AK. CYP2D6 and CYP2C19 genotypes of patients with terodiline cardiotoxicity identified through the yellow card system. Br J Clin Pharmacol 2000; 50(1):77–80.

97. Roden DM. Pharmacogenetics and drug-induced arrhythmias. Cardiovasc Res 2001; 50(2):224–231.

98. Carmeliet E. Use-dependent block and use-dependent unblock of the delayed rectifier K+ current by almokalant in rabbit ventricular myocytes. Circ Res 1993; 73:857–868.

99. Houltz B, Darpo B, Edvardsson N, Blomstrom P, Brachmann J, Crijns HJ et al. Electrocardiographic and clinical predictors of torsades de pointes induced by almokalant infusion in patients with chronic atrial fibrillation or flutter: a prospective study. PACE 1998; 21(5):1044–1057.

100. Carlsson L, Drews L, Duker GD, Schiller-Linhardt G. Attenuation of proarrhythmias related to delayed repolarization by low-dose lidocaine in the anesthetized rabbit. J Pharmacol Exp Ther 1993; 267:1076–1080.

101. Wiesfeld AC, Crijns HJ, Bergstrand RH, Almgren O, Hillege HL, Lie KI. Torsades de pointes with Almokalant, a new class III antiarrhythmic drug. Am Heart J 1993; 126(4):1008–1011.

102. Abrahamsson C, Carlsson L, Duker G. Lidocaine and nisoldipine attenuate almokalant-induced dispersion of repolarization and early afterdepolarizations in vitro. J Cardiovasc Electrophysiol 1996; 7(11):1074–1081.

103. Verduyn SC, Vos MA, Van der Zande J, Kulcsar A, Wellens HJ. Further observations to elucidate the role of interventricular dispersion of repolarization and early afterdepolarizations in the genesis of acquired torsade de pointes arrhythmias: a comparison between almokalant and d-sotalol using the dog as its own control. J Am Coll Cardiol 1997; 30:1575–1584.

104. Kiehn J, Thomas D, Karle CA, Schols W, Kubler W. Inhibitory effects of the class III antiarrhythmic drug amiodarone on cloned HERG potassium channels. Naunyn Schmiedebergs Arch Pharmacol 1999; 359(3):212–219.

105. Kodama I, Kamiya K, Toyama J. Amiodarone: ionic and cellular mechanisms of action of the most promising class III agent. Am J Cardiol 1999; 84(9A):20R–28R.

106. Hii JT, Wyse DG, Gillis AM, Duff HJ, Solylo MA, Mitchell LB. Precordial QT interval dispersion as a marker of torsade de pointes. Disparate effects of class Ia antiarrhythmic drugs and amiodarone. Circulation 1992; 86(5):1376–1382.

107. Hohnloser SH, Klingenheben T, Singh BN. Amiodarone-associated proarrhythmic effects. A review with special reference to torsade de pointes tachycardia. Ann Intern Med 1994; 121:529–535.

108. Merot J, Charpentier F, Poirier JM, Coutris G, Weissenburger J. Effects of chronic treatment by amiodarone on transmural heterogeneity of canine ventricular repolarization in vivo: interactions with acute sotalol. Cardiovasc Res 1999; 44(2):303–314.

109. Drouin E, Lande G, Charpentier F. Amiodarone reduces transmural heterogeneity of repolarization in the human heart. J Am Coll Cardiol 1998; 32(4):1063–1067.

110. Fermini B, Jurkiewicz NK, Jow B, Guinosso PJ, Jr., Baskin EP, Lynch JJ, Jr. et al. Use-dependent effects of the class III antiarrhythmic agent NE-10064 (azimilide) on cardiac repolarization: block of delayed rectifier potassium and L-type calcium currents. J Cardiovasc Pharmacol 1995; 26(2):259–271.

111. Busch AE, Eigenberger B, Jurkiewicz NK, Salata JJ, Pica A, Suessbrich H et al. Blockade of HERG channels by the class III antiarrhythmic azimilide: mode of action. Br J Pharmacol 1998; 123(1):23–30.

112. Yan GX, Wu Y, Liu T, Wang J, Marinchak RA, Kowey PR. Phase 2 early afterdepolarization as a trigger of polymorphic ventricular tachycardia in acquired long-qt syndrome : direct evidence from intracellular recordings in the intact left ventricular wall. Circulation 2001; 103(23):2851–2856.

113. van Opstal JM, Leunissen JD, Wellens HJ, Vos MA. Azimilide and dofetilide produce similar electrophysiological and proarrhythmic effects in a canine model of Torsade de Pointes arrhythmias. Eur J Pharmacol 2001; 412(1):67–76.

114. Connolly SJ, Schnell DJ, Page RL, Wilkinson WE, Marcello SR, Pritchett EL. Dose-response relations of azimilide in the management of symptomatic, recurrent, atrial fibrillation. Am J Cardiol 2001; 88(9):974–979.

115. Kiehn J, Lacerda AE, Wible BA, Brown AM. Molecular physiology and pharmacology of HERG single-channel currents and block by dofetilide. Circulation 1996; 94:2572–2579.

116. Yang T, Roden DM. Extracellular potassium modulation of drug block of I_{Kr}. Implications for torsade de pointes and reverse use-dependence. Circulation 1996; 93:407–411.

117. Buchanan LV, Kabell GG, Brunden MN, Gibson JK. Comparative assessment of ibutilide, D-sotalol, clofilium, E-4031, and UK-68,798 in a rabbit model of proarrhythmia. J Cardiovasc Pharmacol 1993; 22:540–549.

118. Torp-Pedersen C, Moller M, Bloch-Thomsen PE, Kober L, Sandoe E, Egstrup K et al. Dofetilide in patients with congestive heart failure and left ventricular dysfunction. Danish Investigations of Arrhythmia and Mortality on Dofetilide Study Group. N Engl J Med 1999; 341(12):857–865.

119. Yang T, Snyders DJ, Roden DM. Ibutilide, a methanesulfonanilide antiarrhythmic, is a potent blocker of the rapidly activating delayed rectifier K+ current (IKr) in AT-1 cells. Concentration-, time-, voltage-, and use- dependent effects. Circulation 1995; 91:1799–1806.

120. Ellenbogen KA, Stambler BS, Wood MA, Sager PT, Wesley RC, Jr., Meissner MC et al. Efficacy of intravenous ibutilide for rapid termination of atrial fibrillation and atrial flutter: a dose-response study. J Am Coll Cardiol 1996; 28(1):130–136.

121. Glatter K, Yang Y, Chatterjee K, Modin G, Cheng J, Kayser S et al. Chemical Cardioversion of Atrial Fibrillation or Flutter With Ibutilide in Patients Receiving Amiodarone Therapy. Circulation 2001; 103(2):253–257.

122. Po SS, Wang DW, Yang IC, Johnson JP, Jr., Nie L, Bennett PB. Modulation of HERG potassium channels by extracellular magnesium and quinidine. J Cardiovasc Pharmacol 1999; 33(2):181–185.

123. Bauman JL, Bauernfeind RA, Hoff JV, Strasberg B, Swiryn S, Rosen KM. Torsade de pointes due to quinidine: Observations in 31 patients. Am Heart J 1984; 107:425–430.

124. Roden DM, Hoffman BF. Action potential prolongation and induction of abnormal automaticity by low quinidine concentrations in canine Purkinje fibers. Relationship to potassium and cycle length. Circ Res 1985; 56(6):857–867.

125. Sicouri S, Antzelevitch C. Drug-induced afterdepolarizations and triggered activity occur in a discrete subpopulation of ventricular muscle cell (M cells) in the canine heart: Quinidine and Digitalis. J Cardiovasc Electrophysiol 1993; 4:48–58.

126. Carmeliet E. Electrophysiologic and voltage clamp analysis of the effects of sotalol on isolated cardiac muscle and Purkinje fibers. J Pharmacol Exp Ther 1985; 232:817–825.

127. Varro A, Balati B, Iost N, Takacs J, Virag L, Lathrop DA et al. The role of the delayed rectifier component IKs in dog ventricular muscle and Purkinje fibre repolarization. J Physiol (Lond) 2000; 523 Pt 1:67–81.

128. Eckardt L, Breithardt G, Haverkamp W. Electrophysiologic characterization of the antipsychotic drug sertindole in a rabbit heart model of torsade de pointes: low torsadogenic potential despite QT prolongation. J Pharmacol Exp Ther 2002; 300(1):64–71.

129. McKibbin JK, Pocock WA, Barlow JB, Millar RN, Obel IW. Sotalol, hypokalaemia, syncope, and torsade de pointes. Br Heart J 1984; 51(2):157–162.

130. Patterson E, Scherlag BJ, Lazzara R. Early afterdepolarizations produced by d,l-sotalol and clofilium. J Cardiovasc Electrophysiol 1997; 8:667–678.

131. Sicouri S, Moro S, Elizari MV. d-Sotalol induces marked action potential prolongation and early afterdepolarizations in M but not epicardial or endocardial cells of the canine ventricle . J Cardiovasc Pharmacol Ther 1997; 2:27–38.

132. Suessbrich H, Waldegger S, Lang F, Bush AE. Blockade of HERG channels expressed in Xenopus oocytes by the histamine receptor antagonists terfenadine and astemizoles. FEBS Lett 1996; 385:77–80.

133. Delpon E, Valenzuela C, Tamargo J. Blockade of cardiac potassium and other channels by antihistamines. Drug Saf 1999; 21 Suppl 1:11–18.

134. Salata JJ, Jurkiewicz NK, Wallace AA, Stupienski RF, Guinosso PJ, Lynch JJ. Cardiac electrophysiological actions of the histamine H_1-receptor antagonists astemizole and terfenadine compared with chlorpheniramine and pyrilamine. Circ Res 1995; 76:110–119.

135. Sakemi H, VanNatta B. Torsade de pointes induced by astemizole in a patient with prolongation of the QT interval. Am Heart J 1993; 125(5):1436–1438.

136. Tsai WC, Tsai LM, Chen JH. Combined use of astemizole and ketoconazole resulting in torsade de pointes. J Formos Med Assoc 1997; 96(2):144–146.

137. Weissenburger J, Noyer M, Cheymol G, Jaillon P. Electrophysiological effects of cetirizine, astemizole and D-sotalol in a canine model of long QT syndrome. Clin Exp Allergy 1999; 29 Suppl 3:190–196.

138. Pratt CM, Hertz RP, Ellis BE, Crowell SP, Louv W, Moye L. Risk of developing Life-Threatening ventricular arrhythmia associated with terfenadine in comparison with over-the-Counter antihistamines, ibuprofen and clemastine. Am J Cardiol 1994; 73:346–352.

139. Pratt CM, Ruberg S, Morganroth J, Mc Nutt B, Woodward J, Harris S et al. Dose-response relation between terfenadine (Seldane) and the QTc interval on the scalar electrocardiogram: Distinguishing a drug effect from spontaneous variability. Am Heart J 1996; 131:472–480.

140. Monahan BP, Ferguson CL, Killeavy ES, Lloyd BK. Torsades de pointes occurring in association with terfenadine use. JAMA 1990; 264(21):2788–2790.

141. Zimmermann M, Duruz H, Guinand O, Broccard O. Torsades de pointes after treatment with terfenadine and ketoconazole. Eur Heart J 1992; 13(7):1002–1003.

142. Daleau P, Lessard E, Groleau MF, Turgeon J. Erythromycin blocks the rapid component of the delayed rectifier potassium current and lengthens repolarization of guinea pig ventricular myocytes. Circulation 1995; 91:3010–3016.

143. Rampe D, Murawsky MK. Blockade of the human cardiac K+ channel Kv1.5 by the antibiotic erythromycin. Naunyn Schmiedebergs Arch Pharmacol 1997; 355(6):743–750.

144. Antzelevitch C, Sun ZQ, Zhang ZQ, Yan GX. Cellular and ionic mechanisms underlying erythromycin-induced long QT intervals and torsade de pointes. J Am Coll Cardiol 1996; 28:1836–1848.

145. Oberg KC, Bauman JL. QT interval prolongation and torsades de pointes due to erythromycin lactobionate. Pharmacotherapy 1995; 15(6):687–692.

146. Gitler B, Berger LS, Buffa SD. Torsades de pointes induced by erythromycin. Chest 1994; 105:368–372.

147. Fazekas T, Krassoi I, Lengyel C, Varro A, Papp JG. Suppression of erythromycin-induced early afterdepolarizations and torsade de pointes ventricular tachycardia by mexiletine. PACE 1998; 21:147–150.

148. Nattel S, Talajic M, Lemery R, Roy D. Erythromycin induced long QT syndrome: concordance with quinidine and underlying cellular electrophysiologic mechanism. Am J Med 1990; 89:235–238.

149. Zhang S, Zhou Z, Gong Q, Makielski JC, January CT. Mechanism of block and identification of the verapamil binding domain to HERG potassium channels. Circ Res 1999; 84(9):989–998.

150. Hollifield JW, Heusner JJ, DesChamps M, Gray J, Spyker DA, Peace KE et al. Comparison of equal-weight oral dosages of verapamil hydrochloride and diltiazem hydrochloride in patients with mild to moderate hypertension. Clin Pharm 1988; 7(2):129–134.

151. Funck-Brentano C, Coudray P, Planellas J, Motte G, Jaillon P. Effects of Bepridil and Diltiazem on Ventricular Repolarization in Angina Pectoris. Am J Cardiol 1990; 66:812–817.

152. Singh BN. Comparative efficacy and safety of bepridil and diltiazem in chronic stable angina pectoris refractory to diltiazem. The Bepridil Collaborative Study Group. Am J Cardiol 1991; 68(4):306–312.

153. Chouabe C, Drici MD, Romey G, Barhanin J. Effects of calcium channel blockers on cloned cardiac K+ channels IKr and IKs. Therapie 2000; 55(1):195–202.

154. De Cicco M, Macor F, Robieux I, Zanette G, Fantin D, Fabiani F et al. Pharmacokinetic and pharmacodynamic effects of high-dose continuous intravenous verapamil infusion: clinical experience in the intensive care unit. Crit Care Med 1999; 27(2):332–339.

155. Gonzalez-Gomez A, Cires PM, Gamio CF, Rodriguez dl, V, Garcia-Barreto D. Relationships between verapamil plasma concentrations and its antihypertensive action. Int J Clin Pharmacol Ther Toxicol 1988; 26(9):453–460.

156. Boutarin J, Maarek-Charbit M, Aupetit JF, Galey-Arcangioli C, Ritz B. [Efficacy and tolerability of isoptine LP in mild to moderate hypertension. A multicenter study with 50 patients]. Ann Cardiol Angeiol (Paris) 1992; 41(10):587–593.

157. Bril A, Gout B, Bonhomme M, Landais L, Faivre JF, Linee P et al. Combined potassium and calcium channel blocking activities as a basis for antiarrhythmic efficacy with low proarrhythmic risk: experimental profile of BRL-32872. J Pharmacol Exp Ther 1996; 276:637–646.

158. Benardeau A, Weissenburger J, Hondeghem L, Ertel EA. Effects of the T-type Ca(2+) channel blocker mibefradil on repolarization of guinea pig, rabbit, dog, monkey, and human cardiac tissue. J Pharmacol Exp Ther 2000; 292(2):561–575.

159. Glaser S, Steinbach M, Opitz C, Wruck U, Kleber FX. Torsades de pointes caused by Mibefradil. Eur J Heart Fail 2001; 3(5):627–630.

160. Pinto JM, Sosunov EA, Gainullin RZ, Rosen MR, Boyden PA. Effects of mibefradil, a T-type calcium current antagonist, on electrophysiology of Purkinje fibers that survived in the infarcted canine heart. J Cardiovasc Electrophysiol 1999; 10(9):1224–1235.

161. Rowland E, McKenna WJ, Krikler DM. Electrophysiologic and antiarrhythmic actions of bepridil. Comparison with verapamil and ajmaline for atrioventricular reentrant tachycardia. Am J Cardiol 1985; 55(13 Pt 1):1513–1519.

162. Manouvrier J, Sagot M, Caron C, Vaskmann G, Leroy R, Reade R et al. Nine cases of torsade de pointes with bepridil administration. Am Heart J 1986; 111(5):1005–1007.

163. Osaka T, Kodama I, Toyama J, Yamada K. Effects of bepridil on ventricular depolarization and repolarization of rabbit isolated hearts with particular reference to its possible proarrhythmic properties. Br J Pharmacol 1988; 93(4):775–780.

164. Prystowsky EN. Electrophysiologic and antiarrhythmic properties of bepridil. Am J Cardiol 1985; 55(7):59C–62C.

165. Campbell RM, Woosley RL, Iansmith DH, Roden DM. Lack of triggered automaticity despite repolarization abnormalities due to bepridil and lidoflazine. PACE 1990; 13:30–36.

166. Rampe D, Murawsky MK, Grau J, Lewis EW. The antipsychotic agent sertindole is a high affinity antagonist of the human cardiac potassium channel HERG. J Pharmacol Exp Ther 1998; 286(2):788–793.

167. van Kammen DP, McEvoy JP, Targum SD, Kardatzke D, Sebree TB. A randomized, controlled, dose-ranging trial of sertindole in patients with schizophrenia. Psychopharmacology (Berl) 1996; 124(1-2):168–175.

168. Zimbroff DL, Kane JM, Tamminga CA, Daniel DG, Mack RJ, Wozniak PJ et al. Controlled, dose-response study of sertindole and haloperidol in the treatment of schizophrenia. Sertindole Study Group. Am J Psychiatry 1997; 154(6):782–791.

169. Fritze J, Bandelow B. The QT interval and the atypical antipsychotic sertindole. Int J Psych Clinc Pract 1998; 2:265–273.

170. Drolet B, Zhang S, Deschenes D, Rail J, Nadeau S, Zhou Z et al. Droperidol lengthens cardiac repolarization due to block of the rapid component of the delayed rectifier potassium current. J Cardiovasc Electrophysiol 1999; 10(12):1597–1604.

171. Lischke V, Behne M, Doelken P, Schledt U, Probst S, Vettermann J. Droperidol causes a dose-dependent prolongation of the QT interval. Anesth Analg 1994; 79(5):983–986.

172. Guy JM, Andre-Fouet X, Porte J, Bertrand M, Lamaud M, Verneyre H. [Torsades de pointes and prolongation of the duration of QT interval after injection of droperidol]. Ann Cardiol Angeiol (Paris) 1991; 40(9):541–545.

173. Michalets EL, Smith LK, Van Tassel ED. Torsade de pointes resulting from the addition of droperidol to an existing cytochrome P450 drug interaction. Ann Pharmacother 1998; 32(7-8):761–765.

174. Adamantidis MM, Kerram P, Caron JF, Dupuis BA. Droperidol exerts dual effects on repolarization and induces early afterdepolarizations and triggered activity in rabbit purkinje fibers. J Pharmacol Exp Ther 1993; 266:884–893.

175. Mohammad S, Zhou Z, Gong Q, January CT. Blockage of the HERG human cardiac K+ channel by the gastrointestinal prokinetic agent cisapride. Am J Physiol 1997; 273(5 Pt 2):H2534–H2538.

176. Drolet B, Khalifa M, Daleau P, Hamelin BA, Turgeon J. Block of the rapid component of the delayed rectifier potassium current by the prokinetic agent cisapride underlies drug-related lengthening of the QT interval. Circulation 1998; 97(2):204–210.

177. Wysowski DK, Bacsanyi J. Cisapride and fatal arrhythmia [letter]. N Engl J Med 1996; 335:290–291.

178. Di Diego JM, Belardinelli L, Antzelevitch C. Cisapride-induced Transmural Dispersion of Repolarization and Torsade de Pointes in the Canine Left Ventricular Wedge Preparation During Epicardial Stimulation. Circulation 2003; 108:1027–1033.

179. Chen YJ, Lee SH, Hsieh MH, Hsiao CJ, Yu WC, Chiou CW et al. Effects of 17beta-estradiol on tachycardia-induced changes of atrial refractoriness and cisapride-induced ventricular arrhythmia. J Cardiovasc Electrophysiol 1999; 10(4):587–598.

180. Puisieux FL, Adamantidis MM, Dumotier BM, Dupuis BA. Cisapride-induced prolongation of cardiac action potential and early afterdepolarizations in rabbit Purkinje fibres. Br J Pharmacol 1996; 117:1377–1379.

181. Le Grand B, Talmant JM, Rieu JP, Patoiseau JF, Colpaert FC, John GW. Investigation of the mechanism by which ketanserin prolongs the duration of the cardiac action potential. J Cardiovasc Pharmacol 1995; 26(5):803–809.

182. Aldariz AE, Romero H, Baroni M, Baglivo H, Esper RJ. QT prolongation and torsade de pointes ventricular tachycardia produced by Ketanserin. PACE 1986; 9(6 Pt 1):836–841.

183. Zaza A, Malfatto G, Rosen MR. Electrophysiologic effects of ketanserin on canine Purkinje fibers, ventricular myocardium and the intact heart. J Pharmacol Exp Ther 1989; 250:397–405.

184. Antzelevitch C, Belardinelli L, Zygmunt AC, Burashnikov A, Di Diego JM, Fish JM et al. Electrophysiologic effects of ranolazine: A novel anti-anginal agent with antiarrhythmic properties. Circulation 2004; in press.

185. Burashnikov A, Antzelevitch C. A combination of Ikr, Iks, and Ica or Ina block produces a relatively homogeneous prolongation of repolarization of cells spanning the canine left ventricular wall. Pacing and Clinical Electrophysiology 20, II–1216. 1997. Abstract

186. Antzelevitch C, Shimizu W, Yan GX, Sicouri S, Weissenburger J, Nesterenko VV et al. The M cell: its contribution to the ECG and to normal and abnormal electrical function of the heart. J Cardiovasc Electrophysiol 1999; 10(8):1124–1152.

187. Shimizu W, Antzelevitch C. Effects of a K(+) Channel Opener to Reduce Transmural Dispersion of Repolarization and Prevent Torsade de Pointes in LQT1, LQT2, and LQT3 Models of the Long-QT Syndrome. Circulation 2000; 102(6):706–712.

188. Verduyn SC, Vos MA, Van der Zande J, Van der Hulst FF, Wellens HJ. Role of interventricular dispersion of repolarization in acquired torsade-de-pointes arrhythmias: reversal by magnesium. Cardiovasc Res 1997; 34:453–463.

4

hERG Assay, QT Liability,
and Sudden Cardiac Death

Arthur M. Brown, MD, PhD

CONTENTS

INTRODUCTION

Since the late 1990s, several blockbuster, noncardiac drugs including terfenadine (Seldane) *(1,2)*, cisapride (Propulsid) *(3,4)*, and grepafloxacin (Raxar) *(5)* have been associated with prolongation of the QT interval of the electrocardiogram (ECG), polymorphic ventricular tachycardia, torsades de pointes (TdP), and sudden cardiac death. Regulatory agencies such as the Food and Drug Administration (FDA) responded initially with severe labeling restrictions, but ultimately these drugs were withdrawn from the marketplace. Not surprisingly, sudden cardiac death owing to noncardiac drugs has become a major safety issue for the pharmaceutical industry and the agencies that regulate it. TdP is linked to defective repolarization and prolongation of the QT interval of the ECG. At the cellular level, the duration of the cardiac action potential duration (APD) is prolonged. The major membrane currents and channels that are involved are shown in Fig. 1 along with the action potential they generate *(6)*.

When studied in ventricular myocytes, prolongation of APD by noncardiac drugs results from a reduction in the repolarizing cardiac membrane current I_{Kr} *(3,6)*. I_{Kr} is the product of the human ether-a-go-go gene hERG and mutations in hERG have been linked to the LQT2 form of hereditary long QT syndrome (HLQTS) *(7,8)*. HLQTS, like drug-

From: *Cardiac Safety of Noncardiac Drugs:*
Practical Guidelines for Clinical Research and Drug Development
Edited by: J. Morganroth and I. Gussak © Humana Press Inc., Totowa, NJ

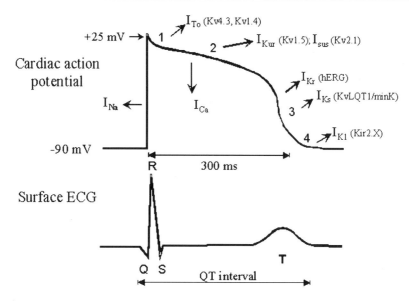

Fig. 1. Relationship among cardiac membrane currents, action potential duration and the QT interval of the ECG. The commonly used gene names are in parentheses.

induced or acquired LQTS (ALQTS) carries the risk of TdP and sudden cardiac death. The logical expansion was for the hERG product to be a molecular target for drug-induced ALQTS *(8)*.

The first direct test of this hypothesis used the poster drug for ALQTS, terfenadine. Terfenadine was the first nonsedating antihistamine and a blockbuster drug used to treat hay fever. Direct application of terfenadine blocked the hERG current transiently expressed in *Xenopus* oocytes *(9)*. Because drug access may be limited in *Xenopus* oocytes, it is preferable to express hERG in mammalian cell lines such as HEK 293 and CHO cells in which access is less problematic. Stable expression with a known passage number for the transfected cells is the preferred method of expression. Under these conditions, hERG produces a current that has the essential pharmacological and biophysical properties of I_{Kr} *(8)*.

At about the same time as terfenadine was raising safety flags, another blockbuster drug, cisapride, used to treat gastroesophageal reflux (GERD) was, like terfenadine, linked to QT prolongation, TdP, and sudden cardiac death. Rampe et al. and Mohammed et al. *(3,4)* used the hERG-mammalian cell system, and whole patch clamp showed that once again hERG was the molecular target. About 100 drugs later it appears that hERG is the only established target for noncardiac drugs carrying the prolonged QT/TdP liability. Table 1 confirms that hERG is by far the most sensitive to drug block of the potassium channels involved in cardiac repolarization *(10)*. Table 1 also shows an absence of class action effects (cf., terfenadine with fexofenadine and risperidone with sertindole). This result is significant for drug design since it indicates that hERG liability can be reduced without loss of efficacy.

To this point, every noncardiac drug that impairs cardiac repolarization has been shown to carry a hERG liability usually *(3),* but not always (see the later discussion on trafficking inhibition) *(11,12)* due to direct block of the hERG current. As a result, the hERG patch clamp assay is now used routinely to test lead compounds for their effects

Table 1
IC50 Values (μM) for Noncardiac Drug Blockade of Cloned Cardiac Potassium Channels

Drug	hERG	Kv1.5	Kv4.3	KvLQT1/mink
Antihistamine				
Terfenadine	0.056	0.367	2.70	4.40
Fexofenadine	13.1	389	112	20.4
Antipsychotic				
Risperidone	0.394	9.50	25.5	9.7
Sertindole	0.005	4.00	8.80	0.880
Prokinetic				
Cisapride	0.044	21.2	9.33	3.39

on hERG current stably expressed in heterologous cell lines. However, the relationship among reduced hERG current, QT prolongation, and TdP may be drug-dependent *(13)*, and not all drugs with a hERG liability impair repolarization *(14,15)*. As a practical matter, placing this triple relationship in context is essential and requires consideration of diverse levels including molecular and systems pharmacology, regulatory guidelines, and the strategies used for drug development by the pharmaceutical industry.

hERG ASSAY

In its customary form gigaseal, whole-cell patch clamp recording is done in HEK293 cells stably transfected with hERG cDNA. Suitable acceptance criteria include: gigaseal, low access resistance, stable leakage current, low voltage error, normal test pulse current waveform (e.g., hERG peak tail current amplitude higher than prepulse current amplitude), small rundown of test pulse current amplitude, and significant inhibition in response to positive controls.

Two pulse protocols may be used, step-pulse or step-ramp (Fig. 2) with the step-ramp giving lower IC_{50}s for drug block *(16)*. Block is gating-dependent and is maximal at conditioning potentials of about +20 mV that fully activate hERG current. Block is measured as the fractional reduction in the tail currents during the test pulse or ramp to potentials of –50 or –80 mV, respectively. For some drugs, e.g., erythromycin, sotalol, block may be strongly temperature-dependent *(16)*.

In all cases to this point, drugs that block hERG access the channel intracellularly. Access is kinetically determined and may vary greatly among drugs. As a result, attaining steady-state block at each concentration of a dose–response curve may be difficult, and failure to do so is probably responsible for much of the IC_{50} variability in the literature (Fig. 3). Thus, experimental data should show that a steady state of block has been reached at each concentration of drug; block should be distinguished from plugging of pipettes or electrodes or a change in access resistance; vehicle and positive controls should be applied along with each drug; pulse protocols should ensure full activation of currents and action potentials; currents should not exceed capacity of voltage clamp amplifier; pulse frequencies should span the physiological range; perfusion lines should be clean; and exchange of drug with test preparation should be complete. When the data satisfy these requirements and proper acceptance criteria for the whole cell gigaseal patch clamp method are used, the 95% confidence limits for IC50s of a number of noncardiac

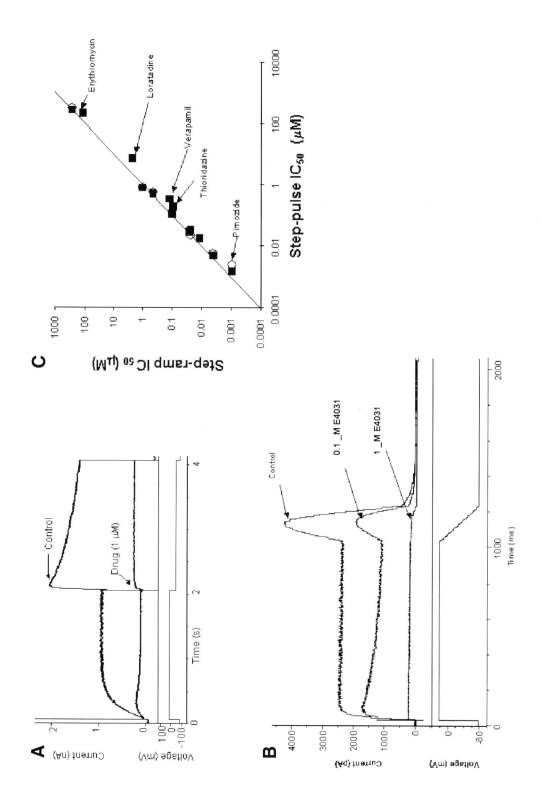

blockers vary by factors of 1.2 to 1.6 rather than the 50- to 100-fold differences that are present in the literature *(16)* (Fig. 3).

IC50 accuracy is critical for at least two reasons: (1) because it provides an estimate of the safety margin *(17)* for potential QT liability described in a subsequent section, and (2) because standard patch clamp is referred to as the gold standard for validating the various high throughput hERG screens that have been and are being introduced in the earlier stages of drug discovery discussed later in this review. The standard should be gold, not brass.

RELATIONSHIP AMONG THE hERG ASSAY, QT LIABILITY, AND TORSADES DE POINTES

Not all drugs with a hERG liability impair repolarization. Drugs may block outward hERG potassium current and inward calcium or sodium currents with similar potencies and the effects may offset each other resulting in no change in APD (Fig. 1) *(14,15)*. The prototypical drugs for these mixed ion channel effects (MICE) *(38)* are the calcium channel blocker verapamil *(14)* and the muscarinic receptor antagonist tolteridine *(15)*. Another drug with polypharmaceutical effects is amiodarone that may cause changes in QT, but is not commonly associated with TdP *(13)*.

For hERG blockers that prolong APD and QT, the adverse event of concern is TdP or monomorphic VT (lumped together as TdP). For the cardiac drug quinidine, the frequency of TdP is about 1:4000 while the frequency of QT prolongation is about 1:20. For noncardiac drugs, each of these frequencies appears to be one to two orders of magnitude lower. The wide range of these frequencies probably reflects their dependence upon voluntary adverse reaction reports from a variety of sources including patients, physicians, and drug companies. A circumstance in which the accuracy of reporting has not been validated.

Because the frequency is so low, TdP is not likely to be detected in clinical trials of noncardiac drugs, and the sudden death liability becomes manifest only during post-marketing surveillance of Phase IV clinical trials. Faced with this dilemma, regulatory bodies have resorted to the use of QT prolongation (ALQTS) as a surrogate for TdP. How good is this surrogate? Not very, for the following reasons: first, the QT interval varies with heart rate and there is neither a mechanistic explanation nor an agreed method of correction for this variability. Second, terfenadine and cisapride, two poster drugs for ALQTS, showed an average QT increase of about 10 ms; this is less than 3% of the regular QT interval and is well within the daily variability of QT in an individual. Third, the relationship between QT prolongation and TdP is a weak power function and has no threshold to identify imminent danger *(39)*. Fourth, the mechanism linking QT prolongation to TdP is unknown; prolongation of APD is associated with early after-depolarizations (EADs) due to reactivation of calcium current. EADs may trigger

---

Fig. 2. Block of hERG by a noncardiac drug. **(A)** hERG currents expressed in stably transfected HEK 293 cells using a conditioning prepulse to +20 mV from -80 mV for 2 s and a test potential of -50 mV done at 22°C at 0.1 Hz. Fractional block is measured from the tail currents (see arrows). Onset and kinetics of block are observed during the prepulse. **(B)** E-4031 block using a step-ramp protocol with a conditioning step to +20 mV for 1 s followed by a test ramp from +20 mV to –80 mV at 0.5 V/s. Fractional block is measured from the ramp peak currents. **(C)** Comparison of $IC_{50}s$ with step-ramp and step-pulse protocols.

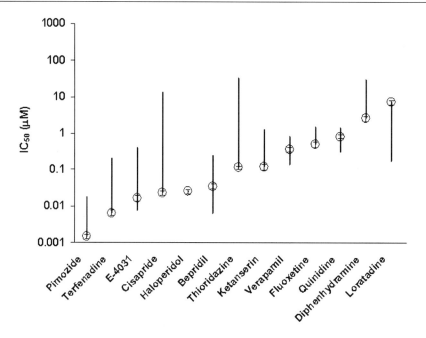

Fig. 3. Comparison of IC_{50} values for hERG/I_{Kr} blockers in mammalian cells. Vertical lines show range of high and low IC_{50}s in the literature *(4,10,18–37)* and open circles show IC_{50}s obtained by Kirsch et al. *(16)* using the step-ramp protocol shown in Figure 2.

arrhythmia, but TdP may occur absent EADs and maintenance of TdP requires increased transmural dispersion of repolarization re-entry pathways that can only be determined phenomenologically at this time. Fifth, the relationship may be drug-dependent; for equivalent QT prolongation drugs may differ in the frequency of TdP (sotalol vs dofetilide, amiodarone vs almokalant) *(39)*. Given all these shortcomings, it is difficult to understand any position that would make clinical QT prolongation the *sine qua non* for risk/ hazard estimates of drug safety as has been suggested *(40)*. Additionally, it would seem that the use of moxifloxacin as a positive control in clinical safety trials is an accident waiting to happen. Since QT prolongation per se reflects defective repolarization involving the currents and channels shown in Fig. 1, it is not surprising that nonclinical measurement of drug effects on channel function provides invaluable information concerning the potential for QT liability will inform the extensiveness of the clinical trials of QT liability, and should be an integral part of the cardiac safety package.

As a practical matter, drug developers cannot wait until phase I clinical trials to determine drug safety. Rather, this determination should be made long before an investigational new drug (IND) submission, preferably during lead development. "Fail early, fail cheap" is the strategy mantra of the pharmaceutical industry these days. A 10% improvement in predicting QT liability might save as much as $100 million per drug in drug development costs. As noted, hERG is the only proven molecular target for noncardiac drugs that carry a defective repolarization liability, and drug block of the hERG current expressed heterologously in cell lines is the most direct test of this propensity. Many drugs will reduce hERG current at sufficiently high concentrations, so the IC_{50} value should be referenced to a realistic drug concentration. This can be achieved using the ratio of the IC_{50} for drug block of hERG (numerator) to the IC50 or EC50 for the drug at its primary target or preferably, the effective therapeutic plasma concentration of the drug (denominator). The ratio is referred to as the safety margin (SM) *(17)*. If the ratio is >100 the SM is adequate; if the ratio is <10 the SM is too low; and between 10 and 100 the interpretation of the SM is indeterminate. SM calculations are limited by their dependence on the accuracy of the IC_{50} value for block and the measurement of free drug in the plasma that is determined by the binding of drug to plasma proteins. If IC_{50} values are taken from the literature, selection must be made critically, because as we have shown in Fig. 3 these values may be suspect. Regarding free concentrations in drug protein, binding is often in the 97–99% range and small differences in the measurement can have large effects on SM. For example, a drug with a hERG IC_{50} of 200 n*M*, a total plasma level of 200 nM, and 99% plasma protein binding, would have an acceptable SM of 100. If binding were 97%, the SM falls to 33.3 and would be less satisfactory.

Judgments must always be made in context. It is possible for drugs such as verapamil and tolterodine to be potent blockers of hERG current, yet avoid repolarization liability by also being potent blockers of inward calcium current, i.e., to have mixed ion channel effects or MICE. Risk analysis is essential. The risk–benefit ratio is very different for drugs used to treat seasonal hay fever or GERD on the one hand, and drugs used to treat cancer or AIDS on the other. For example, the lifetime risk of hay fever to a patient is about zero. Similarly, the lifetime benefit of a drug that treats symptoms of hay fever is about zero. A risk of symptomatic relief as low as 0.001% may not be acceptable when hundreds of millions of prescriptions are being written, especially if an alternative me-too drug with less risk is or becomes available. On the other hand, a drug that prolongs life by months for which there are no alternatives may be acceptable even at high risk for an adverse cardiac reaction.

ACTION POTENTIAL DURATION ASSAY
FOR REPOLARIZATION LIABILITY

This in vitro assay customarily uses APD measurements in Purkinje fibers isolated from the ventricle of a variety of species, the most favored being dog or rabbit. The relative merits of the assay have been described elsewhere *(41)*, but the main shortcoming is access of the drug to the fibers. The rabbit preparation is more sensitive than the dog preparation, probably because access is better. Protocols take the access problem into account by allowing for long periods of stabilization during control and following exposure to drug. In addition to information on repolarization, the assay measures resting potential and rate of rise of the action potential. Potent block of hERG does not necessarily establish QT/TdP liability because, as we have noted, blockers such as verapamil and tolterodine may have mixed ion channel effects and block inward calcium and/or sodium currents with equivalent potency, thereby offsetting the hERG block and maintaining a normal APD. Other drugs, such as cisapride and terfenadine, may block hERG with high potency and sodium and/or calcium currents at lower potency, producing a peak followed by a decrease in the relationship between APD prolongation and drug concentration (Fig. 4).

PRACTICAL ISSUES CONCERNING hERG IC_{50}S
AND APPLICATION OF THE hERG ASSAY TO INDUSTRY'S NEEDS

Although the in vitro patch clamp hERG assay is straightforward, considerable discrepancies in IC_{50}s have been reported (Fig. 3) *(16,17)*. The discrepancies result from unsatisfactory criteria for acceptance of primary gigaseal data and lack of recognition of

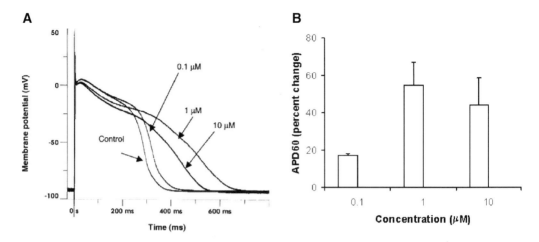

Fig. 4. Biphasic effects of cisapride on dog Purkinje fiber AP. (**A** and **B**) Maximum prolongation of APD occurred at 1 μM. Temperature 36.4°C, basic cycle length 2 s.

factors that may invalidate data collection during exposure to drug. When protocols are standardized and appropriate criteria for satisfying the gigaseal patch clamp method are used and block is measured at steady state with minimal rundown (Fig. 5), the differences between labs are minimal (Table 2). Block may be strongly temperature-dependent (e.g., erythromycin and sotalol) and is most conservatively measured using a pulse-ramp method at physiological temperature. Because block requires channel activation, it may be stronger at higher frequencies. This cumulation effect may not be observed when I_K is measured in cardiomyocytes. In fact, the opposite effect, so-called reverse use-dependence, may be observed due to residual I_{Ks} activation at higher frequencies.

Standard patch clamp is labor intensive and low throughput and is used for drugs that are being considered for IND submissions. This limitation is not a problem for drugs destined for the clinic because the overall numbers of drugs entering the pipeline of the entire biopharmaceutical industry are only in the low thousands per year at most and these numbers can be accommodated by the standard patch clamp hERG assay. Nor is this cost-restrictive given the overall cost of developing an approved drug that satisfies the requirement for cardiac safety. However, the "fail early, fail cheap" mantra means that hundreds of thousands of compounds should be evaluated by industry much earlier during lead optimization. The most direct approach is automation of patch clamp. A number of methods are being implemented generally using planar arrays of chips made from materials as diverse as quartz, silicon, and Sylgard. At present, none of the automated patch clamp methods has the combination of accuracy and throughput that would be desirable for earlier screening during lead development. The device with the highest throughput attains seal resistances in the low hundreds of megohms and suffers from low sensitivity as a result *(42)*. Other devices that attain gigaohm seals have low throughput and fluidics shortcomings *(43)*.

Nonpatch clamp methods with higher throughput do not measure functional hERG current. They include: (1) displacement of high affinity, radioactively labeled ligand blocker; (2) atomic absorption measurement of rubidium flux; and 3. fluorescence detection of voltage-sensitive dyes *(44)*. The first method will only detect compounds that compete for the binding site of the labeled ligand and will miss whole classes of compounds as a result. The second method initiates depolarization with high concentrations

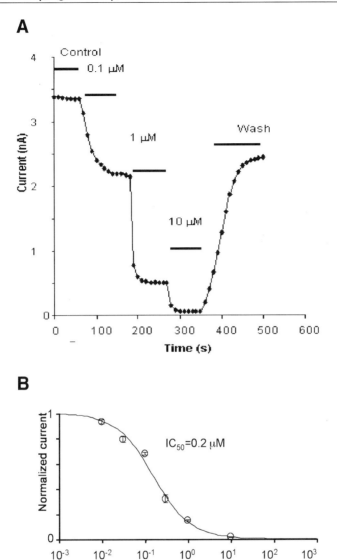

Fig. 5. Measuring steady state block of hERG. (**A**) Step-ramp protocol. When the on- and off-rate of drug block appear equal, i.e., when the change in successive measurements of fractional block is less than 2%, steady state has occurred. (**B**) Concentration-response data are fit by: % Block=$\{1\text{-}1/[1+([\text{Test}]/(\text{IC}_{50})^{N}]\}\cdot 100$ where [Test] is drug concentration, IC_{50} is drug concentration at half-maximal block, % block is fraction of hERG current inhibited at each concentration and N is a slope coefficient. Relationship is measured by non-linear least square fitting. 95% confidence limits are indicated by horizontal bars.

of extracellular potassium that reduce hERG block and decrease sensitivity. It is further limited by the inactivation properties of the hERG channel and contributions from non-hERG channels to resting Rb flux, and the fact that the equilibrium potential of Rb is continually decreasing. The third method has the first two limitations noted for the Rb flux method and may be even more strongly influenced by the relative contributions of other non-potassium ion channel determinants of membrane potential.

Table 2
Test Substances Investigated by ILSI*

	IC50 value (nmol/L)	
Test substance	Chan test*	DSTC
Positive		
Bepridil	24	17
Cisapride	21	26
Haloperidol	27	25
Pimozide	1	2
Thioridazine	74	43
Terfenadine	9	18
Negative		
Amoxicillin	N.A.	> 100000
Aspirin	N.A.	> 100000
Captopril	N.A.	> 100000
Diphenhydramine	1900	997
Propranolol	8200	6658
Verapamil	180	199

* International Life Sciences Institute.
According to Data Summary Graphs of the Cardiovascular Safety Subcommittee presented at ILSI Workshop in Washington, D.C., in June 2003 and DSTC data presented at the Society for Pharmacological Safety meeting, 2003.

Recently, a surface expression method called HERG-Lite® has been introduced *(45)*. This method takes advantage of the fact that direct blockers of hERG rescue trafficking of certain hERG mutations responsible for hereditary long QT syndrome (Fig. 6) *(46)* or inhibit trafficking of the wild type channel (unpublished observations). Like the other nonfunctional assays, this method has reduced sensitivity compared to standard patch clamp. The method has the great advantage that, in addition to detecting drugs that block hERG directly, it detects drugs such as the chemotherapeutic drugs arsenic trioxide and geldamycin *(12)*, that produce hERG/QT liabilities and TdP by inhibition of hERG trafficking.

hERG LIABILITY DUE TO INHIBITION OF TRAFFICKING

Recent reports have identified drugs that produce QT and TdP liabilities not by direct block of hERG, but rather by inhibition of hERG trafficking. Geldanamycin blocks the ATP-ase activity of Hsp 90, a cytoplasmic protein that is important for normal trafficking of hERG *(11)*. As a result, the immature, core-glycosylated form of the protein is retained in the endoplasmic reticulum (ER) and surface expression and hERG currents are reduced. In ventricular myocytes, the APD is prolonged and I_{Kr} is reduced. The effects are specific as other cardiac potassium currents such as I_{Ks} and I_{Kur} are unaffected. A 17-allylamino derivative of geldanamycin is in clinical trials for cancer chemotherapy and may cause hERG block and QT/TdP liabilities.

HERG and QT/TdP liabilities appear to apply to the use arsenic trioxide (AT3) for treatment of refractory or relapsing acute promyelocytic leukemia. AT3 treatment is

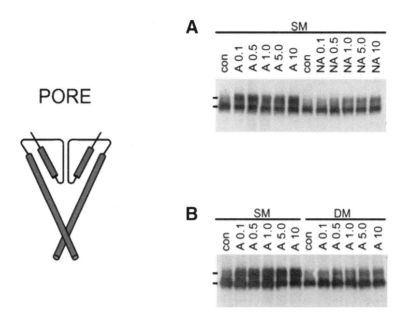

PORE

Fig. 6. Pharmacological rescue of an LQT2 mutant channel *(46)*. **(A)** Western blots of 20 μg amounts of total protein from HEK293 cells stably expressing hERG. SM (single mutant) protein is analyzed with increasing amounts of astemizole (A) and norastemizole (NA). Rescue is more pronounced for A as is potency of block of hERG current. Markers indicate core-glyosylated protein at about 135 kDa (upper band) and fully glycosylated protein at about 155 kDa. **(B)** Rescue of SM by astemizole is abrogated by DM which abolishes the drug binding site.

often accompanied by QT prolongation and TdP has been described *(47,48)*. While direct block of hERG has been reported from one lab *(49)*, two different labs have found no evidence of direct block *(12,50)*. Rather, it appears that AT3 blocks normal trafficking of hERG (Fig. 7). AT3 affects hERG trafficking in a manner similar to geldanamycin, namely that the core-glycosylated, immature form of hERG is retained in the EF and does not progress to the fully glycosylated mature form. Like geldanamycin, AT3 prolongs APD (Fig. 8) and reduces I_{Kr} without affecting I_{Ks} or I_{Kur}. However, unlike geldanamycin, the mechanism by which AT3 inhibits hERG trafficking is unknown. Other drugs have been identified that inhibit hERG trafficking and it is likely that this method of producing hERG liability will be identified more frequently in the future.

SUMMARY

Assessment of potential QT/TdP liability is an essential component in the determination of drug safety. QT liability of noncardiac drugs is uniformly associated with block of the cardiac hERG potassium channel. The in vitro cellular hERG patch clamp assay, when properly done, provides the most accurate, reproducible, quantitative measurement of hERG block. In some instances, hERG block may not cause APD/QT prolongation, e.g., if it is offset by block of sodium and/or calcium currents. The decision to go forward with a lead candidate should be made with this and other considerations, most importantly risk analysis, in mind.

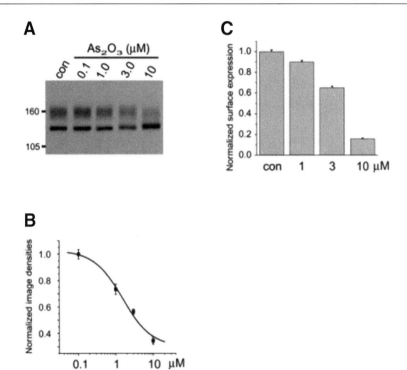

Fig. 7. Arsenic trioxide inhibits maturation and surface expression of hERG. (**A**) Western blot showing effects of overnight exposure to As_2O_3 on hERG WT protein stably expressed in HEK293 cells. (**B**) Concentration-dependent reduction of fully glycosylated 155 kDa hERG after overnight exposure to As_2O_3. IC_{50} is 1.5 μmol/L (n = 4) and is similar to the concentration-dependence of hERG block after overnight incubation. (**C**) Overnight exposure to As_2O_3 reduces surface expression levels of HA_{ex}-tagged hERG protein stably expressed in HEK293 as determined by chemiluminescence measurements (n = 6).

It is now apparent that drug-induced, acquired hERG liability may be produced by inhibition of hERG trafficking rather than direct block. The relative frequency of this mechanism is not yet known.

While it is the reference standard at present, the hERG assay is too labor intensive and too low throughput to be used as a screen early in the discovery/development process. Several indirect high-throughput screens have been used, but none are entirely satisfactory at present.

The link between QT prolongation and TdP is tenuous and QT prolongation is a poorly understood surrogate for adverse cardiac events. A battery of nonclinical tests must complement clinical QT measurements to provide an informed decision concerning the cardiac safety of all drugs.

ACKNOWLEDGMENTS

I am grateful to the study directors, staff scientists, Drs. Barbara Wible, Tony Lacerda, and Glenn Kirsch, and Mrs. Dee Groynom at ChanTest, Inc. and to my colleagues Drs. Eckhard Ficker and Yuri Kuryshev at the MetroHealth campus of Case Western Reserve University. This work was supported in part by NIH grant HL-36930, and ChanTest Inc.

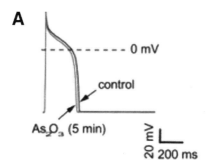

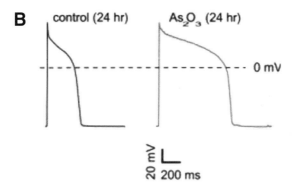

Fig. 8. Arsenic trioxide effects on cardiac action potentials recorded in guinea pig ventricular myocytes. **(A)** Current clamp recordings of action potentials (AP) elicited in a freshly isolated ventricular myocyte under control conditions and 5 min after start of perfusion with 3 μmol/L As_2O_3. **(B)** H.p. was –80 mV, AP recorded in ventricular myocyte cultured overnight under control conditions (left panel) or cultured overnight in the presence of 3 μmol/L As_2O_3 (right panel). H.p. was –80 mV.

REFERENCES

1. Morganroth J, Brown AM, Critz S, et al. Variability of the QT_c interval: impact on defining drug effect and low-frequency cardiac event. Am J Cardiol 1993;72:26B–31B.
2. Woosley RL, Chen Y, Froiman JP, Gillis RA. Mechanism of the cardiotoxic actions of terfenadine. JAMA 1993;269:1532–1536.
3. Rampe D, Roy ML, Dennis A, Brown AM. A mechanism for the proarrhythmic effects of cisapride (Propulsid): high affinity blockade of the human cardiac potassium channel hERG. FEBS Lett 1997;417:28–32.
4. Mohammad S, Zhou Z, Gong Q, January CT. Blockage of the hERG human cardiac K^+ channel by the gastrointestinal prokinetic agent cisapride. Am J Physiol 1997;273:H2534–H2538.
5. Kang J, Wang L. Cai F, Rampe D. High affinity blockade of the hERG cardiac K(+) channel by the neuroleptic pimozide. Eur J Pharmacol 2000;392(3):137–140.
6. Brown AM. Cardiac Potassium Channels in Health and Disease. Trends Cardiovasc Med 1997;7(4): 118–124.
7. Curran ME, Splawski I, Timothy KW, Vincent GM, Green ED, Keating MT. A molecular basis for cardiac arrhythmia: HERG mutations cause long QT syndrome. Cell 1995;80(5):1–20.
8. Sanguinetti MC, Jiang C, Curran ME, Keating MT. A mechanistic link between an inherited and an acquired cardiac arrhythmia: HERG encodes the I_{Kr} potassium channel. Cell 1995;81:299–307.

9. Roy M-L, Dumaine R, Brown AM. HERG, a primary human ventricular target of the nonsedating antihistamine terfenadine. Circulation 1996;94(4):817–823.

10. Lacerda AE, Kramer J, Shen K-Z, Thomas D, Brown AM. Comparison of block among cloned cardiac potassium channels by non-antiarrhythmic drugs. Eur Heart J Supplements 2001;3:K23–K30.

11. Ficker E, Dennis AT, Wang L, Brown AM. Role of the cytosolic chaperones Hsp70 and Hsp90 in maturation of the cardiac potassium channel hERG. Circ Res 2003;92:e87–e100.

12. Ficker E, Kuryshev Y, Dennis AT, et al. Arsenic-induced prolongation of cardiac repolarization and block of hERG trafficking. Mol Pharmacol 2004;66:33–44.

13. Roden DM. Current status of class III antiarrhythmic drug therapy. Am J Cardiol 1993;72:44B–49B.

14. Zhang S; Zhou Z; Gong Q; Makielski JC; January CT. Mechanism of block and identification of the verapamil binding domain to HERG potassium channels. Circ Res 1999;89:989–998.

15. Kang J, Chen XL, Wang H, et al. Cardiac ion channel effects of tolterodine. J Pharmacol Exp Ther. 2004;308:935–940.

16. Kirsch GE, Trepakova ES, Brimecombe JC, et al. Variability in the measurement of hERG potassium channel inhibition: effects of temperature and stimulus pattern. 2004 J Pharmacol Toxicol Methods. Accepted.

17. Redfern WS, Carlsson L, Davis AS, et al. Relationships between non-clinical cardiac electrophysiology, clinical QT interval prolongation and torsade de pointes for a broad range of drugs: evidence for a provisional safety margin in drug development. Cardiovasc Res 2003;58(1):32–45. Review.

18. Chouabe C, Drici MD, Romey G, Barhanin J. Effects of calcium channel blockers on cloned cardiac K^+ channels I_{Kr} and I_{Ks}. Therapie 2000;55:195–202.

19. Crumb WJ. Loratadine blockade of K^+ channels in human heart: comparison with terfenadine under physiological conditions. J Pharmacol Exp Ther 2000;292:261–264.

20. Daleau P, Lessard E, Groleau MF, Turgeon J. Erythromycin blocks the rapid component of the delayed rectifier potassium current and lengthens repolarization of guinea pig ventricular myocytes. Circulation 1995;91:3010–3016.

21. Drolet B, Vincent F, Rail J, et al. Thioridazine lengthens repolarization of cardiac ventricular myocytes by blocking the delayed rectifier potassium current. J Pharmacol Exp Ther 1999;288:1261–1268.

22. Ekins S, Crumb WJ, Sarazan RD, Wikel JH, Wrighton SA. Three-dimensional quantitative structure-activity relationship for inhibition of human ether-a-go-go-related gene potassium channel. J Pharmacol Exp Ther 2002;301:427–434.

23. Hanada E, Ohtani H, Hirota M, et al. Inhibitory effect of erythromycin on potassium currents in rat ventricular myocytes in comparison with disopyramide. J Pharm Pharmacol 2003;55:995–1002.

24. ICH Expert Working Group. Safety Pharmacology Studies for Assessing the Potential for Delayed Ventricular Repolarization (QT Interval Prolongation) By Human Pharmaceuticals. (Accessed in February 2002 at http://www.ich.org).

25. Khalifa M, Drolet B, Daleau P, et al. Block of potassium currents in guinea pig ventricular myocytes and lengthening of cardiac repolarization in man by the histamine H1 receptor antagonist diphenhydramine. J Pharmacol Exp Ther 1999;288:858–865.

26. Kongsamut S, Kang J, Chen XL, Roehr J, Rampe D. A comparison of the receptor binding and HERG channel affinities for a series of antipsychotic drugs. Eur J Pharmacol 2002;450:37–41.

27. Kupershmidt S, Yang IC, Hayashi K, et al. The I_{Kr} drug response is modulated by KCR1 in transfected cardiac and noncardiac cell lines. FASEB Journal 2003;17:2263–2265.

28. Le Grand B, Talmant JM, Rieu JP, Patoiseau JF, Colpaert FC, John GW. Investigation of the mechanism by which ketanserin prolongs the duration of the cardiac action potential. J Cardiovasc Pharmacol 1995;26:803–809.

29. Numaguchi H, Mullins FM, Johnson JP Jr, et al. Probing the interaction between inactivation gating and dl-sotalol block of hERG. Circ Res 2000;87:1012–1018.

30. Po SS, Wang DW, Yang IC, Johnson JP Jr, Nie L, Bennett PB. Modulation of hERG potassium channels by extracellular magnesium and quinidine. J Cardiovasc Pharmacol 1999;33:181–185.

31. Sanguinetti MC, Jurkiewicz NK. Two components of cardiac delayed rectifier K^+ current. Differential sensitivity to block by class III antiarrhythmic agents. J Gen Physiol 1990;96:195–215.

32. Wang J, Della Penna K, Wang H, Karczewski J, et al. Functional and pharmacological properties of canine ERG potassium channels. Am J Physiol 2003;284:H256–H267.

33. Wang JC, Kiyosue T, Kiriyama K, Arita M. Bepridil differentially inhibits two delayed rectifier K^+ currents, I_{Kr} and I_{Ks}, in guinea-pig ventricular myocytes. Br J Pharmacol 1999;128:1733–1738.

34. Weerapura M, Nattel S, Chartier D, Caballero R, Hebert TE. A comparison of currents carried by HERG, with and without coexpression of MiRP1, and the native rapid delayed rectifier current. Is MiRP1 the missing link? J Physiol 2002;540:15–27.
35. Witchel HJ, Milnes JT, Mitcheson JS, Hancox JC. Troubleshooting problems with in vitro screening of drugs for QT interval prolongation using HERG K$^+$ channels expressed in mammalian cell lines and Xenopus oocytes. J Pharmacol Toxicol Methods 2002a;48:65–80.
36. Witchel HJ, Pabbathi VK, Hofmann G, Paul AA, Hancox JC. Inhibitory actions of the selective serotonin re-uptake inhibitor citalopram on HERG and ventricular L-type calcium currents. FEBS Lett 2002b;512:59–66.
37. Zhou Z, Gong Q, Ye B, et al. Properties of hERG channels stably expressed in HEK 293 cells studied at physiological temperature. Biophys J 1998;74:230–241.
38. Hanson, L. Literature Reports of IC50's I_{Kr} Blockade. 2003 Barnett International QT Prolongation Conference 2003.
39. Moss AJ. Measurement of the QT Interval and the Risk Associated with QT$_c$ Interval Prolongation: A Review. Am J Cardiol 1993;72:23B–25B.
40. (Accessed at http://www.eudravigilence.org.)
41. Gintant GA, Limberis JT, McDermott JS, Wegner CD, Cox BF. The canine Purkinje fiber: an in vitro model aystem for acquired long QT syndrome and drug-induced arrhythmogenesis. J Cardiovasc Pharmacol 2001;37:607–618.
42. Kirk Schroeder; Brad Neagle; Derek J. Trezise; Jennings Worley. Ionworks(tm) HT: A New High Throughput Electrophysiology Measurement Platform. J Biomol Screen 2003;1:50–64.
43. Asmild M, Oswald N, Krzywkowski KM, et al. Upscaling and automation of electrophysiology: toward high throughput screening in ion channel drug discovery. Receptors Channels 2003;9:49–58.
44. Tang W, Kang J, Wu X, et al. Development and evaluation of high throughput functional assay methods for HERG potassium channel. J Biomol Screen 2001;6:325–331.
45. Wible BA, Hawryluk P, Ficker E, Brown AM. HERG-Lite(tm), a novel high throughput hERG cardiac safety test. 2003 Society for Biomolecular Screening Annual Meeting, abstract.
46. Ficker E, Obejero-Paz CA, Zhao S, Brown AM. The binding site for channel blockers that rescue misprocessed LQT2 hERG mutations. J Biol Chem 2002;277:4989–4998.
47. Ohnishi K, Yoshida H, Shigeno K et al. Prolongation of the QT interval and ventricular tachycardia in patients treated with arsenic trioxide for acute promyelocytic leukemia. Ann Intern Med 2000;133:881–885.
48. Unnikrishnan D, Dutcher JP, Varshneya N et al. Torsade de pointes in 3 patients with leukemia treated with arsenic trioxide. Blood 2001;97:1514–1516.
49. Drolet B, Simard C, Roden DM. Unusual effects of a QT-prolonging drug, arsenic trioxide, on cardiac potassium currents. Circulation 2004;109:26–29.
50. Imredy JP, Irving WD, Clouse HK; Salata JJ. Electrophysiological and pharmacological characterization of a cell line stably expressing *hKCNQ1* and *hKCNE1* potassium channels. 2004 Biophysical Society Annual Meeting, abstract.

5

Pharmacogenomics in Drug Development

When and How to Apply

Richard Judson, PhD *and* Arthur J. Moss, MD

CONTENTS

INTRODUCTION

Pharmacogenomics research typically aims to find genetic variants that affect the pharmacokinetics or the pharmacodynamics of a drug. Pharmacokinetic effects can be very direct, and are therefore easy to understand. Genetic variants can cause loss of function for a metabolic enzyme that can in turn decrease the rate at which a drug is metabolized. This increases the amount of drug delivered to the active site, as well as the half-life of the drug in the system. There is a wider range of pharmacodynamic effects. A variant can change the binding properties of a receptor to which a drug is targeted, and can therefore affect activity. Alternatively, a variant can simply alter the level of expression of some protein that can lead to an indirect effect on drug action. Variants that cause such expression changes can be *cis*, meaning that a variant in the gene has a direct effect on the gene's expression level. Alternatively, the effect can be *trans*, meaning that variation elsewhere in the genome indirectly affects expression levels for the gene. Genes causing such *trans* effects can be far removed from pathways directly involved in drug action.

The aim of pharmacogenomic research in the cardiac safety area are threefold: (1) to understand variability in safety that is caused by genetics; (2) to develop tools to help evaluate safety of compounds early in clinical trials; and (3) to develop tests to keep

From: *Cardiac Safety of Noncardiac Drugs:*
Practical Guidelines for Clinical Research and Drug Development
Edited by: J. Morganroth and I. Gussak © Humana Press Inc., Totowa, NJ

susceptible patients off of inappropriate drugs, or at safe doses. In almost all therapeutic areas there is large variability in both safety and response, and this variability is driven in part by genetics.

The goals of this chapter are to review current knowledge of the genetic factors that can affect the risk of drug-induced torsades de pointes (TdP), and to describe some possible avenues for further research in this area. As we will show, the range of possible genetic risk factors is large, so that we are far from being able to screen all patients for genetic risk prior to drug prescription. However, a more modest goal seems to be in reach: that of being able to understand the cause for outliers in clinical trials (excessive QT prolongation or TdP). From this, it may then be possible to quantify the risk of seeing significant problems with a drug once it goes into larger clinical trials and onto the market.

Currently, there are about 50 drugs on the market that carry some risk of drug-induced TdP that results from drug-induced QT prolongation. The incidence of TdP ranges from very low (on the order of 1 out of 100,000 users of cisapride) (1), to relatively high (e.g., sotalol, which shows a rate of a few percent) (2–4). These drugs span many classes and indications. However, there are some common risk factors however. Virtually all QT-prolonging drugs block the hERG potassium-ion channel (5). Women are at higher risk than men. Hypokalemia and the use of diuretics increase risk. In addition to these and other "phenotypic" risk factors, there are known "pharmacogenomic" risk factors. We will use the term pharmacogenomic loosely to mean instances where we can directly relate clinical risk to an underlying genetic mechanism. Ultimately, with greater understanding of underlying mechanisms, more of the phenotypic risk factors may change their status to pharmacogenomic.

The most well understood classes of pharmacogenomic risks of TdP involve drug metabolism (pharmacokinetics) and the interaction of drugs, directly or indirectly, with cardiac ion channels (pharmacodynamics) (6). Many QT-prolonging drugs are metabolized by the cytochrome P450 class of enzymes. Some individuals inherit defective versions of these enzymes that can lead them to be poor metabolizers. Most metabolic enzymes can also be inhibited by other drugs that can cause patients on multiple medications to receive higher than desired effective concentrations of the drug at the site of action. Both of these situations are well understood. On the pharmacodynamic side, certain individuals have genetic defects that alter the ability of their cardiac potassium and sodium ion channels to conduct. This can lead to the familial Long QT Syndrome (LQTS). The addition of a hERG blocker can be a second hit that will decrease the conductivity of their IKr channel to the point that significant QT prolongation is seen, which in turn increases the risk of TdP. Although it is now well known that mild prolongation of the QT interval is not always a good surrogate for risk of TdP (7), we will discuss both QT prolongation and TdP risk together.

Cisapride offers an example where both pharmacodynamic and pharmacokinetic genetic risk factors were seen to be important enough to make their way into the label (8). This drug was available from 1993 to 2000, when it was removed from active marketing and placed on a compassionate need program as a result of 341 reports of patients with cardiac events, 80 of whom died. All deaths were associated with drug-induced arrhythmias. These cases were reviewed and analyzed by the Food and Drug Administration (8). In 1999, family history of LQTS was added to the label as a contraindication, based on evidence that the drug could be the critical *second hit* for individuals who had deleterious mutations in the cardiac ion channel genes. At the same time, the ingestion of grapefruit juice was contraindicated. Cisapride is primarily metabolized by CYP3A4, which is inhibited by grapefruit juice. Taking the two together would greatly increase the effective concentration of the drug. A total of 126 of the 341 patients (37%) reported with events also took other medications that were CYP3A4 inhibitors. The median time between the start of use of cisapride and the CYP3A4 inhibitor drug and first event was only 5 d. For patients not on a concomitant CYP3A4 inhibitor, the median time to first event after prescription of cisapride was 14 d. An additional 35 patients with events (10%) had heart ischemia with previous reports of arrhythmias. A further 17 patients (5%) had electrolyte imbalance, and 17 (5%) were simultaneously on a second pro-arrhythmic drug. Finally, 9 patients (3%) suffered a cisapride overdose. Additional serious medical conditions were identified in most other patients, but it is not clear whether these factors were related to the risk of events. In summary, about 60% of patients with events had obvious risk factors, many of which were pharmacogenomic, which could explain the cause of their drug-induced arrhythmia. Therefore, there is significant evidence that genetic factors (pharmacokinetic CYP3A4 inhibition or LQTS) played a major role in putting individuals at risk for drug-induced arrhythmias while taking Cisapride. The overall incidence of TdP among cisapride users is estimated to be about 1 in 100,000 *(1)*. This is much lower than the rates for antiarrhythmic drugs such as sotalol, where the rate of TdP is reported to be in the range of 1.8–4.8% *(2–4)*. There is a significant difference between the patient populations for these drugs. Cisapride was prescribed predominantly for individuals without significant heart disease, whereas sotalol and related drugs are always given to patients with pre-existing cardiac arrhythmias *(9)*. Although cisapride had relatively low risk for TdP given the QT prolongation it caused, other examples are even lower. Ziprasidone causes mild QT prolongation, but even in the presence of metabolic inhibitors or of massive overdoses (as high as 29 times the daily maximum dosage) no cases of TdP have been reported *(10)* even after several years of sales.

THE HYPOTHESES—MULTIPLE HITS (SOME GENETIC) ARE REQUIRED TO TRIGGER TORSADES DE POINTES

More than 20 yr ago, Moss and Schwartz *(11)* proposed that some instances of TdP were actually a manifestation of LQTS that was only uncovered when a QT prolonging drug was added. LQTS is caused by mutations in any one of several ion channel genes, including KCNH2 (hERG), KCNQ1 (KVLQT1), KCNE1 (minK), KCNE2 (MiRP1), and SCN5A. Most LQTS mutations in the potassium channels cause a loss of function, leading to decreased current and longer repolarization times.

The QT interval is the "outer" manifestation of the underlying cardiac action potential (AP). The first phase of the AP is the opening of the sodium channel, SCN5A, causing rapid depolarization of the cell. Several potassium currents, including IKr (produced by the channel composed of KCNH2 and KCNE2) and IKs (produced by the combination of KCNQ1 and KCNE1) open in a synchronized manner to allow the cell to repolarize. If the potassium channels cannot conduct sufficient current to fully repolarize the cell well before the next depolarization step, the synchronization of the cells will fail and an arrhythmia can occur.

Roden *(7,12)* has proposed the concept of "repolarization reserve" to bring together the mechanics of repolarization and the understanding of how multiple hits may be required to cause TdP. Under ordinary conditions, cardiac cells have excess capacity to repolarize. There are more copies of each ion channel in the cell than the absolute minimum needed, and there are multiple pathways for potassium to exit the cell. These lead to a reserve of repolarization capacity. Numerous factors can cause a decrease in this capacity. At some point, the reserve is exhausted and the next factor that is added will cause the QT interval to increase.

Most known cases of TdP have occurred when the QTc interval exceeded 500 ms *(13)*. Although QT prolongation by itself is not clearly associated with increased risk of TdP, a 1997 report by the Center for Proprietary Medicinal Products (CPMP) stated that QTc is a significant risk factor for TdP when it is rises above 500 ms or when an increase of 60 ms or more is seen *(14)* A 60 ms change more reflects that the drug in question is responsible for the observed change rather than spontaneous variability because no data on a change by 60 ms and incidence of TdP are available. Another piece of evidence that demonstrates that multiple factors are needed to cause TdP comes from studies of LQTS and show that there is incomplete penetrance in families that carry even severe LQTS mutations *(15,16)*.

OVERVIEW OF HUMAN GENETIC VARIATION

In the following sections we will discuss specific genetic loci that have been associated with risk of drug-induced QT prolongation and TdP. There are almost certainly more associations to be found with currently known loci and more relevant loci to be discovered. This section briefly describes what is known about human genetic variation and some of the technical issues to be considered in pharmacogenomic studies of cardiac safety issues.

The human population contains an enormous amount of genetic variation. Variation occurs as single nucleotide polymorphisms (SNPs), which are single base pair substitutions; small insertion and deletion polymorphisms, ranging from one to tens or hundreds of bases; whole gene deletions; and whole gene duplications. SNPs are becoming the most widely used type of polymorphism in genetics research. These occur at a rate of approximately one every 200 bases in the human genome, yielding a total of approx 15 million. It is believed that the vast majority of these have no functional effect. The goal of much pharmacogenomic research is to sort through this vast sea of SNPs or other markers to find the few that are relevant for a given clinical phenotype.

Three major approaches are used to define sets of markers to measure in a pharmacogenomic study: known markers, markers in candidate genes or genome-wide marker sets. The known marker category is almost self-explanatory. A series of known, validated markers (e.g., SNPs that define CYP2D6 activity) are measured and directly used as covariates in an association analysis, or as an inclusion/exclusion criterion in a clinical trial. For the other two categories, one is searching for a marker that will help predict a phenotype.

In the candidate gene approach, one selects one or more genes that are suspected to be associated with the phenotype of interest, measures markers of these genes in a patient cohort, and looks for correlations with the phenotype. These genes will typically include the target of the drug, genes in the drug adsorption, distribution, metabolism, excretion (ADME) pathways relevant to the drug, or genes in pathways associated with upstream and downstream processes of the drug or the relevant disease. In a candidate gene study, one commonly genotypes a set of known SNPs in each of the genes, focusing on SNPs that fall in exons, splice regions, and putative promoter regions. The number of SNPs required for this approach is usually in the range of 5–10 per gene. Alternatively, one can resequence the genes in DNA samples from patients, again focusing on the functionally relevant regions. This is typically done when it is expected that the relevant SNPs are rare.

The genome-wide approach is by definition much more expensive and is just now being carried out in a viable way. Obviously, not all 15 million SNPs in the genome can be queried today in a patient population. The first practical approach is to use a selected subset of SNPs that are spaced closely enough to use the linkage disequilibrium properties of the genome. Linkage disequilibrium (LD) is a measure of how correlated a pair of markers are. In general, LD drops off with distance. The current, commercially available genome-wide approach measures one SNP every 2 kb or so, for a total of about 1.5 million. However, the cost is still too high to do this scan on every patient. Instead, the patient cohort must be divided into two pools, representing "cases" and "controls," based on a selected phenotype. These pools are then genotyped for all SNPs, and the frequency of the SNPs in the pools are compared using a simple chi-squared test. For the subset of SNPs that show a significant frequency difference between cases and controls, the samples are tested as individuals. One downside to this approach is that pooling requires one to select a single variable on which to pool. This is ideally suited to finding markers for a well-defined adverse event, but not well suited to finding markers for a series of quantitative traits that are simultaneously examined in the cohort. Because of the extreme number of tests being performed, there is only minimal power to rule out false positive signals. This approach should be viewed as an initial screen to find a large number of candidate markers that can be further evaluated in follow-on trials.

Distribution of Genetic Variation Across Genomic Regions

Most SNPs fall outside of coding regions for the simple fact that these regions make up only a few percent of the genome. Within exons, SNPs that cause radical amino acid changes are less common than ones that cause more conservative changes. This is consistent with the notion that the more radical the amino acid change, the more likely it is to have a functional consequence, and functional changes are more likely to have negative selective consequences than not. In one study *(17),* it was found that the percentage of exonic SNPs in the amino acid change categories (None; Conservative; Moderately Conservative; Moderately Radical; Radical; To Stop Codon) were 44.4, 19.2, 23.6, 8.2, 3.7, 0.9, respectively. Splice site variants are a special case. The splice signal region is somewhat ill defined, but extends 2–6 bases into the intron on either side of an exon. It is well known that there is significant sequence conservation at the first two positions.

Distribution of Genetic Variation Across Populations

The distribution of genetic variation in the human genome is a direct reflection of the history of human evolution. Each of the major population migrations has imposed a genetic bottleneck, which resulted in a decreased level of genetic diversity in the emigrating population. This is especially evident when comparing the three major population groups seen in Africa, Europe, and East Asia. Africans as a group have much more genetic heterogeneity and degree of variation than do either of the other two groups. After the migration out of Africa into Europe and Asia occurred and contact was broken, much new variation sprang up in these groups, which does not occur in Africa. As a consequence, it is relatively easy to find markers (SNPs or otherwise) that easily distinguish between individuals with principal ancestry from Africa, Asia, and Europe. This fact has a significant practical consequence in clinical pharmacogenomic research. If the phenotype of interest is at all correlated with ethnicity, regardless of whether this is caused by underlying genetics, or to cultural factors (diet, climate, etc.) it is possible to find many spurious, confounding associations between irrelevant genetic markers and the phenotype. To manage this, at a minimum, ethnicity must be used as a covariate in genetic association analyses. One can use self-reported ethnicity, or more sophisticated methods such as genomic control *(18)*. The basic approach here is to measure a number of genetic markers that are correlated with ethnicity or ancestry, but known to be uncorrelated with the phenotype. This approach allows one to quantify each individual's genetic background in an unbiased way, and to use this as a covariate in analyses.

Association Analysis

The goal of many genetic studies is to find an association between the presence of a genetic variant and a clinical variable. In most ways, this is no different from analyses carried out using standard clinical or demographic measures as independent variables, and the statistical techniques are similar. However, there are three special situations worthy of note. The first is the issue of multiple comparisons that was mentioned under whole-genome approaches. Because it is relatively inexpensive to measure any given genetic marker, candidate gene and whole-genome studies measure hundreds to hundreds of thousands for each patient. In these cases, the number of independent variables is equal to or potentially far greater than the number of subjects. Some degree of multiple test correction should be used, but standard correction methods (e.g., Bonferonni based on the total set of markers) are usually too conservative because they incorrectly assume that all tests are independent. This is not the case, because there exists some degree of correlation between the SNPs in the gene, as a result of LD. Bonferonni is too conservative because it assumes that all of the markers are independent. A better correction approach uses permutation testing that properly accounts for correlations between markers *(19–21)*.

A second property of most genetic markers is that they are diploid—each person can have zero, one, or two copies of the marker. Because of this, it is often useful to simultaneously consider dominant, recessive, and additive models. An extension of this occurs when multi-SNP haplotypes are used as part of the analysis strategy. In this case, a locus can have many different haplotypes, and each individual has two from that collection *(17,22,23)*.

Third, there is a special situation that occurs in genes such as the cardiac ion channels responsible for LQTS. These genes contain a large number of mutations (hundreds at latest count), any one of which can cause LQTS. So, although there is an association in a population between the gene and the disease, there would be little power to detect an association between a given marker and disease. One must instead use a model where it is not the presence of a given marker that determines risk, but the presence of any one of many potentially pathogenic variants that is the input to the model. An extension to this is to use the number of variants (common or rare) and to calculate a genetic load as an independent variable in a risk model.

PHARMACODYNAMIC FACTORS AND CARDIAC SAFETY

Pharmacodynamic effects leading to drug-induced arrhythmias arise in several ways. The best characterized cause of this are LQTS and related syndromes that are caused by mutations in several key cardiac ion channel genes which regulate the heart rhythm. The majority of these mutations cause a loss of function in potassium channels, meaning that the baseline current needed to repolarize the cells is decreased. LQTS mutations decrease the repolarization reserve that in turn leads to an enhanced effect on the QT interval of a hERG-blocking drug. Many specific LQTS mutations have been functionally characterized in vitro (for examples, see Table 1). The variants can affect the expression of the channels, the formation of multimeric channels, the current, or the opening/closing dynamics. Second, variants in the ion channel genes that do not cause LQTS may increase drug binding, which can increase the degree of channel block. Also, there are subclinical variants in these genes, which may only manifest their effect in the presence of an additional stress such as a drug challenge. Although the main action of almost all QT-prolonging drugs is the block of hERG, in vitro studies have shown binding of certain drugs to the other cardiac ion channels (24). Finally, variants in regulatory pathways could affect a patient's response to the drug.

A number of case studies have shown that specific LQTS mutations are associated with TdP. Some of these mutations have been functionally characterized to better understand their molecular effects. Table 1 lists a sampling of variants in the LQTS-related ion channel genes that have been reported to cause TdP, or have been functionally characterized for drug binding or LQTS. Each of these variants has been classified into one or more of five categories: L, causes LQTS; D, causes TdP; B, site demonstrated to be important for drug binding in vitro; F, functionally characterized in vivo; C, common, i.e., seen in a reference population of healthy individuals. A more extensive compilation of variants associated with LQTS, Brugada Syndrome, and TdP are given at the web site of the Study Group on Molecular Basis of Arrhythmias of Fondazione Salvatore Maugeri at: http://pc4.fsm.it:81/cardmoc/.

Variants That Cause Long QT Syndrome

It is well documented that patients with LQTS have an elevated risk of TdP because of their reduced repolarization reserve (16,25–28). Moss and Schwartz (11) proposed this link as early as 1982. Many LQTS variants cause a decrease in function (like partial blocking) so that normal drug blocking can have an increased relative effect. It has been estimated that 56–71% of patients who suffer from TdP may have prolonged baseline QT intervals (29). Sesti et al. (30) and Abbott et al. (31) examined several variants in KCNE2 that were associated with TdP and showed that these variants decreased baseline current, meaning that they are really LQTS variants that lead to TdP upon drug challenge. Similar findings have been reported for KCNQ1 by Jongbloed et al. (32), Donger et al. (26), and Yang et al. (25); Makita et al. (33) have reported similar findings for SCN5A.

Variants Can Affect Drug Binding

Sites of drug binding in the cardiac ion channel genes have been mapped out, so that it is possible to predict that mutations in these regions could lead to patient-specific levels of binding and secondary effects of the drug. For instance, Mitcheson and coworkers (34,35) worked out the binding sites in hERG for a particular drug, MK-499. They found that mutating any one of a few variants could greatly decrease the binding of the drug. Ficker et al. (36) and Lees-Miller et al. (37) have also reported specific residues in hERG that if altered will decrease drug binding. All of these residues lie in either the S6 transmembrane domain or the pore helix. Although there are currently no reported naturally occurring variants at these positions, such mutations would change the effect of hERG-blocking drugs in vivo. Recall that drugs causing TdP primarily block hERG. However,

Table 1
Sample of Variants That are Characterized to be Associated With Functional Changes in Key Cardiac Ion Channel Genes

Gene	Site or variant	Class	Drug	Functional effect	Clinical Effect	Minor allele freq. (AA : CA : AS : HL)	Reference(s)
KCNH2	P347S	D,C	cisapride clarithromycin		TdP	0.0 : 0.0025 : 0.0 : 0.0	47,67
KCNH2	N470D	L,B	E4031, astemizole, cisapride	Trafficking deficient, rescued in vitro by E4031, astemizole, cisapride	LQTS		36
KCNH2	D540K	B	MK-499	Increase speed of channel opening and decreases drug block			35
KCNH2	G601S	L,B	E4031, astemizole, cisapride	Trafficking deficient, rescued in vitro by E4031, astemizole, cisapride	LQTS		36,68
KCNH2	S620T	B	Dofetilide	Critical for high-affinity binding			69
KCNH2	T623	B	MK-499	Critical for high-affinity binding			34
KCNH2	V625	B	MK-499	Critical for high-affinity binding			34
KCNH2	S631A	B	Dofetilide	Critical for high-affinity binding			37
KCNH2	G648	B	MK-499	Critical for high-affinity binding			34
KCNH2	Y652	B	MK-499, terfenadine, cisapride	Critical for high-affinity binding			34,70
KCNH2	F656V	B	dofetilide, quinidine, MK-499, terfenadine, cisapride	Necessary but not sufficient for binding			34,37,70

Gene	Mutation		Drug	Description	Phenotype	Ratio	Refs
KCNH2	R784W	D		TdP			25
KCNH2	K897T	F,C	Amiodarone	Changes activation and deactivation parameters	Increased baseline QTc, Potential TdP	0.0041 : 0.166 : / 0.038 : 0.034	47,48,67
KCNE2	T8A	L,D,F,C	TMP/SMX, quinidine, amiodarone	Slight decrease in baseline current; similar or increased drug block relative to WT	TdP, QTP, LQTS(?)	0.0 : 0.0055 : 0.0 : 0.0	30,31,47,67
KCNE2	Q9E	D,F,C	erythromycin	Clarithromycin shows increased block relative to WT	TdP	0.015 : 0.0 : 0.0 : 0.0	31,47
KCNE2	M54T	L,D,F	procainamide	Decrease in baseline current; drug block similar to WT	TdP, LQTS		30,31
KCNE2	I57T	L,D,F	Oxatomide	Decrease in baseline current	TdP, LQTS		30,31
KCNE2	A116V	D,F	quinidine sulfamethoxazole	Decrease in baseline current	TdP		30
KCNQ1	R259C	L,F		Reduced current relative to WT	hypokalemia-induced TdP, LQTS		32,71
KCNQ1	T312	L,B	novel IKs blockers	Drug-binding site	LQTS		72–74
KCNQ1	Y315C	L,D,F	Cisapride	No current in mutant channel	TdP, LQTS		26,27,32,75
KCNQ1	I337	B	novel IKs blockers	Drug-binding site	LQTS		24
KCNQ1	F339	B	novel IKs blockers	Drug-binding site	LQTS		24,76
KCNQ1	F340	B	novel IKs blockers	Drug-binding site	LQTS		24
KCNQ1	A344	B	novel IKs blockers	Drug-binding site	LQTS		24,26
KCNQ1	R555C	L,D	terfenadine, disopyramide, meflaquine, diuretics		TdP, LQTS		26
KCNQ1	R583C	L,D,F	Dofetilide	Reduced current	TdP, LQTS		25,77

(continued)

Table 1 (*continued*)

Gene	Site or variant	Class	Drug	Functional effect	Clinical Effect	Minor allele freq. (AA : CA : AS : HL)	Reference(s)
KCNQ1	G589D	L,F		Site required for binding of complex involved in beta-adrenergic modulation	LQTS		51,52
KCNQ1	Residues 588-616	F		Leucine zipper motif in C-terminus—beta-adrenergic modulation			51
KCNE1	G38S	L,D,C			potential TdP, LQTS	0.18 : 0.22 : 0.082 : 0.24	47,67
KCNE1	Residues 39-43	B	stilbene, fenamate	Drug interaction site			38
KCNE1	D76N	L,F	stilbene, fenamate	Decreased baseline current, activity rescued by drug	LQTS		38
KCNE1	D85N	D,C	sotalol, quinidine		TdP	0.0035 : 0.0055 : 0.0035 : 0.0	67
SCN5A	H558R	D,C			Potential TdP	0.29 : 0.20 : 0.092 : 0.23	47,67
SCN5A	G615E	D,F	Quinidine	No effect seen in vitro relative to WT	TdP		25

Gene	Variant	Category	Drug	In vitro effect		Clinical	Ref
SCN5A	L618F	D,F	Quinidine	No effect seen in vitro relative to WT		TdP	25
SCN5A	S1102Y	L,F,C		Small change in current	0.063 : 0.0 : 0.0 : 0.0	LQTS (weak)	49
SCN5A	F1250L	D,F	Sotalol	No effect seen in vitro relative to WT		TdP	25
SCN5A	D1790G	L,F	Flecainide	Decreased current relative to WT with drug		LQTS, unusual flecanide block	78,79
SCN5A	Y1795C	L,F	Flecainide	Decreased current relative to WT with drug		LQTS, unusual flecainide block	78
SCN5A	Y1795H	L,F	flecainide	Decreased current relative to WT with drug		BrS, unusual flecainide block	78
SCN5A	L1825P	D,F	cisapride	Decreased current relative to WT; drug has no effect on current of mutant or WT		TdP	33

Each of these variants has been classified into one or more of five categories: L, Causes LQTS; D, Causes TdP; B, Site demonstrated to be important for drug binding in vitro; F, Functionally characterized in vitro; C, common, i.e., seen in a reference population of healthy individuals.

in vitro screens have shown that some of these drugs can also bind to KCNQ1 and KCNE1. Seebohm et al. *(24)* investigated several LQTS mutants in KCNQ1, and showed that they were potential drug binding sites. Abitbol et al. *(38)* performed similar experiments to find potential drug binding sites in KCNE1. In particular, they showed that conformational effects of mutations can cause decreased function and that the binding of a drug can overcome the molecular defect. A particular exception to the rule that drugs only bind hERG is amiodarone, which interacts with both hERG and calcium channels. The calcium channel block may in fact be protective against TdP *(12)*.

Variants Can Affect Channel Formation or Expression

Mutations can lead to changes in expression of the cardiac ion channel genes and their incorporation into working multi-unit channels *(12)*. Obviously, decreased channel expression will have effects similar to that seen when channels are defective. It is known that ion channel expression decreases in patients with ischemic heart disease, which is one risk factor for sensitivity to QT-prolonging drugs *(9)*. Variants have been shown to affect the transport of the immature protein to the cell membrane *(39,40)*, and it is almost certain that regulatory variants will be found that affect the expression of mRNA for these genes.

Spatial Distribution of Gene Expression or Drug Action Can Affect Risk

The spatial distribution of ion channels throughout the myocardium can modulate the risk of TdP *(9,41–44)*. hERG and KCNQ1 are the major potassium ion channels. KCNQ1 expression levels are lower in the Purkinje fibers and M-cells than in other layers of the myocardium, so that the effect on repolarization reserve in these layers is larger *(45)*. A drug that is effectively transported to these layers will have a strong effect here on the action potential duration and hence the local QT interval. It is possible that the difference between two drugs that cause the same apparent QT prolongation but that have greatly differing risks of TdP is because of this spatial inhomogeneity in drug distribution and action *(12,42–44,46)*. The mechanism of drug transport through the layers of the myocardium may be under genetic control and could offer a set of candidate genes to examine as risk loci.

Subclinical LQTS Common Polymorphisms May Be Functionally Important in Drug Risk

Most of the ion channel variants that have been characterized are rare mutants found in LQTS patients. However, these genes also contain common polymorphisms that lead to changes in the protein *(47)*. One can speculate that these variants have functional effects, but ones that are not large enough to give rise to the LQTS phenotype. However, these variants may have enough of an impact on channel function to play a role in risk of drug-related arrhythmias. The variants in these genes cover a spectrum ranging from the very rare and deleterious to the very common and benign. In the middle of this spectrum almost certainly lie variants that are relatively common, but functionally dangerous in the right circumstances.

There are case reports of variants thought to be responsible for LQTS or TdP but that appear at 1% and higher frequency in the general population for at least one ethnic group *(47)*. This is unexpected because the prevalence of LQTS is typically reported to be 1/5000, and no more than 1/1000–1/1300 *(25)*. However, relatively frequent variants may still have a phenotypic effect when combined with other risk factors. A possible confounding effect is that some of these polymorphisms are ethnic specific and were characterized as mutations because the control cohort did not include enough genetic diversity. Examples include KCNE2:T8A *(30,31)*, KCNE2:Q9E *(31)*, and KCNH2:K897T *(48)*. These were suggested as possible causes of cases of TdP. However, in the absence of any negative evidence, it is possible that these variants cause mild changes in channel function that contribute to a reduction in repolarization reserve and increase in risk of arrhythmias. For instance, the T8A variant in KCNE2 is seen in about 1% of Caucasians *(47)*, but has been associated with LQTS. In vitro studies show that this variant has slightly decreased current relative to wild-type (WT) *(30,31)*. In addition, this variant has been associated with TdP in cases involving TMP/SMX, quinidine, and amiodarone. The Q9E variant in KCNE2 has been associated with TdP associated with use of erythromycin *(31)*. This variant is seen in 3% of African-Americans. A final interesting example of such a polymorphism is the S1103Y variant in SCN5A. It is seen in approx 13% of African-Americans, but less than 0.5% of Caucasians. It was shown to have a slight effect in vitro relative to WT and has been assigned an LQTS phenotype based on a case report *(49)*.

It is already known that even among members of families who are carriers of LQTS mutations that there is variable penetrance *(15)*, so differences in the effect size of a genetic variant across population is not surprising. In summary, these common polymorphisms are phenotypically weaker than typical LQTS mutations, but may be one hit in a multistep process leading to a drug-induced arrhythmia.

Pharmacogenomic Effects of Regulatory Pathways

Another class of pharmacodynamic effect comes from signaling pathways that help modulate the action of the ion channel genes. In particular, the ion channel dynamics are regulated by the beta-adrenergic system. The effect of polymorphisms in the β_1 and β_2-adrenergic receptors on the risk of TdP was examined *(50)*. A modest association was seen linking a 2-SNP haplotype including Gly16 and Gln27 in the β_2-adrenergic receptor with risk of TdP. These SNPs have also been implicated in variable response to albuterol in asthmatics *(22)*. A number of intermediate molecules are involved in the signaling pathway, ending with the interaction of ACAP9 (yotiao) with residues 588–616 of KCNQ1 *(51)*. The result of this interaction is phosphorylation and inactivation of KVLQT1. At least one LQTS mutation has been discovered in this region *(51,52)*. These findings show that regulation of these ion channel genes can play a role in channel function, so that effects even in upstream parts of the regulatory pathways can have a functional effect, including putting patients at risk from a drug challenge. There are also polymorphisms in AKAP9, the PKA (protein kinase A) molecule to which it binds, as well as other proteins in this cascade. These are candidate modifiers of the strength of drug-induced QT prolongation.

Sex hormones are known to play a role in regulating the QT interval both at baseline and in response to drugs *(53,54)*. Women have higher baseline QTc than men *(55)*. To the extent that these hormones are under genetic control, this is another avenue to look for genetic variants that predispose to risk. It has been shown that although the phase of the menstrual cycle does not affect the QTc interval *(56)*, the effect on the QTc of ibutilide does correlate with the phase *(54)*. The greatest increase is seen in the first half of the cycle. One speculation is that sex hormones estradiol and progesterone may play a role in setting the QT interval, and genetic factors that alter levels of these hormones could be involved in risk *(54)*. This factor may be related to the increased incidence of events among female carriers of LQTS mutations in the postpartum period *(57)*. In rabbits, sex hormones play a role in altering the levels of expression of cardiac potassium channels *(58)*.

PHARMACOKINETIC FACTORS AND CARDIAC SAFETY

Pharmacokinetic factors ultimately drive the effective concentration that is seen at the site of action of the drug. Although there is conflicting evidence that the risk of TdP is dependent on the dose that a patient is given, it is almost certainly true that as the concentration of the drug at the hERG channels increases, that the amount of hERG block will go up accordingly. Dose is seen as a risk factor for certain drugs, including terfenadine (59), cisapride (8), and sotalol (4). QT-prolonging drugs are principally metabolized by CYP2D6 and CYP3A4. There are a few drugs metabolized by alternative routes including aldehyde oxidase, glucuronyl transferase, quinone oxidoreductase, and through beta-oxidation and N-acetylation. Note that some drugs are excreted unchanged. Table 2 lists the route of metabolism for several drugs showing risk of TdP. The basic pharmacogenomic risk factor is straightforward here—if a patient's metabolism for the drug is compromised then the effective concentration at the target is increased, as is the risk for an event. Metabolism can be compromised by in-born defects in metabolic enzymes, reduced expression of the enzymes caused by a condition such as disease or advanced age, or inhibition of the enzyme by another drug.

Pharmacokinetics covers not only drug metabolism, but also the entire ADME process. There are likely person-to-person differences in how these drugs are processed in the other ADME steps, and candidate gene pharmacogenomic studies often will include polymorphisms in these pathways when looking at variable drug action. However, little is known currently about how the other ADME pathways affect the potential for TdP among QT-prolonging drugs.

Inborn Defects in Metabolic Enzymes

The prototypical example of a pharmacokinetics/pharmacogenomic link is offered by CYP2D6. The protein expressed by this gene metabolizes a wide variety of pharmaceutical compounds, among which are several drugs associated with QT prolongation and risk of TdP (Table 2).

The CYP2D6 gene exists in a wide variety of forms, a summary of which can be found at www.imm.ki.se/CYPalleles/cyp2d6.htm. Most forms are distinguished by the presence of one or more SNPs. In addition to single nucleotide changes, individuals can have the entire gene deleted (one or both copies) and can have the gene duplicated one or more times. As is typical, most of the SNPs seen in CYP2D6 are nonfunctional and simply lead to increased complexity of the gene taxonomy. The principle functional SNPs are those responsible for the *3, *4, *6, *7, and *8 alleles. Each of these is distinguished by a SNP that causes the resulting protein to be nonfunctional. The *10 allele has reduced activity relative to the fully functional *1 version of the gene. The whole gene deletion is designated by the *5 allele. Frequencies of these SNPs vary widely between ethnic groups—for instance there is a lower rate of poor metabolizers (individuals with two nonfunctional copies of CYP2D6) in Japan than in Caucasian populations (60,61). For the most part then an individual can have zero, one, or two working copies of the gene, so that their metabolic activity can nominally be in one of these three levels. Typically, the log of the metabolic ratio (amount of parent compound divided by amount of metabolite) is roughly linear with the number of active copies of the gene that an individual carries. There is still considerable spread in in vivo activity, however, because the level of protein expression varies among individuals, and because there is typically a backup pathway that can metabolize drugs even in the absence of any CYP2D6 activity.

Table 2
Major Route of Metabolism for Selected Drugs With High Risk of Causing TdP

Drug	Metabolized by	Inhibits
Amiodarone	3A4 2C8	1A2 2C9 2D6 3A4
Bepridil	3A4	
Chloroquine	2D6 3A4 2C8	2D6
chlorpromazine	2D6 GT	2D6 AO FMO3 GT QO
Cisapride	3A4	
clarithromycin	3A4	3A4
disopyramide	3A4	
Dofetilide	3A4 (MINOR)	
Droperidol	3A4	
erythromycin	3A4	1A2 3A4
Halofantrine	3A4 3A5	2D6
Haloperidol	3A4	2D6 QO
Ibutilide	BO	
levomethadyl	3A4	
Methadone	3A4	2D6
Pimozide	3A4	2D6
procainamide	2D6 NA	
Quinidine	3A4	2D6 3A4
Sotalol	Not metabolized	
Sparfloxacin	GT	
Thioridazine	2D6	2D6

Drug list taken from www.torsades.org.
CYPs are abbreviated by their unique designation, e.g., 2D6, CYP2D6; AO, aldehyde oxidase; GT, glucuronyl transferase; QO, quinone oxidoreductase. BO, β-oxidation; NA, N-acetylation.

Because the link between genotype and activity is so clear for CYP2D6, it is possible to carry out a genotyping assay and use the results to tailor the dosage of CYP2D6 metabolized drugs to the particular patient. This is especially valuable in situations where the patient is on multiple drugs that are substrates for this gene.

A more complex example is provided by CYP3A4. This gene is responsible for metabolizing even more compounds than CYP2D6—perhaps 60% of all prescription drugs. It also shows variable metabolic efficiency, but the specific alleles responsible for this variability have not been identified. CYP3A4 has several variant forms owing to relatively common SNPs, but none of these is associated with differential in vivo activity. Instead, this functional variability is driven by changes in expression that can be induced, or by activity changes caused by inhibition (62). A specific *cis*-acting element in the CYP3A4 gene enhancer has been identified (63). This may control the induction of gene expression, and is a candidate region for polymorphisms that could cause variability in metabolic rates. Expression levels for CYP3A4 and CYP2D6 are also reduced in elderly patients that can lead to correspondingly reduced metabolism and increased effective concentrations.

Inhibition of the Enzyme by Another Drug

Both CYP2D6 and CYP3A4 can be inhibited by a variety of other drugs as well as by common foods. For instance, grapefruit juice is a CYP3A4 inhibitor and should not be consumed while taking certain drugs. Table 2 shows not only what enzymes metabolize this selection of drugs, but also which enzymes are inhibited strongly by these. Although this mechanism of drug–drug interaction is well understood, and should be well known among physicians, there are many case reports of incidents of TdP where a patient was simultaneously taking a hERG-blocking drug and a corresponding enzyme inhibitor. Curtis *(64)* and Roe *(65)* have both documented this large-scale inappropriate double prescription.

DISCUSSION

Two goals of this chapter were to describe the pharmacogenomic factors that can affect the risk of TdP and to outline areas of further research. These risk factors were broken down into pharmacodynamic factors, mainly involving cardiac ion channel genes and pharmacokinetic factors, which centered on drug metabolizing enzymes. Most individuals have sufficient repolarization reserve to be able to tolerate decreased potassium current caused by a hERG-blocking drug at normal doses. However, if the patient has inborn defects in their potassium channels (as in LQTS) or has decreased expression of the channels (as can happen as a result of the presence of heart disease), then the effect of the drug can be significantly enhanced. Likewise, if the effective concentration of the drug is greatly increased because the normal routes of metabolism are ineffective, then the patient is again at increased risk. The main metabolic enzymes (CYP2D6 and CYP3A4) have inborn variation in activity, and both can be inhibited by certain other medications and foods. Table 3 summarizes these and other pharmacogenomic risk factors. Several phenotypic factors are well documented. These include female gender, advanced age, renal or hepatic impairment, hypokalemia, hypomagnesia, use of diuretics, certain cardiac disorders (congestive heart failure, cardiac hypertrophy, bradycardia), recent conversion from atrial fibrillation, drug overdose, and baseline ECG abnormalities such as a long QT interval or T-wave liability *(12,66)*. It may be that a mild, and usually benign pharmacogenomic factor when combined with one of these phenotypic factors, can finally lead to an arrhythmia.

For both patients in the clinic and clinical trial subjects, CYP2D6 testing is readily available. It is widely used in clinical trials, but still rarely used in clinical practice. This is unfortunate because it could greatly help in the management of patients taking multiple medications that include a CYP2D6-metabolized hERG-blocker (see Table 2). Unfortunately, no similar test currently exists for CYP3A4. One can control risks here mainly by watching for concomitant prescription of CYP3A4 inhibitors.

In the case of cardiac ion channel genes, it is possible to test clinical trial subjects for the presence of LQTS mutations. This requires sequencing the five major channel genes. This is an expensive test today, so it is not possible to test all clinical trial subjects. However, potentially all subjects in cardiac safety trials could be tested, as could any outliers (individuals with excessive QT prolongation as a result of the experimental drug) in other trials. If it is found that most outliers in these situations actually had LQTS, then estimates of risk could be made. Because as many as one in a few thousand patients will carry these mutations, the risk of events in the general population could be this high. The likelihood of seeing any LQTS patients in a particular clinical trial is low, but integrated over all drugs tested in all companies; a number of these individuals will be enrolled in clinical trials in any given year.

The cardiac ion channels also contain a number of common polymorphisms, some of which have been implicated as risk factors for TdP in cases studies. To our knowledge,

Table 3
Candidate Genes or Factors That Potentially Increase Risk of TdP
and Should be Considered in Pharmacogenomic Studies Involving Cardiac Safety

Gene class	Example gene or effect
Cardiac ion channel genes	Variants that
	Increase drug binding
	Decrease potassium current
	Increase sodium current
	Alter ion channel expression
	Alter channel opening/closing dynamics
	Disrupt protein-protein interactions leading to formation of multi-subunit channels
	Disrupt binding of regulatory molecules to channel proteins
	High drug dose leading to increased HERG block
	Potential binding of drug to proteins other than HERG
Regulatory genes	Beta-adrenergic receptors
	Components of the beta-adrenergic signaling pathway
Other cardiac genes	Ryanodine receptor
	Ankyrin receptor
	Calcium channels
	Potassium channels other than those associated with LQTS
Metabolism / ADME genes	Activity-reducing mutations, e.g., CYP2D6, leading to poor metabolizer phenotype
	Drug–drug interactions—simultaneous use of relevant enzyme inhibitor
	Drug transport variation, subject-to-subject variability in bioavailability
	Heterogeneous distribution of drug through layers of myocardium
	Other ADME effects

no prospective trial has been reported which quantitatively assessed the effects of these polymorphisms on QT prolongation. Such trials will help answer the question of how much of a risk these polymorphism impose. Short of running prospective trials, one could gather information from ongoing clinical trials by simply genotyping the handful of common polymorphisms in any trial in which ECG data is also gathered. One could then perform meta-analyses spanning the collection of trials in a drug development program and look for trends. Because actual events will be rare with any new drug that proceeds very far in human trials, this type of analysis will only help identify a link between genotype and QT prolongation, but not the risk of events. This is still important for the following reason. Many trials (at least for noncardiac drugs) will not enroll a significant number of patients with the full spectrum of clinical risk factors (e.g., female sex, elderly, individuals with renal insufficiency, or heart disease, individuals taking multiple concomitant medications). Therefore, the degree of quantitative risk caused by these real world factors may not be evaluated until the drugs is marketed. The genetic risk factor is one that can potentially be quantified in the clinical trial cohort. One factor to be considered if this strategy is carried out is the ethnic-specific nature of some of these polymorphisms. For instance, the S1103Y polymorphism in SCN5A, which has been implicated in LQTS, is present in 13% of African-Americans but in only 0.2% of

Caucasians. If the clinical trial population is not ethnically mixed effects of such polymorphisms may be unmeasured. A question that will only be answered with time is if the risk associated with these polymorphisms and one drug can be generalized to apply to other drugs in the same classes or to other classes of drugs.

Finally, there are other avenues for research on the pharmacogenomics of cardiac safety. There are other ion channels and related proteins in the heart that are not implicated in familial LQTS, but that may play a role in risk of QT prolongation and TdP. Likewise, variations in the β-adrenergic and other signaling pathways could also be involved in risk. If prospective trials were run to assess the quantitative effect of the cardiac ion channel genes, then genes in these other pathways should also be included as candidates.

REFERENCES

1. Barbey JT, Lazzara R, Zipes DP. Spontaneous adverse event reports of serious ventricular arrhythmias, QT prolongation, syncope, and sudden death in patients treated with cisapride. J Cardiovasc Pharmacol Ther 2002; 7:65–76.
2. Haverkamp W, Martinez-Rubio A, Hief C, Lammers A, Muhlenkamp S, Wichter T et al. Efficacy and safety of d,l-sotalol in patients with ventricular tachycardia and in survivors of cardiac arrest. J Am Coll Cardiol 1997; 30:487–495.
3. Lehmann MH, Hardy S, Archibald D, quart B, MacNeil DJ. Sex difference in risk of torsade de pointes with d,l-sotalol. Circulation 1996; 94:2535–2541.
4. Hohnloser SH. Proarrhythmia with class III antiarrhythmic drugs: types, risks, and management. Am J Cardiol 1997; 80:82G–89G.
5. Fermini B, Fossa AA. The impact of drug-induced QT interval prolongation on drug discovery and development. Nat Rev Drug Discov 2003; 2:439–447.
6. Shah RR. Pharmacogenetic aspects of drug-induced torsade de pointes : potential tool for improving clinical drug development and prescribing. Drug Saf 2004; 27:145–172.
7. Roden DM. Drug-induced prolongation of the QT interval. N Engl J Med 2004; 350:1013–1022.
8. Wysowski DK, Corken A, Gallo-Torres H, Talarico L, Rodriguez EM. Postmarketing reports of QT prolongation and ventricular arrhythmia in association with cisapride and Food and Drug Administration regulatory actions. Am J Gastroenterol 2001; 96:1698–1703.
9. Haverkamp W, Breithardt G, Camm AJ, Janse MJ, Rosen MR, Antzelevitch C et al. The potential for QT prolongation and pro-arrhythmia by non-anti-arrhythmic drugs: clinical and regulatory implications. Report on a Policy Conference of the European Society of Cardiology. Cardiovasc Res 2000; 47:219–233.
10. FDA - Psychological Drugs Advisory Committee. Briefing Document for Zeldex Capsules (ziprasidone hydrochloride). 7-19–2000.
11. Moss AJ, Schwartz PJ. Delayed repolarization (QT or QTU prolongation) and malignant ventricular arrhythmias. Mod Concepts Cardiovasc Dis 1982; 51:85–90.
12. Roden DM. Taking the "idio" out of "idiosyncratic": predicting torsades de pointes. Pacing Clin Electrophysiol 1998; 21:1029–1034.
13. Bednar MM, Harrigan EP, Anziano RJ, Camm AJ, Ruskin JN. The QT interval. Prog Cardiovasc Dis 2001; 43:1–45.
14. CPMP - Committee for Proprietary Medicinal Products. Points to Consider: The assessment of the potential for QT prolongation by non-cardiovascular medicinal products. 1997. London. Ref Type: Report
15. Priori SG, Napolitano C, Schwartz PJ. Low penetrance in the long-QT syndrome: clinical impact. Circulation 1999; 99:529–533.
16. Priori SG, Napolitano C. Genetic defects of cardiac ion channels. The hidden substrate for torsades de pointes. Cardiovasc Drugs Ther 2002; 16:89–92.
17. Stephens JC, Schneider JA, Tanguay DA, Choi J, Acharya T, Stanley SE et al. Haplotype variation and linkage disequilibrium in 313 human genes. Science 2001; 293:489–493.
18. Marchini J, Cardon LR, Phillips MS, Donnelly P. The effects of human population structure on large genetic association studies. Nat Genet 2004.

19. Pitman EJG. Significance tests which may be applied to samples from any populations. Journal of the Royal Statistical Society (Series B) 1937; 4:119–130.
20. Brown CC, Fears TR. Exact significance levels for multiple binomial testing with application to carcinogenicity screens. Biometrics 1981; 37:763–774.
21. Heyse J, Rom D. Adjusting for multiplicity of statistical tests in the analysis of carcinogenicity studies. Biometric Journal 1988; 30:883–896.
22. Drysdale CM, McGraw DW, Stack CB, Stephens JC, Judson RS, Nandabalan K et al. Complex promoter and coding region beta 2-adrenergic receptor haplotypes alter receptor expression and predict in vivo responsiveness. Proc Natl Acad Sci U S A 2000; 97:10483–10488.
23. Judson R, Stephens JC, Windemuth A. The predictive power of haplotypes in clinical response. Pharmacogenomics 2000; 1:15–26.
24. Seebohm G, Chen J, Strutz N, Culberson C, Lerche C, Sanguinetti MC. Molecular determinants of KCNQ1 channel block by a benzodiazepine. Mol Pharmacol 2003; 64:70–77.
25. Yang P, Kanki H, Drolet B, Yang T, Wei J, Viswanathan PC et al. Allelic variants in long-QT disease genes in patients with drug-associated torsades de pointes. Circulation 2002; 105:1943–1948.
26. Donger C, Denjoy I, Berthet M, Neyroud N, Cruaud C, Bennaceur M et al. KVLQT1 C-terminal missense mutation causes a forme fruste long-QT syndrome. Circulation 1997; 96:2778–2781.
27. Napolitano C, Schwartz PJ, Brown AM, Ronchetti E, Bianchi L, Pinnavaia A et al. Evidence for a cardiac ion channel mutation underlying drug-induced QT prolongation and life-threatening arrhythmias. J Cardiovasc Electrophysiol 2000; 11:691–696.
28. Roden DM, Woosley RL, Primm RK. Incidence and clinical features of the quinidine-associated long QT syndrome: implications for patient care. Am Heart J 1986; 111:1088–1093.
29. Zehender M, Hohnloser S, Just H. QT-interval prolonging drugs: mechanisms and clinical relevance of their arrhythmogenic hazards. Cardiovasc Drugs Ther 1991; 5:515–530.
30. Sesti F, Abbott GW, Wei J, Murray KT, Saksena S, Schwartz PJ et al. A common polymorphism associated with antibiotic-induced cardiac arrhythmia. Proc Natl Acad Sci USA 2000; 97:10613–10618.
31. Abbott GW, Sesti F, Splawski I, Buck ME, Lehmann MH, Timothy KW et al. MiRP1 forms IKr potassium channels with hERG and is associated with cardiac arrhythmia. Cell 1999; 97:175–187.
32. Jongbloed R, Marcelis C, Velter C, Doevendans P, Geraedts J, Smeets H. DHPLC analysis of potassium ion channel genes in congenital long QT syndrome. Hum Mutat 2002; 20:382–391.
33. Makita N, Horie M, Nakamura T, Ai T, Sasaki K, Yokoi H et al. Drug-induced long-QT syndrome associated with a subclinical SCN5A mutation. Circulation 2002; 106:1269–1274.
34. Mitcheson JS, Chen J, Lin M, Culberson C, Sanguinetti MC. A structural basis for drug-induced long QT syndrome. Proc Natl Acad Sci U S A 2000; 97:12329–12333.
35. Mitcheson JS, Chen J, Sanguinetti MC. Trapping of a methanesulfonanilide by closure of the hERG potassium channel activation gate. J Gen Physiol 2000; 115:229–240.
36. Ficker E, Obejero-Paz CA, Zhao S, Brown AM. The binding site for channel blockers that rescue misprocessed human long QT syndrome type 2 ether-a-gogo-related gene (hERG) mutations. J Biol Chem 2002; 277:4989–4998.
37. Lees-Miller JP, Duan Y, Teng GQ, Duff HJ. Molecular determinant of high-affinity dofetilide binding to hERG1 expressed in Xenopus oocytes: involvement of S6 sites. Mol Pharmacol 2000; 57:367–374.
38. Abitbol I, Peretz A, Lerche C, Busch AE, Attali B. Stilbenes and fenamates rescue the loss of I(KS) channel function induced by an LQT5 mutation and other IsK mutants. EMBO J 1999; 18:4137–4148.
39. Roti EC, Myers CD, Ayers RA, Boatman DE, Delfosse SA, Chan EK et al. Interaction with GM130 during hERG ion channel trafficking. Disruption by type 2 congenital long QT syndrome mutations. Human Ether-a-go-go-Related Gene. J Biol Chem 2002; 277:47779–47785.
40. Valdivia CR, Tester DJ, Rok BA, Porter CB, Munger TM, Jahangir A et al. A trafficking defective, Brugada syndrome-causing SCN5A mutation rescued by drugs. Cardiovasc Res 2004; 62:53–62.
41. El Sherif N, Caref EB, Yin H, Restivo M. The electrophysiological mechanism of ventricular arrhythmias in the long QT syndrome. Tridimensional mapping of activation and recovery patterns. Circ Res 1996; 79:474–492.
42. Akar FG, Yan GX, Antzelevitch C, Rosenbaum DS. Unique topographical distribution of M cells underlies reentrant mechanism of torsade de pointes in the long-QT syndrome. Circulation 2002; 105:1247–1253.
43. Shimizu W, McMahon B, Antzelevitch C. Sodium pentobarbital reduces transmural dispersion of repolarization and prevents torsades de Pointes in models of acquired and congenital long QT syndrome. J Cardiovasc Electrophysiol 1999; 10:154–164.
44. Keating MT, Sanguinetti MC. Molecular and cellular mechanisms of cardiac arrhythmias. Cell 2001; 104:569–580.

45. Liu DW, Antzelevitch C. Characteristics of the delayed rectifier current (IKr and IKs) in canine ventricular epicardial, midmyocardial, and endocardial myocytes. A weaker IKs contributes to the longer action potential of the M cell. Circ Res 1995; 76:351–365.

46. Houltz B, Darpo B, Edvardsson N, Blomstrom P, Brachmann J, Crijns HJ et al. Electrocardiographic and clinical predictors of torsades de pointes induced by almokalant infusion in patients with chronic atrial fibrillation or flutter: a prospective study. Pacing Clin Electrophysiol 1998; 21:1044–1057.

47. Ackerman MJ, Tester DJ, Jones GS, Will ML, Burrow CR, Curran ME. Ethnic differences in cardiac potassium channel variants: implications for genetic susceptibility to sudden cardiac death and genetic testing for congenital long QT syndrome. Mayo Clin Proc 2003; 78:1479–1487.

48. Bezzina CR, Verkerk AO, Busjahn A, Jeron A, Erdmann J, Koopmann TT et al. A common polymorphism in KCNH2 (hERG) hastens cardiac repolarization. Cardiovasc Res 2003; 59:27–36.

49. Splawski I, Timothy KW, Tateyama M, Clancy CE, Malhotra A, Beggs AH et al. Variant of SCN5A sodium channel implicated in risk of cardiac arrhythmia. Science 2002; 297:1333–1336.

50. Kanki H, Yang P, Xie HG, Kim RB, George AL, Jr., Roden DM. Polymorphisms in beta-adrenergic receptor genes in the acquired long QT syndrome. J Cardiovasc Electrophysiol 2002; 13:252–256.

51. Marx SO, Kurokawa J, Reiken S, Motoike H, D'Armiento J, Marks AR et al. Requirement of a macromolecular signaling complex for beta adrenergic receptor modulation of the KCNQ1-KCNE1 potassium channel. Science 2002; 295:496–499.

52. Piippo K, Swan H, Pasternack M, Chapman H, Paavonen K, Viitasalo M et al. A founder mutation of the potassium channel KCNQ1 in long QT syndrome: implications for estimation of disease prevalence and molecular diagnostics. J Am Coll Cardiol 2001; 37:562–568.

53. Hara M, Danilo P, Jr., Rosen MR. Effects of gonadal steroids on ventricular repolarization and on the response to E4031. J Pharmacol Exp Ther 1998; 285:1068–1072.

54. Rodriguez I, Kilborn MJ, Liu XK, Pezzullo JC, Woosley RL. Drug-induced QT prolongation in women during the menstrual cycle. JAMA 2001; 285:1322–1326.

55. Stramba-Badiale M, Locati EH, Martinelli A, Courville J, Schwartz PJ. Gender and the relationship between ventricular repolarization and cardiac cycle length during 24-h Holter recordings. Eur Heart J 1997; 18:1000–1006.

56. Burke JH, Goldberger JJ, Ehlert FA, Kruse JT, Parker MA, Kadish AH. Gender differences in heart rate before and after autonomic blockade: evidence against an intrinsic gender effect. Am J Med 1996; 100:537–543.

57. Rashba EJ, Zareba W, Moss AJ, Hall WJ, Robinson J, Locati EH et al. Influence of pregnancy on the risk for cardiac events in patients with hereditary long QT syndrome. LQTS Investigators. Circulation 1998; 97:451–456.

58. Drici MD, Burklow TR, Haridasse V, Glazer RI, Woosley RL. Sex hormones prolong the QT interval and downregulate potassium channel expression in the rabbit heart. Circulation 1996; 94:1471–1474.

59. Monahan BP, Ferguson CL, Killeavy ES, Lloyd BK, Troy J, Cantilena LR, Jr. Torsades de pointes occurring in association with terfenadine use. JAMA 1990; 264:2788–2790.

60. Garte S, Gaspari L, Alexandrie AK, Ambrosone C, Autrup H, Autrup JL et al. Metabolic gene polymorphism frequencies in control populations. Cancer Epidemiol Biomarkers Prev 2001; 10:1239–1248.

61. Nakamura K, Goto F, Ray WA, McAllister CB, Jacqz E, Wilkinson GR et al. Interethnic differences in genetic polymorphism of debrisoquin and mephenytoin hydroxylation between Japanese and Caucasian populations. Clin Pharmacol Ther 1985; 38:402–408.

62. Thummel KE, Wilkinson GR. In vitro and in vivo drug interactions involving human CYP3A. Annu Rev Pharmacol Toxicol 1998; 38:389–430.

63. Tirona RG, Lee W, Leake BF, Lan LB, Cline CB, Lamba V et al. The orphan nuclear receptor HNF4alpha determines PXR- and CAR-mediated xenobiotic induction of CYP3A4. Nat Med 2003; 9:220–224.

64. Curtis LH, Ostbye T, Sendersky V, Hutchison S, Allen LaPointe NM, Al Khatib SM et al. Prescription of QT-prolonging drugs in a cohort of about 5 million outpatients. Am J Med 2003; 114:135–141.

65. Roe CM, Odell KW, Henderson RR. Concomitant use of antipsychotics and drugs that may prolong the QT interval. J Clin Psychopharmacol 2003; 23:197–200.

66. Haddad PM, Anderson IM. Antipsychotic-related QTc prolongation, torsade de pointes and sudden death. Drugs 2002; 62:1649–1671.

67. Paulussen AD, Gilissen RA, Armstrong M, Doevendans PA, Verhasselt P, Smeets HJ et al. Genetic variations of KCNQ1, KCNH2, SCN5A, KCNE1, and KCNE2 in drug-induced long QT syndrome patients. J Mol Med 2004; 82:182–188.

68. Swan H, Viitasalo M, Piippo K, Laitinen P, Kontula K, Toivonen L. Sinus node function and ventricular repolarization during exercise stress test in long QT syndrome patients with KvLQT1 and hERG potassium channel defects. J Am Coll Cardiol 1999; 34:823–829.

69. Ficker E, Jarolimek W, Kiehn J, Baumann A, Brown AM. Molecular determinants of dofetilide block of hERG K+ channels. Circ Res 1998; 82:386–395.

70. Chen J, Seebohm G, Sanguinetti MC. Position of aromatic residues in the S6 domain, not inactivation, dictates cisapride sensitivity of hERG and eag potassium channels. Proc Natl Acad Sci U S A 2002; 99:12461–12466.

71. Kubota T, Shimizu W, Kamakura S, Horie M. Hypokalemia-induced long QT syndrome with an underlying novel missense mutation in S4-S5 linker of KCNQ1. J Cardiovasc Electrophysiol 2000; 11:1048–1054.

72. Seebohm G, Scherer CR, Busch AE, Lerche C. Identification of specific pore residues mediating KCNQ1 inactivation. A novel mechanism for long QT syndrome. J Biol Chem 2001; 276:13600–13605.

73. Wang Q, Curran ME, Splawski I, Burn TC, Millholland JM, VanRaay TJ et al. Positional cloning of a novel potassium channel gene: KVLQT1 mutations cause cardiac arrhythmias. Nat Genet 1996; 12:17–23.

74. Shalaby FY, Levesque PC, Yang WP, Little WA, Conder ML, Jenkins-West T et al. Dominant-negative KvLQT1 mutations underlie the LQT1 form of long QT syndrome. Circulation 1997; 96:1733–1736.

75. Splawski I, Shen J, Timothy KW, Vincent GM, Lehmann MH, Keating MT. Genomic structure of three long QT syndrome genes: KVLQT1, hERG, and KCNE1. Genomics 1998; 51:86–97.

76. Ackerman MJ, Schroeder JJ, Berry R, Schaid DJ, Porter CJ, Michels VV et al. A novel mutation in KVLQT1 is the molecular basis of inherited long QT syndrome in a near-drowning patient's family. Pediatr Res 1998; 44:148–153.

77. Splawski I, Shen J, Timothy KW, Lehmann MH, Priori S, Robinson JL et al. Spectrum of mutations in long-QT syndrome genes. KVLQT1, hERG, SCN5A, KCNE1, and KCNE2. Circulation 2000; 102:1178–1185.

78. Liu H, Tateyama M, Clancy CE, Abriel H, Kass RS. Channel openings are necessary but not sufficient for use-dependent block of cardiac Na(+) channels by flecainide: evidence from the analysis of disease-linked mutations. J Gen Physiol 2002; 120:39–51.

79. Abriel H, Wehrens XH, Benhorin J, Kerem B, Kass RS. Molecular pharmacology of the sodium channel mutation D1790G linked to the long-QT syndrome. Circulation 2000; 102:921–925.

III

Clinical Methodologies and Technical Aspects of Assessing Cardiac Safety of Investigational Drugs: Focus on Cardiac Repolarization

6

Assessment of Ventricular Repolarization From Body-Surface ECGs in Humans

Jean-Philippe Couderc, PhD
and Wojciech Zareba, MD, PhD

CONTENTS

INTRODUCTION

In 1887, the first recording of electrical activity of the human heart was done using Waller's capillary meter. The recorded signal included four waves called A, B, C, and D. Einthoven mathematically modified this signal to correct the inertia associated with the movement of the mercury column in the capillary electrometer. To avoid confusion with Waller's recording, Einthoven named the five identified deflections P, Q, R, S, and T having used the O point as the origin of the time scale (by mathematical convention O is used for the origin of the Cartesian coordinates). The interval QT was defined as the interval between the beginning of the QRS complex and the end of the T wave. The ventricular repolarization process of the heart begins in the early-activated myocardial cells while the rest of the ventricle is still depolarizing. This is why the entire duration of the ventricular repolarization is commonly associated with a measure including the QRS complex. It is also during the late 19th century that new discovery, including the electrical triggering of contraction during late refractory period, would open an entire field of quantitative electrocardiology focusing on a better understanding of the cardiac repolarization.

From: *Cardiac Safety of Noncardiac Drugs:*
Practical Guidelines for Clinical Research and Drug Development
Edited by: J. Morganroth and I. Gussak © Humana Press Inc., Totowa, NJ

This chapter aims to help the reader understand why the QT interval has become the most accepted biomarker for evaluating a potential risk of torsade de pointes (TdP) in drug development and clinical studies. Also, it provides some insight into the problematic linked to the measurement of the QT-interval duration. The chapter is organized in five parts: (1) a brief description of the current understanding of the T wave genesis on the surface electrocardiograms (ECGs); (2) an overview of the various mechanisms involved in the triggering and maintaining of TdP. Findings from the cellular, genetic, and clinical fields are reviewed; (3) the third part focuses on the problematic of QT interval and QT prolongation measurements with an emphasis on the effect of physiological confounding factors such as heart rate, repolarization adaptation, and the autonomic regulation. The advantages and drawbacks of current manual and automatic methods for QT measurements are presented; (4) this section reviews the interest of QT dispersion in drug cardiotoxicity assessment; and (5) an introduction to novel methods that could potentially improve the quality of drug safety evaluation in the future.

GENESIS OF THE T WAVE

The T wave represents the ventricular repolarization or recovery phase of the ventricles. Based on the dipolar theory, the T wave is an averaging of all existing local differences in repolarization forces within the ventricles. But there are clinical findings demonstrating that the T wave may have nondipolar content as well *(1)*. Zabel et al. *(2)* emphasized that there is *a combined contribution of local and global repolarization forces to the T wave* on the body surface that may significantly vary between clinical situations. Based on a wedge preparation, Antzelevitch et al. *(3)* demonstrated that transmural dispersion of myocardium may also play a role in the morphology and duration of the T wave. This was recently supported by Rudy et al. *(4)*, who presented an ECG imaging technique that can accurately reconstruct epicardial electrograms noninvasively from body surface ECG potentials. Their model supports the hypothesis that the components of the electrocardiographic signal mostly reflect local activity *(proximity effect)* and small contribution of the other regions of the heart.

It is clear that more research work is required to clarify the contribution of local and global electrical forces to the T wave. Presently, the genesis of the T wave from the surface ECG remains an unsolved problem of modern electrocardiography.

QT PROLONGATION: AN ACCEPTED MARKER
OF VENTRICULAR ARRHYTHMIC EVENTS

QT interval prolongation is used as a surrogate biomarker for the assessment of the risk of TdP in all drug-safety studies. Testing for drug-induced QT prolongation has been recommended by the European Agency for the Evaluation of Medical Products and the Food and Drug Administration, and research organizations such as the International Society for Holter and Non-invasive Electrocardiography *(5)*. QT interval analysis for drug-safety evaluation should report changes in QT interval duration in the presence of the tested compound vs QT intervals recorded at baseline (off drug), and should address possible dose-dependency while monitoring plasma drug concentration; finally, it may require positive controls (moxifloxacin being recommended for positive control substance) to document ability of an ECG core lab to detect minimal drug-related QT changes.

The understanding of the cellular and ionic mechanisms underlying arrhythogenesis has progressed considerably over the past decade. The main ionic currents involved in the repolarization of the cardiac cells have been described and abnormalities of these currents have been associated to inherited channelopathies like the long QT syndrome (LQTS) *(6)*, abnormal electrolyte/metabolic disorders, and cardiac/noncardiac drugs *(7)*.

Mechanisms Involved in the Occurrence of Torsade de Pointes: A Brief Review

Torsade de Pointes

The TdP, literally translated from French as *twisting of the pointes*, describes ventricular tachycardia with the cardiac axis rotating, changing from one direction to another and back again. It is an uncommon polymorphic ventricular tachycardia that by definition is associated with baseline QT prolongation. First reported in 1966 by Dessertenne *(8)* in a 80-yr-old woman, the specific morphology of the malignant arrhythmias was suspected to be generated by two competing foci leading to presentation with changing QRS morphology. This hypothesis was confirmed 15 yr later in a canine model where the TdP could be recorded from both the left and right ventricular sites at a similar, but periodically changing rate *(9)*.

Triggering Cardiac Arrhythmias and Early After-Depolarizations (EADs)

Abnormal repolarization leading to abnormal impulse formation as well as re-entry systems are two mechanisms involved in the triggering of cardiac arrhythmia *(10)*. In the long QT syndrome (congenital or acquired), the TdP is known to be induced by EADs *(11,12)*, which has been observed in monophasic action potential (MAP) recordings from clinical models *(13)* and has been largely documented in animal models *(14,15)*. In 1988, Cranefield and Aronson *(16)* defined EADs as "depolarizing afterpotentials that begin prior to the completion of repolarization and cause (or constitute) an interruption or retardation of normal repolarization." EAD activity has also been associated with arrhythmias in hypertrophy and heart failure in which downregulation of ionic currents have been documented. Other mechanisms are discussed in details in the Chapter 3.

The Prominent Role of Rapid Delayed Rectifier Potassium Current

One of the major discoveries in basic electrophysiology was the identification of the different types of myocardial cells across the ventricular wall, as well as the description of their electrical characteristics: the epicardial, midmyocardium (M), and endocardial cells *(17)*. The differences between the shapes of the action potentials of these three types of cells reside in the differences in phase 1 and phase 3. Epicardial and M cells have a prominent dome during phase 1 explained by more pronounced outward I_{to} currents. M cells have action potential prolonging more than epicardial and endocardial cells when the heart rate slows down or in reaction to agent that prolong action potential duration *(18,19)*.

As evidenced in animals *(20–22)* and in humans *(12,23,24)*, the response to various pharmacological agents of these three types of myocardial layers are different. The action potential of the adult ventricular human myocyte reflects the coordinated action of several ion channels that open and close in an orderly fashion. The rapid upstroke of the phase 0 is caused by a large Na^+ inward current, the following phases 1 to 3 depends on subtle balance between voltage-gated inward (Na^+ and Ca^+) and outward (I_k^+) repolarizing currents. The repolarizing I_k^+ currents are the most diverse ones: fast and slow outward

I_{to} currents are contributing the most to phase 1, while delayed rapid and slow rectifier current (I_{kr}, I_{ks}) play a more important role in latter phase 3. Both inward and outward ionic repolarizing currents impact the duration of the ventricular action potentials, and as a result the modification of their normal properties may have dramatic effects on refractory periods and cardiac rhythms. Nearly all the drugs associated with human TdPs have been associated with blockade of the I_{kr} current.

INTER-VENTRICULAR DISPERSION OF REPOLARIZATION

Studies conducted in hearts of canine models with chronic atrioventricular (AV) blocks and after almokalant revealed spontaneous triggering of TdP following a consistent mechanism: increase of dispersion of action potential duration (APD) between the left and right ventricles, occurrence of EADs increasing further endocardial inter-ventricle dispersion, and finally genesis of ventricular ectopic beats initiating TdP *(25)*. The role of the inter-ventricle dispersion in the mechanisms of acquired TdP arrhythmias is crucial, as it was demonstrated by experiments involving drugs such as sotalol and almokalant *(26)*. The study revealed that the occurrence of spontaneous TdP is lower with sotalol; and sotalol was associated with significantly lower inter-ventricle dispersion (80 ± 45 ms) than almokalant (110 ± 60 ms, $p < 0.05$).

TRANSMURAL DISPERSION OF REPOLARIZATION

Another important myocardial dysfunction that is likely to play a crucial role in the triggering of TdP is the transmural dispersion of repolarization. Documented by Weissenburger et al. *(27)* in anesthetized dogs receiving sotalol, TdP was observed only in animals anesthetized using halothane but not pentobarbital. Halothane was associated with significant increased transmural dispersion of repolarization in comparison to pentobarbital (88 ± 17 vs 53 ± 7 ms, $p < 0.005$). Similar observations were reported with other compounds in wedge preparations: d-sotalol, ATX-II, erythromycin, and anthopleurin-A *(28,29)*.

Detailed descriptions of the various mechanisms involved in the triggering of the drug-induced cardiac arrhythmias are discussed in Chapter 3.

Congenital Long QT Syndrome

Undoubtedly, the parallel progress of clinical, molecular, and genetic research has been key to the current state-of-the-art of arrhythmogenesis. The database of the International Long QT Syndrome registry is one important stone of this edifice. The LQTS is characterized by a prolongation of QT intervals on the ECGs and is associated with an increased risk for ventricular arrhythmias that can degenerate in cardiac arrest and sudden death *(30,31)*. The mutation of genes encoding cardiac ion channels has been identified in patients with congenital form of LQTS *(6)*. These mutations lead to dysfunction of ionic channels in LQT3 patients, mutations of the SCN5A channel gene, the sodium inward current (I_{Na}) has been shown to be leaking during the repolarization phase (1 to 3) leading to a prolongation of the repolarization process. In LQT2 patients, a reduction of the I_{kr} current is caused by the mutation in *HERG* gene regulating pore-forming subunit. In LQT1 patients, the mutation of the *KVLQT1* gene encoding a α-subunit of potassium channel protein produces a reduction in the slowly activating I_{ks}. Reduction in I_{ks} and I_{kr} current leads to a prolongation of the repolarization process. It is noteworthy that pore mutations are associated with several-fold higher risk for cardiac events than nonpore mutations of *HERG*. This observation indicates that I_{Kr}, affected by many drugs is likely to be the current underlying high risk of TdP *(32)*. I_{ks} and I_{Na} are of interest in drug development because of their involvement in the prolongation of QT in the congenital syndrome.

In clinical studies, an increased risk of arrhythmic events is associated with heart-rate corrected QT (QTc) prolongation. In a prospective longitudinal study of 328 families with the LQTS, it was shown that for every 10-ms increase in QTc duration there is a 5% exponential increase of the risk of cardiac events *(30)*. In a study of LQTS family members (without β-blockers) from the International LQTS Registry the odds ratio of cardiac events by QTc duration were 1.43 for QTc between 0.45 and 0.46, 2.42 for QTc between 0.47 and 0.50, and 4.84 for QTc > 0.50 when compared to QTc = 0.44 *(31)*.

Acquired Form of the Long QT Syndrome

Noncardiac drugs that prolong the QT/QTc interval include various classes: opoids, antimigraine, antimalarial, anti-asthmatic, antihistamines, anti-infectives, antineoplatics, antilipemic, diuretics, gastrointestinal, hormones, antidepressants, and antipsychotics *(33)*. As stated earlier, most of the drugs with a QT prolonging effect have a direct blocking effect on the I_{kr} ion current, the others lead to QT prolongation when administrated with other drugs affecting functions of the cytochrome P-450 enzymatic system. An exhaustive list of the drugs that prolong the QT/QTc interval or induce TdP is provided on www.qtdrugs.org.

Based on clinical data in LQTS patients, a QTc interval above 500 ms is associated with a significant increased risk of TdP. When evaluating drug-safety based on QTc prolongation this threshold remains valid: a QTc prolongation longer than 500 ms may lead to TdP and may jeopardize the commercialization of a new compound. A relative QTc prolongation of at least 30 ms should raise concerns; these concerns would be, of course, greater if this prolongation exceeds 60 ms in individually compared ECGs.

It is noteworthy that among the millions of patients taking drugs blocking cardiac ion channels and prolonging QT interval, only rarely is TdP observed *(34)*. This rarity of drug-induced TdP is explained by the need for combining the drug-induced prolongation with other predisposing factors such as gender, genetic make-up, electrolyte imbalance, hypothermia, clinically significant bradycardia, and impaired hepatic of renal function.

Difference in QTc Between Gender

Two-thirds of the cases of reported drug-induced TdP occur in women *(35–38)*. Repolarization is known to be longer in adult women than in men. Women have longer early phase of repolarization and a steeper ascending slope of the T wave *(39,40)*. The QT/RR slope is also steeper in women than in men *(40–42)*. Also, there is evidence for drug-induced variation in QTc prolongation with menstrual cycle, menstruation, and ovulatory phase associated with longer QTc interval than during the luteal phase *(43)*. Studies looking at differences in QTc values between genders during childhood are negative, however, after puberty the QTc is longer in females than in males *(4445)*. The protective role of androgens or the predisposing nature of estrogenes are two potential explanations that are still to be elucidated.

Genetic Predisposition and Torsade de Pointes

The genetic make-up of an individual may favor the triggering of TdP following a drug-induced QT/QTc prolongation. This interesting concept has been supported by small studies. Fifteen percent decrease in ionic function was reported in subject with polymorphism of MiRP1 involved in the encoding of proteins regulating function of the I_{kr} current. It is expected that the association of a I_{kr}-blocking agent effect with such genetic polymorphism may lead to harmful ionic dysfunction *(46)*. In 2002, a study from

Yang et al. *(46a)* investigated the prevalence of ion cardiac channel gene polymorphisms in patients with drug-induced TdP in comparison with control subjects. No difference was found between patients and subjects. That same year Splawski et al. *(47)* reported the presence of a variant of sodium channel gene SCN5A, the so-called allele Y1102 accelerated channel activation, increasing the probability for arrhythmias through abnormal repolarization functions. The Y1102 allele was found in 13.2% of a group of African-Americans (group of 205 subjects). If the variant is not sufficient for justifying spontaneously triggering arrhythmic events, it may contribute to an increased predisposition to arrhythmias in the context of additional acquired risk factors such as noncardiac QT-prolonging drugs *(47)*. Further research is needed to determine causative role of polymorphism and drug-related QT prolongation.

The current knowledge of the mechanisms involved in the development of potentially lethal polymorphic ventricular arrhythmias was substantially advanced over the last decade. The role of ion current in triggering TdP and the association between ion dysfunctions and QT prolongation justify the use of the QT interval as a surrogate biomarker for the assessment of the risk of TdP. The following will review the challenges associated with measurements of the QT intervals and its prolongation.

HOW TO MEASURE THE QT INTERVAL ON THE SURFACE ELECTROCARDIOGRAM

Measuring the QT interval is a challenging task requiring careful consideration of several technical, clinical, and physiological factors (Fig. 1). Among these factors, the recording technique *(48)* (*see* Chapter 7), the lead choice *(49)*, the subject age, and gender *(50)* are easy to control. The effect of other factors, such as the autonomic balance *(51)*, the repolarization adaptation *(52)*, QT hysteresis *(53)*, and the heart-rate dependency are more difficult to assess mainly because their levels are likely to be different between individuals. Nevertheless, these factors have to be controlled in order to minimize their impact on the QT measurements.

The presence of a U wave adds another level of complexity to this measurement. The origin and the definition of U wave is unclear and where certain cardiologists would identify U waves others would see an abnormal T wave morphology. It seems important to distinguish them. Studies using wedge preparation have evidence that large amplitude secondary T wave components could be produced following the same mechanism producing the T wave. These should be referred as T2 waves, or notched T wave if merged inside the first component of the T wave. Other low-amplitude components may be called U waves.

From 12-lead ECGs, the clinical definition of the QT interval is the interval between the earliest beginning of QRS complex and the latest end of the T wave from all measurable leads. Because of cost issues or technical limitations, the QT interval measurement is often limited to two or three leads (manual) or to mathematically combined leads (computer-based measurements). This approach usually underestimates QT intervals when comparing to the analysis based on the earliest onset and latest offset in any lead.

Correcting the QT Interval for Heart Rate

Correcting QT intervals for heart rate allows for comparing repolarization measurements obtained at different heart rates, either between subjects or within the same subject. The most popular correction is the Bazett's formula. It is implemented in all commercial ECG systems, but its validity is highly criticized *(54,55)*. Bazett's formula underesti-

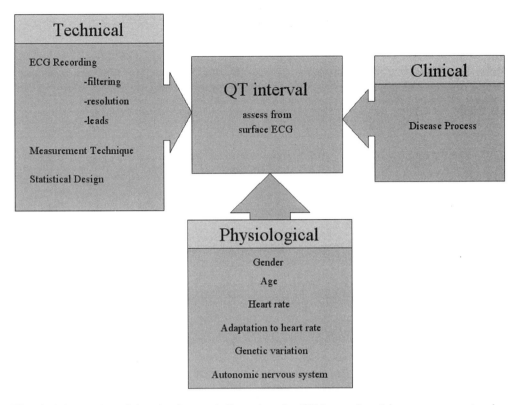

Fig. 1. Schema describing the factors influencing the QT interval and its measurements when measured from surface ECGs.

mates the QT interval at slow heart rate and overestimates it at fast ones. The need for a better correction method is crucial for the safety evaluation process of a new drug, because the correction may hide a prolongation *(56,57)*. The Bazett's correction may lead to both false-positive and false-negative observations *(55)*.

Among a large set of published correction formulae, Fridericia's (QTc = QT.RR$^{-1/3}$) is one that seems better than Bazett's (QTc = QT.RR$^{-1/2}$) *(56,58)*. Nevertheless, the use of a mathematical function characterizing QT/RR relationship and generalized to any patient is a questionable approach, because the QT/RR relationship was reported to be subject dependent *(58)*. Today, there are three alternatives to a general predefined mathematical formula. The first one compares the QT interval for matched heart rate; the so-called *bin method* does not use any correction model *(59)*. This method is described in depth in Chapter 9. The second alternative is a population-based formula (or pool formula) based on a QT/RR model designed on measurements from all subjects of the study population *(56)*. This alternative may be the best one when a limited number of short ECGs is available for each subject *(58)*. The third option is an individual-based formula. This method relies on the computation of a QT/RR correction model in each subject. The resulting model is used to correct the QT measurements for this subject.

The stability of the individual-based correction model has been assessed *(58)*. Our group investigated the stability of this correction model as a function of three factors: (1) the number of measurements (N) used to design this model, (2) the heart rate range (and its variance), and (3) the T wave amplitude that is known to effect the quality of the QT measurements *(60)*. The study was based on 305 Holter recordings from healthy subjects *(41)*. All the factors had an important impact on the stability of the QT/RR regression slope (linear and exponential models). We demonstrated that (1) QT measurements should be done using the lead where the amplitude is the highest, (2) at least a few hours of continuous ECG were needed to obtain enough QT/RR measurement, and (3) reducing the range of the heart rate covered by the QT/RR measurements decreases the stability of the QT/RR model. The study concludes that the use of individual formula based on QT/RR regression analysis in drug safety evaluation should be used with caution because an inappropriate design of the correction model may lead to large errors on QTc values.

Controlling for QT Adaptation to Heart Rate: Restitution Curve

The time of adaptation to heart rate of the QT interval have been documented using endocardial action potential duration recordings under specific pacing protocol by Franz et al. *(61)* in 17 subjects. Their pacing protocol included abrupt sustained rate acceleration and deceleration that evidenced nonsteady-state and steady-state APD. The time of steady-state adaptation was found to be several minutes (2–3 min). Any ECG recorded within few minutes following a rapid heart rate change (deceleration or acceleration) would provide QT interval in nonsteady state. Repolarization restitution time was shown to be different between individuals *(62)*. Also, the repolarization adaptation is faster when the heart rhythm is increased than when it is decreased leading to a "hysteresis" effect *(63)*. These observations on the QT adaptation to heart rate should be taken into consideration when measuring QT interval, a direct consequence being that a valid QT measurement can be ensured only if there is a stable heart rate during at least the previous two minutes.

The QT intervals measured during nonsteady-state of repolarization should not be discarded, we will see at the end of this chapter that they may contain relevant information.

Autonomic Nervous System and QT Intervals

The results from the literature describing the role of the autonomic nervous system on the QT interval are difficult to reconcile. Based on pharmacological autonomic blockade, it was found that sympathetic stimulations prolong the interval QT, and vagal stimulation shortens it *(64)*. Opposite results were found by Browne *(65)* and Bellavere et al. *(66)*. Most likely, the explanation for such inconsistency is explained by the differences between study designs. Other authors compared QT intervals between diurnal and nocturnal periods at similar heart rates (60 bpm). This difference was consistently close to 18 ms between studies when subtracting nocturnal from diurnal values *(65)*. Thus, the predominance of the sympathetic tone within the vago-sympathetic balance seems to be associated to an increased QT interval.

When considering the analysis of the QT/RR slope between day and night, studies have shown that the slope is steeper during daytime This results may be easily confirmed using 24-h ECG signals and an appropriate selective method for removing QT/RR values in nonsteady-state such as the one our group developed in our software for COMPrehensive Analysis of repolarization Signal (COMPAS) *(41)*. Our group reported slope values between day and time equal to 0.16 ± 0.08 vs 0.12 ± 0.12 ($p = 0.0001$) based on one of the largest group of 24-h Holter ECGs, 204 healthy subjects. Experts in the field provide the following explanation, the rate-dependence of ventricular repolarization may be explained by two components: (1) intrinsic characteristics of myocardial fibers, and/or (2) its modulation by the autonomic nervous system *(67)*.

Manual Measurements of the Interval QT

Manual measurements done in 12-lead ECGs are usually considered a standard of care *(56,68–70)*. Manual measurements can be obtained on paper ECGs using simple caliper or digipad technology *(68)*. Papercopy of ECG strips may also be scanned into a digital image and onscreen calipers software can be used *(69)*. Another option is to use digital ECG signal and use onscreen caliper software. The assessment of the level of agreements between digipad and onscreen measurement have been investigated by Sarapa et al. *(69)*. The same study also addresses the agreement between QT measurements obtained from 12-lead ECGs and Holter digital Holter ECGs. Chapter 9 provides an in-depth description of this important study. Briefly, the study investigated the QT/QTc prolongation induced by sotalol when measured by these methods. The average mean drug-induced changes were comparable between these techniques.

The leads usually considered for measuring the QT interval are lead II (or lead V5 if lead II must be avoided). If high heart rate is present like in pediatric ECGs, the use of average measurements is recommended (four to five beat averages of RR and QT intervals). Same techniques should be used on patients with atrial fibrillation.

With the digital era, the quantitative electrocardiography welcomed the birth of computer algorithms providing fast and reproducible analysis of the ECG signal *(71)*.

Automatic Measurements

The use of automatic methods for assessing QT prolongation in drug-safety study is not yet well accepted. The current guidance does not reject automatic measurement of QT interval but recommend visual confirmation of the accuracy of the computer-measured QT interval. Most of the comparison between automatic and manual QT measurements were based on clinical data. Willems et al. *(72)* concluded on a similar quality between QT measured by 11 different algorithm and manual measurements: the standard deviation of difference between QTs varied between 8 and 28 ms. The inter-observer difference was 15 ms. Salieva et al. *(70)* reported a shorter QT interval measurements when based on automatic method (least-square fit technique, *see* Fig. 2) in comparison to manual measurements. In Lead V1, automatic measurements were 25 ms shorter than manual measurements *(70)*. Obviously, these results are dependent on the method of measurements and the quality of the QT algorithm, and for drug-related studies the potential errors that the algorithm may generate are of concern. Figure 2 illustrates the automatic identification of the end of the T wave.

For drug-safety evaluation, it seems important to have a positive control group for demonstrating the ability of an algorithm to detect changes and to have the ability to manually check and correct the QT measurements. Our group has developed a software allowing for automatic measurements of the QT intervals on short- and long-term ECGs, and providing the ability to quickly identify potential erroneous detection that can be manually adjusted (Fig. 3) *(41,56)*.

The pioneers in developing concepts for the measurements of QT intervals were Lepeschkin et al. *(73)*, Puddu et al. *(74)* , O'Donnell et al. *(75,76)*, Pisani et al. *(77)*, and Algra et al. *(78)*. Later, others and sometimes more complex techniques were implemented. Table 1 provides a list of automatic methods used for the measurement of the QT interval from surface ECGs.

Comparing the quality of all these methods is challenging because they have been validated on different study populations including the PhysioNet repolarization database

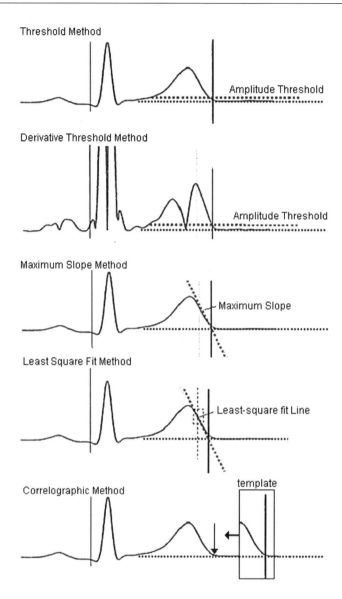

Fig. 2. Description of several methods used for the identification of the end of the T-wave. From upper to lower panels: 1. the threshold method, 2. the derivative method, 3. the maximum slope method, 4. the least square fit method, and 5. the correlographic method.

(79) the CSE database *(72),* or other smaller ECG databases. Majority of automatic methods are based on amplitude threshold, T wave area-based, slope fitting techniques. The most recent techniques involve neural-network and wavelet-based techniques (Table 1). The validity of these new techniques needs to be evaluated on large clinical populations. The errors of measurements of automatic method have been associated with low-amplitude T wave, mainly *(80,81)* abnormal morphology of T wave (biphasic and notched T wave), and the presence of a U wave.

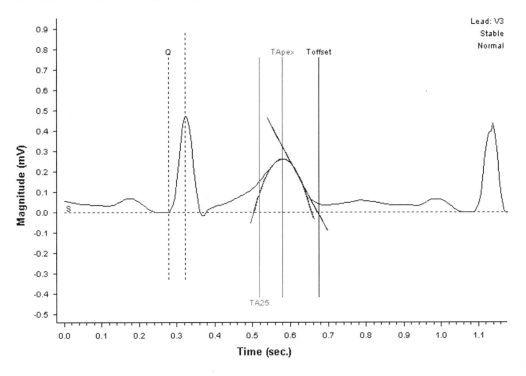

Fig. 3. A snapshot from the COMPAS software. From 12-lead Holter ECG signal (lead V3), the software allows the users to visually verify the location of the T-wave apex and offset and to modify manually it if needed. The software provide an evaluation of the stability of the measurement based on the previous variation of heart rate as well as a class annotation of the repolarization wave (normal in this example). The first vertical line inside the T-wave marks the T25% point namely, the time needed to reach 25% of the total cumulated area under the T wave.

Statistical Consideration: Sample Size Issue

One important question that has to be addressed when designing a study for evidencing the effect of a drug on the QT interval is to define how many subjects should be included in a study to ensure enough statistical power for detecting the repolarization change. The relevant parameter for the power calculation is the ratio of the change in means (effect size) to the standard deviation of the change for a given subject. For instance, for $N = 20$ subjects, this ratio needs to be between 0.63 and 0.80 in order to achieve 80–95% power, with $N = 30$ subjects the same level of power is obtained for a ratio value between 0.51 and 0.62. In drug-induced QTc prolongation, moxifloxacin has been accepted as a reference (or positive control). For a 400 mg moxifloxacin dose, QT interval changes varied from 2.3 to 4% depending on heart rate with a standard deviation ranging from 3 to 5% *(82)*, thus 95% power may be achieved using 20–30 subjects to detect effect using a one-sided *t*-test at the 0.05 level of significance.

THE QT DISPERSION

A certain level of repolarization heterogeneity is present in the normal myocardium. Differences in repolarization morphology between anterior, inferior, and posterior walls create this basal level required to the normal functioning of the heart. An increase in the

Table 1
List of Studies Proposing Automatic Methods Designed
for the Measurement of the QT Interval From Surface ECGs

Author	Ref.	Year	Method
Mirvis, D.M.	127	1985	Threshold crossing on moving fitting-slope value
Merri, M.	40	1989	Area-based quantification of T wave
Van Bemmel, J.H.	128	1990	Template matching technique
Laguna, P.	129,130	1990/1994	Slope-adaptative threshold method
Ferretti G.F.	131	1992	Tangent method
Xue, Q.	132	1996	Amplitude threshold and least square-curve fitting technique
Sosnowski, M	133	1998	FFT-based QT measurement (high resolution ECG)
Bystricky,W	134	2002	Neural-network technique
Hayn, D.	135	2003	Coarse T-offset detection (ranges on amplitude in T portions)
Almeida, R.	136	2003	Wavelet-based technique
Couderc, J.P.	56	2003	Modified area method from ref. 31
Schreier, G.	137	2003	Threshold, tangent and model-based methods combined

magnitude of these regional heterogeneities may create opportunities for re-entrant circuits responsible for the perpetuation of arrhythmias. These have been described in experimental and clinical studies (83–85) The transmural (local) dispersion is a more recent concept; it has been presented as another factor contributing to the triggering and development of TdP (10). How these heterogeneities are reflected on the surface ECGs is an unsolved question. QT dispersion (QTD) was considered as one of possible measures of repolarization heterogeneity (80,86).

The number of publications related to QTD has remained constant during the past five years (approx 130 publications per year). QTD has been reported as useful parameters predicting cardiac events in post-infraction patients (87), in patients with congestive heart failure (88), in LQTS patients (89), and in patients exposed to certain proarrhtyhmic drugs (90). Chapter 15 reviews QTD in detail. Among the most recent publications, QTD was found to be a poor independent predictor of cardiovascular mortality in 37,579 male veterans (91), but QTc dispersion was significantly increased in children with ventricular ectopic beats compared to control subjects (92), as well as in post-myocardial infarction adults (93).

Which Leads to Use

Based on a simple mathematical relationship, two limb leads are sufficient to reconstruct the remaining four using Einthoven's law (III = II-I) and aVR = -1/2(I+II), aVL = I-1/2II and aVF = II-1/2I. Thus, only two limb leads are necessary when evaluating the contribution of all limb leads to the overall QTD (94). It is why most authors measured QTD between eight leads (the six precordial leads and two limb leads). Of course, such reasoning stands under the assumption that the effect of body size and internal thoracic structure is negligible.

QTD Measurement Methods

First, the range of QT intervals within all available leads was used to quantify QTD. Then, the standard deviation of QT duration between leads allowed to reduce the effect of outlying measurements *(95)*. Lee et al. *(96)* and Macfarlane et al. *(97)* demonstrated that QTD is dependent on the number of leads included in its measurement by measuring a larger QTD in reconstructed 12-lead ECGs than in 3-orthogonal leads. Following this observation and because all QT interval cannot systematically be measured in all leads (because of noise, low-amplitude T wave, etc.), several authors such as Day et al. *(98)* used a corrected QTD value for the number of lead included in its computation (using a weighting factors equal to the square root of the number of measured leads). Others used a combination of both factors: numbers of leads as well as T-wave amplitude *(80)*.

According to the dipole theory, the QTD occurrence could be explained by a projection phenomenon dependent on the lead placement *(99)*. However, studies of body surface mapping have proven that the nature of repolarization has nondipolar contents as well *(100)*. So, the fundamental question is: does the difference in QT interval duration between leads reflect the presence of repolarization heterogeneity within the ventricular myocardium? A recent study by Rautaharju *(101)* on the analysis of the various components of QT dispersion concluded on the meaningless information related to QT dispersion, and the possibly more attractive measurement of nondipolar voltage as potential marker of localized dispersion and heterogeneity of ventricular repolarization for the evaluation of the risk of adverse cardiac events. Similar conclusions were published by Lund et al. *(80)* based on a population of 247 post-infarction patients.

Presently, experts in the field are still undecided on the relative contribution of measurement errors, projection, and repolarization heterogeneity to QTD measured in surface ECGs *(2,102)*. Nevertheless, QTD is not a recommended measure of repolarization despite the fact that it might reflect abnormalities in T-wave morphology.

Drug-Induced QT Dispersion

What about drug-induced dispersion of repolarization? Again, experimental and clinical studies investigated the role of antiarrhythmic drugs on the ventricular dispersion when using both endocardial MAPs and ECGs. Zabel at al. *(103)* reported important results on the effect of quinidine, D-sotalol, and amiodarone in perfused rabbit heart. Quinidine and D-sotalol were associated with an increased ventricular dispersion, whereas amiodarone did not induce any changes in ventricular dispersion. The dispersion was measured by both endo- and epicardial MAP recordings. This absence of effect of amiodarone on ventricular dispersion was confirmed in humans and strengthened the role of ventricular dispersion in the development of TdP *(90)*.

Regardless how the differences in QT intervals between leads are addressed, the remaining and indisputable limitation of 12-lead or 3-lead QTD is to be dependent on the quality of the QT measurements *(86)*. Consequently, researchers have investigated other techniques to quantify the ventricular repolarization heterogeneity.

NEW POTENTIAL REPOLARIZATION SURROGATE MARKERS FOR TORSADE DE POINTES

Morphology of the T Wave on Scalar ECGs

In the current process of drug-safety evaluation, QT interval prolongation is the only accepted marker for the assessment of an increased risk for TdP. However, several studies

Baseline, HR=71 bpm, QT=383 ms, SPC= 0 ng/ml

SPC= 582 ng/ml, HR=74 bpm, QT=416 ms

SPC= 1430 ng/ml, HR=71 bpm, QT=454 ms

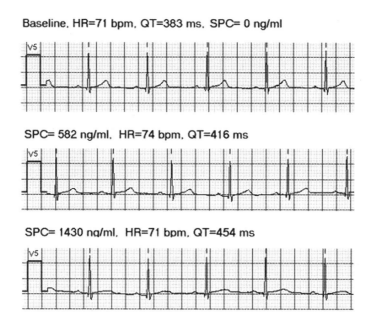

Fig. 4. The repolarization changes induced by sotalol in the same patient for very similar heart rates on the surface ECGs. During baseline, the T waves have high amplitude and QT interval is normal, after dosing the sotalol plasma concentration (SPC) rise to 682 ng/mL and the QT interval is prolonged, after double dosing the SPC rise to 1430 ng/ml and both T-wave morphology and QT intervals are drastically modified.

have shown that ion channel dysfunction in patients with the congenital LQTS or with certain drugs are associated with T-wave morphology changes and increased repolarization heterogeneity *(41,56,103–106)*

Some drugs leading to small QT prolongation in specific conditions (stress tachycardia, ventricular premature beats with short–long–short series) may trigger TdP *(107),* but all drugs causing QT prolongation are not arrhythmogenic. For instance, amiodarone causes QTc prolongation with minimal evidence of TdP. It is believed that these specific drugs have a homogeneous prolonging effect in all layers of the myocardial muscle leading to a smaller transmural heterogeneity of repolarization (and refractoriness) that may play an important role in the continuation of TdP by creating re-entrant circuits *(108).*

Our group has investigated the changes in morphology in T wave induced by sotalol. This study evidenced changes in T wave morphology induced by sotalol as described in Fig. 4. This figure shows the ECG from lead V5 from the same patient for three levels of plasma concentration of the drug. During baseline, the T wave looks normal when the plasma concentration increases the QT prolongs and T-wave base becomes broader (amplitude decrease). We studied this phenomenon using a T wave area-based technique *(40,56,105,109),* and identified changes in morphology within the overall repolarization. Table 2 describes the values of QT and area-based parameters during baseline and at three levels of sotalol plasma concentration (population-based heart rate correction was used). The drug modified the overall T wave (25%, 50%, and 97% of the total cumulated area under the T wave; *see* Fig. 3). Recent work on the role of transmural dispersion of repolarization and its role in the genesis of ventricular arrhythmias have hypothesized that only the final portion of the T wave (QT apex to QT end) may be relevant. Our results do not support such hypothesis.

Table 2
QT Repolarization Measurements Associated With Three Doses
of Sotalol Plasma Concentrations

SPC (ng/ml)	N	RR	QTc slope	QTac 25%	QTac 50%	QTac 97%
0	558	899 ± 128	359 ± 32	220 ± 25	261 ± 27	346 ± 34
> 0–300	69	1001 ± 122	393 ± 35	**240 ± 29**	**288 ± 30**	**384 ± 36**
≤ 300–600	135	**1000 ± 129**	393 ± 34	**236 ± 26**	285 ± 28	**380 ± 36**
≤ 600	649	**1052 ± 134**	**434 ± 43**	**249 ± 31**	**308 ± 34**	**419 ± 46**

Comparing mean values in reference to plasma concentration free of sotalol, the values in bold are significantly higher ($p > 0.001$) than baseline values. Sotalol plasma concentration (SPC) is expressed in ng/ml, all other parameters are in ms. QTacn% are the HR-corrected intervals between Q onset and the point at which n% of the total area under the T-wave is reached. The QTac25%, QTac50%, and QTac97% are area-based parameters reflecting changes in duration and morphology of the T wave. Modified from ref. 56.

Values in bold $p > 0.001$.

Morphology of the T Loop

The use of vectocardiographic approach to evaluate T wave loop has been shown to be independent from the projection phenomenon and from the determination of the end of the T wave. Few clinical studies have investigated the prognostic significance of T wave and T loop dispersion in patients with LQTS. These studies were based on body-surface mapping *(110,111)*, 12-lead ECGs (112), and Holter ECG recordings *(113,114)*. These studies have demonstrated regional electrical disparities in the ventricular recovery process that are believed to play an important role in the triggering and continuation of ventricular tachycardia. The most popular method to analyze the T-wave loop morphology is based on the principal components analysis (PCA) of the repolarization signal *(115,116)*. Briefly, the method quantifies the three-dimensional structure of the T-wave loop in a space defined by its principal axes of inertia. In this space, the morphology of the loop is defined by the three eigenvalues relative to the principal axes: λ_1, λ_2, and λ_3. The maximum energy of the loop is concentrated in the so-called preferential plan defined by the two first eigenvectors, the third axis (related to λ_3) is small with respect to that of λ_1 and λ_2. The normal loop in the preferential plan is narrow ($\lambda_2/\lambda_1 < 1$), having a more round T-wave loop is associated with an increased repolarization heterogeneity *(117)*.

In patients with LQTS, Priori et al, *(118)* identified abnormal morphology (also called T-wave complexity) of the repolarization segment. In patients with hypertrophic cardiomyopathy, indexes quantifying T-wave loop morphology were also increased and significantly higher in symptomatic patients *(119)*. T wave complexity has been found to be independent of QTD suggesting that PCA measures provide different information about the repolarization process. Also, there are studies demonstrating the association between quantitative measures of T-wave morphology and the risk of arrhythmic events in clinical data *(120–122)*, but there is no study demonstrating an association between drug-induced repolarization morphology changes and the occurrence of cardiac events. One would foresee the role of PCA-based technique for the evaluation of repolarization heterogeneity from surface ECGs playing a crucial role in future drug-safety evaluation.

Other interesting methods were developed by Acar et al. *(123)*, among them the so-called TCRT parameter defined as a measure of the vector deviation between the depolarization and the repolarization waves. This parameter has the particularity of being correlated with none of the others usually investigated (PCA parameters, lead dispersion QTc interval, etc.). In a group of 63 patients with hypertrophic cardiomyopathy, total cosine R to T (TRCT) was 0.35 ± 0.52 vs 0.52 ± 0.27 for a comparison group of 76 normal subjects. The change in sign corresponds to an increased deviation between the principal directions of repolarization and depolarization waves. This method was also relevant for predicting arrhythmic events in patients with ischemic heart disease. From 12-lead ECGs of post-infarction patients, TCRT has predictive power for sudden cardiac death in Cox regression analysis after adjustment for left ventricular ejection, age, and heart rate among others (124). Even if TCRT is predictive in patients with diseases modifying profoundly the balance of electric forces within the overall myocardium, it would be worth investigating its potential in studies evaluating the safety of new pharmacological compounds.

Abnormalities of Repolarization Adaptation to Heart Rate Changes

Analyzing the effect of rapid changes of heart rate on QT intervals is a new and interesting dynamic aspect of repolarization. Examples in preclinical model and in Long QT syndrome patients (LQT2) demonstrated that predictor of arrhythmic events may be identified in this transitory phase (125), and this adaptation period may be abnormal, and thus predispose an individual to arrhythmic events (126).

The benefit of such phenomenon for both clinical and drug-safety studies is currently being investigated by several research groups.

QT/RR Relationship

The Holter ECG recordings may be extremely useful for the assessment of potential cardiotoxicity of a new drug in phase I study. It provides a large set of information allowing for the comparison of QT intervals at similar heart rate as it is done in the bin analysis. Analyzing the QT/RR relationship may also provide relevant information about drug-induced QT prolongation. We developed a method extracting steady-state QT interval from Holter recordings, and computing the QT/RR relationship for specific periods of the recordings (before and after dosing). This method provides a comprehensive method identifying both drug-induced prolongation and its dose-dependency over time as shown in Fig. 5. This method is currently evaluated on large databases.

CONCLUSION

The QT interval is an accepted biomarker for identifying an increased risk for TdP, as supported by cellular and clinical studies. Various factors influence the duration of the QT interval. Hence, it seems that the assessment of drug-safety based on few QT intervals measured in one or two leads of a standard 12-lead ECG recorded at discrete time may poorly document the true risk of a new drug. Acquiring 12-lead ECG data in a continuous way (Holter ECG) in phase I/II may help to better assess the drug-induced QT prolongation, and thus ensure pharmaceutical companies that they invest in the right and safe compound. Automatic measurements of QT intervals could play a more important role in studies evaluating drug safety. Automatic QT measurements are more reproducible and reliable than manual measurements and, because a large set of data can be analyzed, a better identification of relevant findings can be made. Finally, further emphasis needs to be put on dynamic features of repolarization and the analysis of its adaptation to rapid heart rate changes.

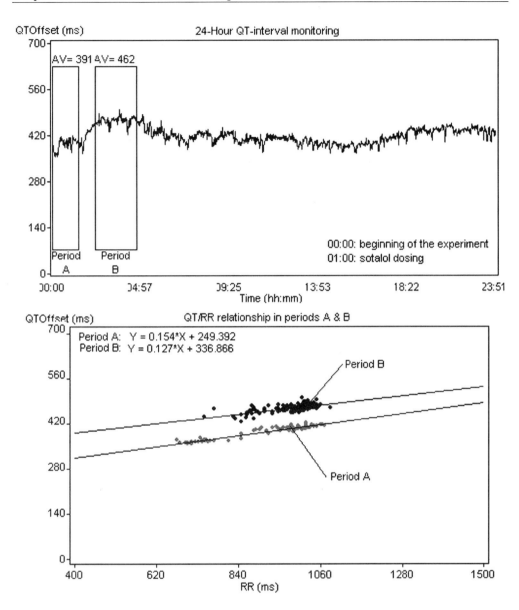

Fig. 5. Example of changes in QT/RR relationship from an Holter ECG recording from a healthy volunteer who received a single dose of sotalol 1-h after the beginning of the recording. The upper panel is the 24-h QT interval monitoring. Period (A) is located before dosing (from 8:00 to 9:00, 00:00 to 01:00 on the graph). It corresponds to the baseline period and it is used as a reference. The second period (B) is located after dosing (from 10:00 to 13:00). The lower panel is the QT/RR relationship for two specified periods (A and B). Only stable QT measurements (repolarization steady-state) are included in the lower panel. The QT/RR regression lines for the two periods have similar slopes, the drug-induced QT prolongation shifts up the regression line for period B.

Unfortunately, the QT prolongation is not a perfect surrogate of an increased risk for arrhythmic events. First, QT prolongation is not systematically associated with an increased risk for arrhythmic events. Second, identifying the QT measurement is challenging. It suffers from a lack of standardization and it requires to be corrected for heart rate among other factors. These limitations explain partially why QTD, when measured from surface ECGs, has lost its clinical appeal. Currently, other more complex methods are investigated that focus on T wave and loop morphology. Changes in morphology of T loop has been associated with an increased heterogeneity and associated with an increased risk for ventricular arrhythmias. These methods should be investigated to evaluate their ability to identify increased drug-induced risk for TdP.

REFERENCES

1. Taccardi B, Punske B B, Lux RL, MacLeod RS, Ershler PR, Dustman TJ, Vyhmeister Y. Useful lessons from body surface mapping. JCardiovasc Electrophysiol 1998;9:773–786.
2. Zabel M, Franz MR. The electrophysiological Basis of QT dispersion: global or local repolarization? Circulation 6-27-2000;101:E235–E236.
3. Antzelevitch C, Neterenko VV. Contribution of electrical heterogeneity of repolarization to the ECG. In Cardiac Repolarization: Bridging Basic and Clinical Sciences. Gussak I, Antzelevitch C, eds. Totowa, NJ: Humana Press 2004; 111–126.
4. Ghanem RN, Ramanathan C, Jia P, Rudy Y. Heart-surface reconstruction and ECG electrodes localization using fluoroscopy, epipolar geometry and stereovision: application to noninvasive imaging of dardiac electrical activity. IEEE Trans.Med.Imaging 2003;22:1307–1318.
5. Moss AJ, Zareba W, Benhorin J, Couderc JP, Kennedy H, Locati-Heilbron E, Maison-Blanche P. ISHNE guidelines for electrocardiographic evaluation of drug-related QT prolongation and other alterations in ventricular repolarization: task force summary. A report of the task force of the International Society for Holter and Noninvasive Electrocardiology (ISHNE), Committee on Ventricular Repolarization. Ann. Noninvasive Electrocardiol 2001;6:333–341.
6. Zareba W, Moss AJ, Schwartz PJ, Vincent GM, Robinson JL, Priori SG., et al. Influence of genotype on the clinical course of the long-QT syndrome. International Long-QT Syndrome Registry Research Group. N Engl J Med 1998;339:960–965.
7. De Ponti F, Poluzzi E, Cavalli A, Recanatini M, Montanaro N. Safety of non-antiarrhythmic drugs that prolong the QT interval or induce Torsade de Pointes: an overview. Drug Saf 2002;25:263–286.
8. Dessertenne F. La tachycardie ventriculaire a deux foyers opposes variables. Arch Mal Coeur 1966;59:263–272.
9. D'Alnoncourt CN, Zierhut W, Bluderitz B. "Torsade de Pointes" tachycardia. Re-entry or focal activity? Br Heart J 1982;48:213–216.
10. Antzelevitch C, Burashnikov A, Di Diego JM. Cellular and ionic mechanisms underlying arrhythmogenesis. In Cardiac Repolarization: Brodging Basic and Clinical Sciences. Gussak I, Antzelevitch C, eds. Totowa, NJ: Humana Press 2004:201–251.
11. Roden DM, Lazzara R, Rosen M, Schwartz PJ, Towbin J, Vincent GM. Multiple mechanisms in the long-QT syndrome. Current knowledge, gaps, and future directions. The SADS oundation Task Force on LQTS. Circulation 1996;94:1996–2012.
12. Antzelevitch C, Nesterenko VV, Yan GX. Role of M cells in acquired long QT syndrome, U waves, and Torsade de Pointes. J Electrocardiol 1995;28:131–138.
13. Jackman WM, Friday KJ, Anderson JL., Aliot EM, Clark M, Lazzara R. The long QT syndromes: a critical review, new clinical observations and a unifying hypothesis. Prog Cardiovasc Dis 1988;31:115–172.
14. Asano Y, Davidenko JM, Baxter WT, Gray RA, Jalife J. Optical mapping of drug-induced polymorphic arrhythmias and Torsade fd Pointes in the isolated rabbit heart. J Am Coll Cardiol. 1997;29:831–842.
15. Ben David J, Zipes DP. Differential response to right and left ansae subclaviae stimulation of early afterdepolarizations and ventricular tachycardia induced by cesium in dogs. Circulation 1988;78: 1241–1250.
16. Koumi S, Backer CL, Arentzen CE. Characterization of inwardly rectifying K+ channel in human cardiac myocytes. Alterations in channel behavior in myocytes isolated from patients with idiopathic dilated cardiomyopathy. Circulation 1995;92:164–174.
17. Antzelevitch C, Sicouri S, Litovsky SH, Lukas A, Krishnan SC, Di Diego JM, Gintant GA, Liu DW. Heterogeneity within the ventricular wall. Electrophysiology and pharmacology of epicardial, endocardial, and M cells. Circ Res 1991;69:1427–1449.
18. Liu DW, Antzelevitch C. Characteristics of the delayed rectifier current (IKr and IKs) in canine ventricular epicardial, midmyocardial, and endocardial myocytes. A weaker IKs contributes to the longer action potential of the M cell. Circ Res 1995;76:351–365.

19. Sicouri S, Antzelevitch C. A subpopulation of cells with unique electrophysiological properties in the deep subepicardium of the canine ventricle. The M cell. Circ Res 1991;68:1729–1741.

20. Gilmour RF, Jr., Zipes DP. Different electrophysiological responses of canine endocardium and epicardium to combined hyperkalemia, hypoxia, and acidosis. Circ Res 1980;46:814–825.

21. Litovsky SH, Antzelevitch C. Differences in the electrophysiological response of canine ventricular subendocardium and subepicardium to acetylcholine and isoproterenol. A direct effect of acetylcholine in ventricular mMyocardium. Circ Res 1990;67:615–627.

22. Liu DW, Gintant GA, Antzelevitch C. Ionic bases for electrophysiological distinctions among epicardial, midmyocardial, and endocardial myocytes from the free wall of the canine left ventricle. Circ Res 1993;72:671–687.

23. Drouin E, Charpentier F, Gauthier C, Laurent K, Le Marec H. electrophysiologic characteristics of cells spanning the left ventricular wall of human heart: evidence for presence of M cells. J Am Coll Cardiol 1995;26:185–192.

24. Anyukhovsky EP, Sosunov EA, Rosen MR. Regional differences in electrophysiological properties of epicardium, midmyocardium, and endocardium. In vitro and in vivo correlations. Circulation 1996;94:1981–1988.

25. Vos MA, Cora Verduyn S, Wellens HJ. Early afterdepolarization in the In situ canine heart: Mechanistic insights into acquired torsades de pointes arrhythmias. In Monophasic Action Potentials: Bridging cell and Bedside. (Franz MR, ed.). Armonk, NY: Futura Publishing Company, Inc. 2000:553–569.

26. Verduyn SC, Vos MA., van der Zande J, Kulcsar A, Wellens HJ. Further observations to elucidate the role of interventricular dispersion of repolarization and early afterdepolarizations in the genesis of acquired Torsade de Pointes arrhythmias: a comparison between almokalant and D-sotalol using the dog as its own control. J Am Coll Cardiol 1997;30:1575–1584.

27. WeissenburgerJ, Nesterenko VV, Antzelevitch C. Transmural heterogeneity of ventricular tepolarization under naseline and long QT vonditions in the canine heart in vivo: Torsades fe Pointes fevelops with halothane but not pentobarbital snesthesia. J Cardiovasc Electrophysiol 2000;11: 290–304.

28. Antzelevitch C, Sun ZQ, Zhang ZQ, Yan GX. Cellular and ionic mechanisms underlying erythromycin-induced long QT intervals and Torsade de Pointes. J Am Coll Cardiol 1996;28:1836–1848.

29. Shimizu W, Antzelevitch C. Sodium channel block with mexiletine is effective in reducing dispersion of repolarization and preventing Torsade de Pointes in LQT2 and LQT3 models of the long QT syndrome. Circulation 1997;96:2038–2047.

30. Moss AJ, Schwartz PJ, Crampton RS, Tzivoni D, Locati EH, MacCluerJ, et al. The long QT syndrome. prospective longitudinal study of 328 families. Circulation 1991;84:1136–1144.

31. Zareba W, Moss AJ, le Cessie S, Locati EH., Robinson JL, Hall WJ, Andrews ML. Risk of cardiac events in family members of patients with long QT syndrome. J Am Coll Cardiol 1995;26:1685–1691.

32. Moss AJ, Zareba W, Kaufman ES, Gartman E, Peterson DR, Benhorin J, et al. Increased risk of arrhythmic events in long-QT syndrome with mutations in the pore region of the human ether-a-go-go-related gene potassium channel. Circulation 2002;105:794–799.

33. Zareba W, Moss AJ. QT interval and its drug-induced prolongation. In Cardiac Repolarization: Bridging Basic and Clinical Science. Gussak I, Antzelevitch C, eds. Totowa, NJ: Humana Press 2004:311–328.

34. Zareba W, Moss AJ, Rosero SZ, Hajj-Ali R, Konecki J, Andrews M. Electrocardiographic findings in patients with diphenhydramine overdose. Am J Cardiology 1997;80:1168–1173.

35. Drici MD, Clement N. Is gender a risk factor for adverse drug reactions? The example of drug-induced long QT syndrome. Drug Saf 2001;24:575–585.

36. Drici MD, Baker L, Plan P, Barhanin J, Romey G, Salama G. Mice display sex differences in halothane-induced polymorphic ventricular tachycardia. Circulation 2002;106:497–503.

37. Lehmann MH, Hardy S, Archibald D, Quart B, MacNeil DJ. Sex difference in risk of Torsade de Pointes with D,l-sotalol. Circulation 1996;94:2535–2541.

38. Lehmann MH, Hardy S, Archibald D, MacNeil DJ. JTc prolongation with D,l-sotalol in women versus men. Am J Cardiol 1999;83:354–359.

39. Lehmann MH., Yang H. Sexual dimorphism in the electrocardiographic dynamics of human ventricular repolarization: characterization in true time domain. Circulation 2001;104:32–38.

40. Merri M, Benhorin J, Alberti M, Locati E, Moss AJ. Electrocardiographic quantitation of ventricular repolarization. Circulation 1989;80:1301–1308.

41. Couderc JP, Zareba W, Moss AJ. Assessment of the stability of the individual-based correction of QT interval for heart rate. Ann Noninvasive Electrocardiol 2004; in press.

42. Stramba-Badiale M, Locati EH, Martinelli A, Courville J, Schwartz PJ. Gender and the relationship between ventricular repolarization and cardiac cycle length during 24-h Holter recordings. Eur Heart J 1997;18:1000–1006.

43. Rodriguez I, Kilborn MJ, Liu XK, Pezzullo JC, Woosley RL. Drug-induced QT prolongation in women during the menstrual cycle. JAMA 2001;285:1322–1326.

44. Surawicz B, Parikh SR. Differences between ventricular repolarization in men and women: description, mechanism and implications. Ann Noninvasive Electrocardiol 2003;8:333–340.

45. Locati EH, Zareba W, Moss AJ, Schwartz PJ, Vincent GM, Lehmann MH, et al. Age- and sex-related differences in clinical manifestations in patients with congenital long-QT syndrome: findings from the International LQTS Registry. Circulation 1998;97:2237–2344.

46. Sesti F, Abbott GW, Wei J, Murray KT, Saksena S, Schwartz PJ, et al. A common polymorphism associated with antibiotic-induced cardiac arrhythmia. Proc Natl Acad Sci USA 2000;97:10613–10618.

46a. Yang P, Kanki H, Prolet B, Yang T, Wei J, Viswanathan PC, et al. Allelic variants in Long-QT disease genes in patients with drug-associated Torsades de Vointes. Circulation 2002;105:1943–1948.

47. Splawski I, Timothy KW, Tateyama M, Clancy CE, Malhotra A, Beggs AH, et al. Variant of SCN5A sodium channel implicated in risk of cardiac arrhythmia. Science 2002;297:1333–1336.

48. McLaughlin NB, Campbell RW, Murray A. Comparison of automatic QT measurement techniques in the normal 12 lead electrocardiogram. Br Heart J 1995;74:84–89.

49. McLaughlin NB, Campbell RW, Murray A. Accuracy of four automatic QT measurement techniques in cardiac patients and healthy subjects. Heart 1996;76:422–426.

50. Stramba-Badiale M, Locati EH, Martinelli A, Courville J, Schwartz PJ. Gender and the relationship between ventricular repolarization and cardiac cycle length during 24-h Holter recordings. Eur Heart J 1997;18:1000–1006.

51. Magnano AR, Holleran S, Ramakrishnan R, Reiffel JA, Bloomfield DM. Autonomic nervous system influences on QT interval in normal subjects. J Am Coll Cardiol 2002;39:1820–1826.

52. Franz MR, Swerdlow CD, Liem LB, Schaefer J. Cycle length dependence of human action potential duration in vivo. Effects of single extrastimuli, sudden sustained rate acceleration and deceleration, and different steady-state frequencies.. J Clin Invest 1988;82:972–979.

53. Krahn AD, Klein GJ, Yee R. Hysteresis of the RT interval with exercise: a new marker for the long-QT syndrome? Circulation 1997;96:1551–1556.

54. Funck-Brentano C, Jaillon P. Rate-corrected QT interval: techniques and limitations. Am J Cardiol 1993;72:17B–22B.

55. Malik M. Problems of heart rate correction in assessment of drug-induced QT interval prolongation. J Cardiovasc Electrophysiol 2001;12:411–420.

56. Couderc JP, Zareba W, Moss AJ, Sarapa N, Morganroth J, Darpo B. Identification of sotalol-induced changes in repolarization with T wave area-based repolarization duration parameters. J Electrocardiol 2003;36 Suppl:115–120.

57. Malik M. The imprecision in heart rate correction may lead to artificial observations of drug induced QT interval changes. Pacing Clin Electrophysiol 2002;25:209–216.

58. Malik M, Farbom P, Batchvarov V, Hnatkova K, Camm AJ. Relation between QT and RR intervals is highly individual among healthy subjects: implications for heart rate correction of the QT interval. Heart 2002;87:220–228.

59. Badilini F, Maison-Blanche P, Childers R, Coumel P. QT interval analysis on ambulatory electrocardiogram recordings: a selective beat averaging approach. Med Biol Eng Comput 1999;37:71–79.

60. Murray A, McLaughlin NB, Bourke JP, Doig JC, Furniss SS, Campbell RW. Errors in manual measurement of QT intervals. Br Heart J 1994;71:386–390.

61. Franz MR, Swerdlow CD, Liem LB, Schaefer J. Cycle length dependence of human action potential duration in vivo. Effects of single extrastimuli, sudden sustained rate acceleration and deceleration, and different steady-state frequencies. J Clin Invest 1988;82:972–979.

62. Pueyo E, Smetana P, Laguna P, Malik M. Estimation of the QT/RR hysteresis lag. J Electrocardiol 2003;36:187–190.

63. Lau CP, Freedman AR, Fleming S, Malik M, Camm AJ, Ward DE. Hysteresis of the ventricular paced QT interval in response to abrupt changes in pacing rate. Cardiovasc Res 1988;22:67–72.

64. Extramiana F, Tavernier R, Maison-Blanche P, Neyroud N, Jordaens L, Leenhardt A, Coumel P. Ventricular repolarization and Holter monitoring. Effect of sympathetic blockage on the QT/RR ratio. Arch Mal Coeur Vaiss 2000;93:1277–1283.

65. Browne KF, Prystowsky E, Heger JJ, Zipes DP. Modulation of the Q-T interval by the autonomic nervous system. Pacing Clin Electrophysiol 1983;6:1050–1056.

66. Bellavere F, Ferri M, Guarini L, Bax G, Piccoli A, Cardone C, Fedele D. Prolonged QT period in diabetic autonomic neuropathy: a possible role in sudden cardiac death? Br Heart J 1988;59:379–383.

67. Coumel P, Maison-Blanche P. Neuro-mediated repolarization abnormalities. In Cardiac Repolarization: Bridging Basic and Clinical Science. Totowa, New-Jersey: Humana Press 2003:329–350.

68. Malik M, Bradford A. Human precision of operating a digitizing board: implications for electrocardiogram measurements. Pacing Clin Electrophysiol 1998;21:1656–1662.

69. Sarapa N, Morganroth J, Couderc JP, Francom SF, Darpo B, Fleishaker JC, et al. Electrocardiographic identification of drug-induced QT prolongation: assessment by different recording and measurement methods. Ann Noninvasive Electrocardiol 2004;9:48–57.

70. Savelieva I, Yi G, Guo X, Hnatkova K, Malik M. Agreement and reproducibility of automatic versus manual measurement of QT interval and QT dispersion. Am J Cardiol 1998;81:471–477.

71. Kors JA, van Herpen G. The coming of age of computerized ECG processing: can it replace the cardiologist in epidemiological studies and clinical trials? Medinfo 2001;10:1161–1167.

72. Willems JL. Common standards for quantitative electrocardiography. Leuven: ACCO Publ; 1986. Report No.: CSE 86-12-08. (CSE 6th Progress Report;vol.)

73. Lepeschkin E, Surawicz B. The measurement of the Q-T interval of the electrocardiogram. Circulation 1952;6:378–388.

74. Puddu PE, Bernard PM, Chaitman BR, Bourassa MG. QT interval measurement by a computer assisted program: a potentially useful clinical parameter. J Electrocardiol 1982;15:15–21.

75. O'Donnell J, Knoebel SB, Lovelace DE, McHenry PL. Computer quantitation of Q-T and terminal T wave (aT-ET) intervals during exercise: methodology and results in normal men. Am J Cardiol 1981;47:1168–1172.

76. O'Donnell J, Lovelace DE, Knoebel SB, McHenry PL. Behavior of the terminal T wave during exercise in normal subjects, patients with symptomatic coronary artery disease and apparently healthy wubjects with abnormal ST segment depression. J Am Coll Cardiol 1985;5:78–84.

77. Pisani E, Pelligrini E, Ansuini G. Performances of algorithms for QT interval measurements in ambulatory ECG monitoring. Los Alamitos, CA: IEEE Computer Society Press, 1985, Computers in Cardiology 11:459–462.

78. Algra A, Le Brun H, Zeelenberg C. An algorithm for computer measurements of the QT intervals in the 24 hour ECG. IEEE Computer Society Press, 1987 Computers in Cardiology 13:117–119.

79. Moody GB, Mark RG, Goldberger AL. PhysioNet: a web-based resource for the study of physiologic signals. IEEE Eng Med Biol Mag 2001;20:70–75.

80. Lund K, Nygaard H, Pedersen A. Weighing the QT intervals with the slope or the amplitude of the T wave. Ann Noninvasive Electrocardiol 2002;7:4–9.

81. Murray A, McLaughlin NB, Bourke JP, Doig JC, Furniss SS, Campbell RW. Errors in manual measurement of QT intervals. Br Heart J 1994;71:386–390.

82. Demolis JL, Kubitza D, Tenneze L, Funck-Brentano C. Effect of a single oral dose of moxifloxacin (400 mg and 800 mg) on ventricular repolarization in healthy subjects. Clin Pharmacol Ther 2000;68:658–666.

83. Kuo CS, Munakata K, Reddy CP, Surawicz B. Characteristics and possible mechanism of ventricular arrhythmia dependent on the dispersion of action potential durations. Circulation 1983;67:1356–1367.

84. Kuo, C. S., Reddy, C. P., Munakata, K., and SURAWICZ, B. Mechanism of Ventricular Arrhythmias Caused by Increased Dispersion of Repolarization. Eur.Heart J. 1985;6 Suppl D:63–70.

85. Vassallo JA, Cassidy DM, Kindwall KE, Marchlinski FE, Josephson ME. Nonuniform recovery of excitability in the left ventricle. Circulation 1988;78:1365–1372.

86. Lund K, Lund B, Brohet C, Nygaard H. Evaluation of electrocardiogram T-wave dispersion measurement methods. Med Biol Eng Comput 2003;41:410–415.

87. Zabel M, Klingenheben T, Franz MR, Hohnloser SH. Assessment of QT dispersion for prediction of mortality or arrhythmic events after myocardial infarction: results of a prospective, long-term follow-up study. Circulation 1998;97:2543–2550.

88. Fu GS, Meissner A, Simon R. Repolarization dispersion and sudden cardiac death in patients with impaired left ventricular function. Eur Heart J 1997;18:281–289.

89. Priori SG, Napolitano C, Diehl L, Schwartz PJ. Dispersion of the QT interval. A marker of therapeutic efficacy in the idiopathic Long QT syndrome. Circulation 1994;89:1681–1689.

90. Hii JT, Wyse DG, Gillis AM, Duff HJ, Solylo MA, Mitchell LB. Precordial QT interval dispersion as a marker of Torsade de Pointes. Disparate effects of class Ia antiarrhythmic drugs and amiodarone. Circulation 1992;86:1376–1382.

91. Shah BR, Yamazaki T, Engel G, Cho S, Chun SH, Froelicher VF. Computerized QT dispersion measurement and cardiovascular mortality in male veterans. Am J Cardiol 2004;93:483–486.

92. Das BB, Sharma J. Repolarization abnormalities in children with a structurally normal heart and ventricular ectopy. Pediatr Cardiol 2004.

93. Jain H, Avasthi R. Correlation between dispersion of repolarization (QT dispersion) and ventricular ectopic beat frequency in patients with acute myocardial infarction: a marker for risk of arrhythmo-genesis? Int J Cardiol . 2004;93:69–73.

94. Kors JA, van Herpen G. Measurement error as a source of QT dispersion: a computerised analysis. Heart 1998;80:453–458.

95. de Bruyne MC, Hoes AW, Kors JA, Dekker JM, Hofman A, van Bemmel JH., Grobbee DE. Prolonged QT interval: a tricky diagnosis? Am J Cardiol 1997;80:1300–1304.

96. Lee KW, Kligfield P, Okin PM, Dower GE. Determinants of precordial QT dispersion in normal subjects. J Electrocardiol 1998;31 Suppl:128–133.

97. Macfarlane PW, McLaughlin SC, Rodger JC. Influence of lead selection and population on automated measurement of QT dispersion. Circulation 1998;98:2160–2167.

98. Day CP, McComb JM, Matthews J, Campbell RW. Reduction in QT dispersion by sotalol following myocardial infarction. Eur Heart J 1991;12:423–427.

99. Kors JA, van Herpen G. Measurement error as a source of QT dispersion: a computerised analysis. Heart 1998;80:453–458.

100. Taccardi B, Punske BB, Lux RL, MacLeod RS, Ershler PR., Dustman TJ, Vyhmeister Y. Useful lessons from body surface mapping. J Cardiovasc Electrophysiol 1998;9:773–786.

101. Rautaharju PM. Why did QT dispersion die? Card Electrophysiol Rev 2002;6:295–301.

102. Di Bernardo D, Langley P, Murray A. Dispersion of QT intervals: a measure of dispersion of repolarization or simply a projection effect? Pacing Clin Electrophysiol 2000;23:1392–1396.

103. Zabel M, Hohnloser SH, Behrens S, Woosley RL, Franz MR. Differential effects of D-sotalol, quinidine, and amiodarone on dispersion of ventricular repolarization in the isolated rabbit heart. J Cardiovasc Electrophysiol 1997;8:1239–1245.

104. Moss AJ, Zareba W, Benhorin J, Locati EH, Hall WJ, Robinson JL, et al. H. ECG T-wave patterns in genetically distinct forms of the hereditary Long QT syndrome [see comments]. Circulation 1995;92:2929–2934.

105. Couderc JP, Burratini L, Konecki JA, Moss AJ. Detection of abnormal time-frequency components of the QT interval using wavelet transformation technique. Computers in Cardiology 1999;24:661–664.

106. Zareba W, Moss AJ, Konecki J. TU wave area-derived measures of repolarization dispersion in the Long QT syndrome. J Electrocardiol 1998;30 Suppl:191–195.

107. Monahan BP, Ferguson CL, Killeavy ES, Lloyd BK, Troy J, Cantilena L. R, Jr. Torsades de Pointes occurring in association with terfenadine use. JAMA 1990;264:2788–2790.

108. Antzelevitch C, Fish J. Electrical heterogeneity within the ventricular wall. Basic Res Cardiol 2001;96:517–527.

109. Couderc JP, Nomura A, Zareba W, Moss AJ. Heterogeneity of venticular repolarization morphology measured using orthogonal wavelet time-sale decomposition of the surface ECG. Computers in Cardiology 1999;26:61–64.

110. De Ambroggi L, Bertoni T, Locati E, Stramba-Badiale M, Schwartz PJ. Mapping of body surface potentials in patients with the idiopathic Long QT syndrome. Circulation 1986;74:1334–1345.

111. Taccardi B, Punske BB, Lux RL, MacLeod RS, Ershler PR, Dustman TJ, Vyhmeister Y. Useful lessons from body surface mapping. J Cardiovasc Electrophysiol 1998;9:773–786.

112. Day CP, McComb JM, Campbell RW. QT dispersion: an indication of arrhythmia risk in patients with Long QT intervals. Br Heart J 1990;63:342–344.

113. Priori SG, Mortara DW, Napolitano C, Diehl L, Paganini V, Cantu F, Cantu G, Schwartz PJ. Evaluation of the spatial aspects of T-wave complexity in the Long QT syndrome. Circulation 1997;96: 3006–3012.

114. Kallert T, Couderc JP, Voss A, Zareba W. Semi-automatic method quantifying T wave loop morphology: relevance for assessment of heterogenous repolarization. Computers in Cardiology 1999;26: 153–156.

115. Fayn J, Rubel P, Mohsen N. An improved method for the precise measurement of serial ECG changes in QRS duration and QT interval. Performance assessment on the CSE moise-testing database and a healthy 720 case-set population. J Electrocardiol 1992;24 Suppl:123–127.

116. Zareba W, Couderc JP, Moss AJ. Automatic detection of spatial and temporal heterogeneity of repolarization. Ann Noninvasive Electrocardiol 2000;5:1–3.

117. Kors JA, van Herpen G, van Bemmel JH. QT dispersion as an attribute of T-loop morphology. Circulation 1999;99:1458–1463.
118. Priori SG, Mortara DW, Napolitano C, Diehl L, Paganini V, Cantu F, Cantu G, Schwartz PJ. Evaluation of the spatial aspects of T-wave complexity in the Long QT syndrome. Circulation 1997;96: 3006–3012.
119. Yi G, Prasad K, Elliott P, Sharma S, Guo X, McKenna WJ, Malik M. T wave complexity in patients with hypertrophic cardiomyopathy. Pacing Clin Electrophysiol 1998;21:2382–2386.
120. Zabel M, Acar B, Klingenheben T, Franz MR, Hohnloser SH, Malik M. Analysis of 12-lead T-wave morphology for risk stratification after myocardial infarction. Circulation 2000;102:1252–1257.
121. Zabel M, Malik M. Predictive value of T-wave morphology variables and QT dispersion for postmyocardial infarction risk assessment. J Electrocardiol 2001;34 :27–35.
122. Zabel M, Malik M, Hnatkova K, Papademetriou V, Pittaras A, Fletcher RD, Franz MR. Analysis of T-wave morphology from the 12-lead electrocardiogram for prediction of long-term prognosis in male US veterans. Circulation 2002;105:1066–1070.
123. Acar B, Yi G, Hnatkova,K, Malik M. Spatial, temporal and wavefront direction characteristics of 12-lead T-wave morphology. Med Biol Eng Comput 1999;37:574–584.
124. Zabel M, Acar B, Klingenheben T, Franz MR, Hohnloser SH, Malik M. analysis of 12-lead T-wave morphology for risk stratification after myocardial infarction. Circulation 2000;102:1252–1257.
125. Burashnikov A, Antzelevitch C. Acceleration-induced action potential prolongation and early afterdepolarizations. J Cardiovasc Electrophysiol 1998;9:934–948.
126. Schwartz PJ, Priori SG, Locati EH, Napolitano C, Cantu F, Towbin JA, et al. S. Long QT syndrome patients with mutations of the SCN5A and HERG genes have differential responses to Na+ channel blockade and to increases in heart rate. Implications for gene-specific therapy. Circulation 1995;92:3381–3386.
127. Mirvis DM. Spatial variation of QT intervals in normal persons and patients with acute myocardial infarction. J Am Coll Cardiol 1985;5:625–631.
128. van Bemmel JH, Zywietz C, Kors JA. Signal analysis for ECG interpretation. Methods Inf Med 1990;29:317–329.
129. Laguna P, Thakor NV, Caminal P, Jane R, Yoon HR, Bayes de Luna A, Marti V, Guindo J. New algorithm for QT interval analysis in 24-hour Holter ECG: performance and applications. Med Biol Eng Comput 1990;28:67–73.
130. Laguna P, Jane R, Caminal P. Automatic detection of wave boundaries in multilead ECG signals: validation with the CSE database. Comput Biomed Res 1994;27:45–60.
131. Ferretti GF. A New Method for the Simultaneous Automatic Measurments of the RR and the QT Intervals in Ambulatory ECG Recordings. Durham, NC: IEEE Computer Society Press, 1992.
132. Xue Q, Reddy S. Algorithms for computerized QT analysis. J Electrocardiol 1998;30 Suppl:181–186.
133. Sosnowski M, Czyz Z, Leski J, Petelenz T, Tendera, M. High resolution electrocardiography-its application for the measurement of the QT interval in the presence of low-amplitude T-wave. Ann Noninvasive Electrocardiol 1998;3:304–310.
134. Bystricky W, Safer A . Modelling T-end in Holter ECGs by 2-layer Perceptrons: IEEE Computer Society; 2002, 29:105–108.
135. Hayn D, Schreier G, Lobodzinski S. Development and evaluation of a QT interval algorithm using different ECG databases. Intl J Bioelectromagnetism 2003;5:122–123.
136. Almeida R, Martinez JP, Olmos S., Rocha AP, Luguna P Doblare, M, Cerrolaza M, Rodrigues H. Automatic Delineation of T and P Waves Using a Wavelet-Based Multiscale Approach. Proc. Int. Congr. Comput. Bioeng. Madrid, Spain, 2003, pp. 243–247.
137. Schreier G, Hayn D, Lobodzinski S. Development of a new QT algorithm with heterogenous ECG databases. J Electrocardiol 2003;36 Suppl:145–50.

7

ECG Acquisition and Signal Processing

12-Lead ECG Acquisition

Justin L. Mortara, PhD

INTRODUCTION

The birth of electrocardiography can be traced back more than a century to the laboratories of Dutch physician and physiologist Willem Einthoven. In 1895, Einthoven published one of his seminal papers in which he identified and labeled five electrocardiogram waves P, Q, R, S, and T *(1)*. By 1900 he developed the string galvanometer that was to become the first electrocardiograph (ECG) *(2)*. Acknowledgment of Einthoven's essential contribution to electrocardiography is made everyday all over the world as clinicians and scientists speak of his curiously named waves in terms of QT intervals, PR, QRS durations, etc. *(3)*[a]. In 1924, his work earned him the Nobel Prize for the invention of the electrocardiograph.

In 1934, Frank Wilson introduced the notion of "unipolar" leads that would ultimately become the basis for the today's precordial leads *(4)*. Differing from the limb leads that were derived from bipolar combinations of the limb electrodes, the unipolar leads were thought of as referenced to a common terminal constructed from the limb lead electrodes and an associated *V* electrode that could be placed anywhere on the body surface. The creation of the Wilson Central Terminal, as this common terminal became known, provided the reference voltage for what Wilson called the *V* leads. Shortly thereafter, the standard placements and labels were established for the chest leads V1–V6 utilized today in electrocardiography *(5)*. In 1942, Emanuel Goldberger introduced the augmented limb leads aVR, aVL, and aVF. In conjunction with the chest leads of Wilson and the three Einthoven leads, the 12-leads of 12-lead electrocardiography were established.

---

[a] Lacking any other motivation for assignment of the wave names. Einthoven or others might have adopted an alphabetical approach to their appearance resulting in A, B, C, D, E assignments for P, Q, R, S, T waves.

From: *Cardiac Safety of Noncardiac Drugs:*
Practical Guidelines for Clinical Research and Drug Development
Edited by: J. Morganroth and I. Gussak © Humana Press Inc., Totowa, NJ

131

12-LEAD ELECTROCARDIOGRAPHY

Much has changed since the days of Einthoven and Wilson. Today, we are focused on acquisition, transmission, and analysis of 12-lead digital data. We have various means to acquire variable length ECG records, different options to transmit this data, and a variety of technologies with which to analyze it. This compares to Einthoven's original electro-cardiographs which occupied a sizeable room, collected limited leads of ECG data, and recorded that data on photographic paper in an indisputably clever,[b] but decisively pre-digital manner.

What is a 12-Lead Digital Electrocardiograph?

The 12-lead ECG is one of the most common diagnostic procedures used today. It is acquired in a wide range of clinical care settings from pre-hospital sites to critical care units, from primary care offices to home healthcare visits. Across all these settings, the defining characteristics of this procedure are the acquired leads and the electrode place-ment utilized to generate them. The 12-leads of a 12-lead ECG are leads I, II, III, aVR, aVL, aVF, V1, V2, V3, V4, V5, and V6. A typical resting 12-lead electrocardiograph recording is shown in Fig. 1.

To understand what a "digital" ECG is, it is important to distinguish digital from analog. The heart signals measured from the body surface are continuous analog signals. These signals can be converted to a series of quantized, time ordered numbers or "digi-tized." This concept is illustrated in Fig. 2. The continuous line represents the analog signal and the bars represent the digital conversion of that analog signal. The conversion process quantizes both the amplitude and sampling rate as suggested in Fig. 2. The result is a series of time ordered numbers that correspond to particular amplitudes at particular moments in time. Converted to a digital signal, the ECG can be transmitted and analyzed as digital data within various computational environments.

The 12-lead digital ECG is the extension of the digital ECG concept to incorporate all 12-leads. Hence, a digital 12-lead ECG is defined by two fundamental aspects: (1) the recorded signals are obtained with 10 electrodes and 12 leads as previously defined, and (2) the recorded data is digital in nature. The 12-lead digital ECG data itself can be of variable duration from a few seconds to several hours. Different 12-lead acquisition technologies yield variable duration recordings for use in different subject environments and drug development phases. These different technologies will be discussed later in the chapter.

Motivation for Utilizing 12-Lead Digital Electrocardiograph

Digital management of the 12-lead ECG data collected for both patient care and clinical research purposes provides enormous benefits over paper-based methods. These advantages can be grouped into three basic categories including accuracy, access, and analyzability.

The Association for the Advancement of Medical Instrumentation (AAMI) standard for the time base accuracy for paper outputs is set at $\pm 5\%$ *(6)*. This tolerance range reflects the expected variation of mechanically printed outputs, and can be translated directly into

---

[b]It should not be ignored that Einthoven himself executed what is likely the first transmission of the ECG over telephone lines in 1905. Analog ECG signals were transmitted over a distance greater than a 1 kilometer from the hospital to his nearby laboratory.

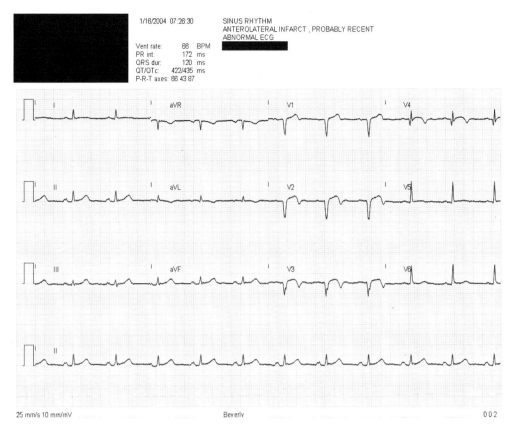

1/16/2004 07:26:30

SINUS RHYTHM
ANTEROLATERAL INFARCT , PROBABLY RECENT
ABNORMAL ECG

Vent rate: 66 BPM
PR int: 172 ms
QRS dur: 120 ms
QT/QTc: 422/435 ms
P-R-T axes: 66 43 87

25 mm/s 10 mm/mV   Beverly   002

Fig. 1. Standard 12-lead electrocardiograph in four channel print format showing automatic measurements and interpretive statements.

a potential fluctuation of the time base on the printed ECG. Expressed in terms of a typical cardiac cycle with a QT interval of 400 ms, such variation could manifest itself in absolute fluctuations of up to ± 20 ms without lying outside the standards for such recording devices. In light of the fact that studies are intended to detect much smaller QT effects, it is unreasonable to accept this potential systematic variation in a study design.[c] Digital ECG records, which are not subject to the mechanical fluctuations of writer outputs, simply do not exhibit such fluctuations and are inherently more accurate. Onscreen computer visualization of these digital ECG records can completely avoid the use of paper and the associated challenges that come with it.

With 12-lead digital ECG data, access can be easily granted to responsible parties for the review and/or analysis of the data provided a recognized open standard for the data format exists. Such an open standard exists for annotated ECG waveforms and is pro-

---

[c]Internal tests of third-party electrocardiographs have suggested that paper speed variation depends on the amount of paper loaded in the electrocardiographs. Hence, an ECG taken when the ECG was fully loaded with paper could exhibit a different time base than an ECG taken with the same machine hours later as the paper is depleted. This could give rise to a systematic error correlated with dose or other study parameters in paper-based collection of ECG data.

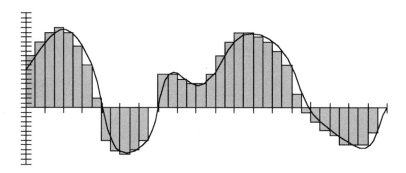

Fig. 2. Representation of digitization of analog signal (continuous curve).

vided under HL7 version 3.[d] Multiple medical device manufacturers, core laboratories, and software tool designers have already implemented solutions for viewing and annotating ECGs using the HL7 V3 annotated ECG (aECG) standard. Widespread adoption of the aECG standard now allows for data access across broad platforms in either clinical research or, in some cases, in clinical care environments. Digital ECG data formatted according the aECG standard can be rendered by a variety of different systems from ECG analysis workstations to clinical trial management systems, with access possible on a global scale. In contrast, paper ECG records are necessarily cumbersome to provide broad access to. High fidelity copies of the original paper ECG record are difficult to obtain and in any case the paper copy must be transported. A small study processed in this manner is difficult, a large study nearly impossible. Finally, the aECG standard enables the FDA Center for Drugs to receive and review digital ECG data as part of new drug application submissions, which was a stated objective in late 2001 *(7)*.

With 12-lead digital data collected and available in a defined open format, there is enormous potential for more detailed analysis of various ECG parameters. One clear analysis advantage the digital ECG presents is the ability to superimpose data on top of one another for visual comparison purposes as show in Fig. 3, where the superimposition of median beats is demonstrated.

Such visual superimposition is nearly impossible with paper-based ECGs. Furthermore, with the digital data available, all of the ECG signal can be viewed independent of print format. A standard print format such as the four-channel format shown in Fig. 1 only provides complete rendering of the 10 s of lead II, while the other channels have only 2.5 s displayed. With a digital ECG, the same ECG can be redisplayed in a 12-channel format so that all 10 s of all leads is visible as shown in Fig. 4. Finally, with the underlying digital data available, extensive quantitative analysis on enormous datasets collected as part of clinical trials will become possible. Such extended analysis may result in a better characterization of repolarization response to compounds, including the development of a measure other than the always used, often criticized, QT interval.

---

[d]Annotated ECG (aECG) standard was developed and fully approved by HL7 membership in January 2004.

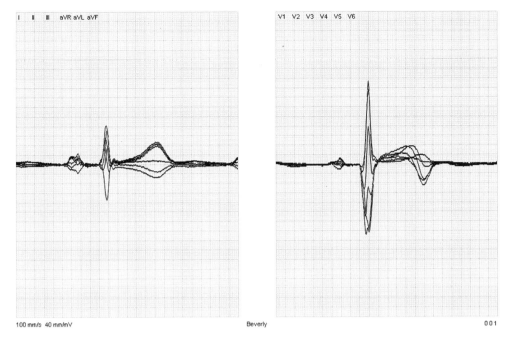

Fig. 3. Superimposition of median complexes formed from 12-lead ECG. Limb leads at left, chest leads at right.

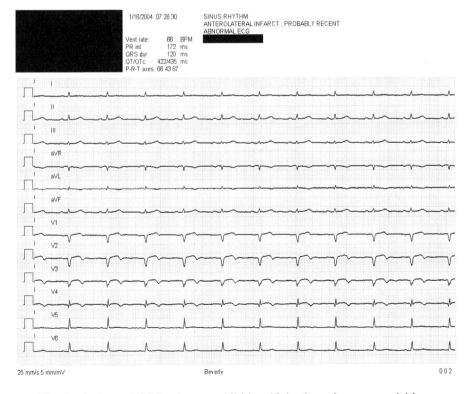

Fig. 4. 12-channel ECG printout exhibiting 12-lead continuous acquisition.

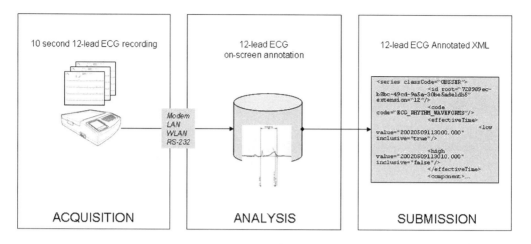

Fig. 5. Process flow for 12-lead electrocardiograph acquisition, analysis, and submission.

12-LEAD ECG ACQUISITION TECHNOLOGIES

Traditional 12-lead ECG data collection is obtained with resting electrocardiographs. However, as data collection requirements become more intensive alternative data acquisition technologies have emerged as important components in 12-lead ECG data collection.

Resting Electrocardiograph

The resting electrocardiograph typically records a 10 s "snapshot" of the 12-lead ECG. This snapshot is output on paper and in some models can be stored digitally within the electrocardiograph memory.

Depending on the electrocardiograph model, the 12-lead recording can be simultaneous or sequenced. Sequenced recordings do not capture simultaneous data in all 12-leads. Historically, this was linked to the number of writer "channels" available to couple the analog signal to the paper output. With only one writer channel, it was possible to record to paper only a single lead at a time. The different leads were then recorded by switching through the different leads recorded on the single channel. Today, the majority of digital electrocardiographs capture 12-lead simultaneous data. The simultaneous lead recordings provide greater information content and allow for a complete view of all leads over the entire 10 s recording.

"Interpretive" electrocardiographs will also generate an automatic interpretation of the 10 s record. This automatic interpretation is generally presented in two parts: (1) global measurements and (2) interpretive statements. Global measurements consist of PR, QRS, QT intervals, ventricular rate, and P-QRS-T axis. The interpretative statements are text statements (e.g., NORMAL SINUS RHYTHM) derived from the automatic measurements obtained by the analysis algorithm.

The typical process flow associated with a digital 12-lead ECG record is shown in Fig. 5. After the acquisition of one or more digital 12-lead ECG records, the records can be transmitted in a variety of ways for subsequent analysis and review. Transport mediums supported by some electrocardiographs include modem, LAN, WLAN, and serial data transfer. Digital data is typically transferred from the collection site to a centralized laboratory with 26 CFR Part 11 compliant data management and analysis tools to process the 12-lead digital data. These tools enable the onscreen measurement and annotation of the digital ECG data and can be used to export the resulting aECG XML file.

Holter Recording

For historical reasons, Holter is generally thought of as limited to two or three bi-polar channels. In 1994, with the introduction of the H-12 Holter recorder (Mortara Instrument, Inc., Milwaukee, WI) this limitation was no longer true. Both the Holter recorder and its subsequent version H12+ provided full 12-lead digital ECG recording capabilities with leads acquired in the same manner as a resting electrocardiograph. With these devices it became possible to record continuous 12-lead digital data for 24 h.

In the case of 12-lead Holter, the limb lead placement is slightly modified from that of the traditional resting ECG. A Mason-Likar placement, also utilized in stress exercise testing, is used with 12-lead Holter technology. The Mason-Likar placement locates the limb leads on the torso at appropriate locations to minimize artifact associated with ambulatory movement *(8)*.

With the 12-lead Holter technology, continuous digital data is recorded to a removable memory card. The removable card is subsequently analyzed within a Holter scanning system that allows for creation of both a Holter arrhythmia report and selection of discrete 12-lead periods for subsequent interval duration and/or amplitude measurements. The advantage of the continuous 12-lead digital record, when contrasted with the discrete 12-lead resting ECC, is that it provides the ability to retrospectively select any time segment for analysis during a dosing period.

Figure 6 outlines a generalized process flow for 12-lead Holter data. Contrasted with Fig. 5, the 12-lead Holter recording differs in that the continuous digital data is recorded to a removable memory card that is subsequently analyzed in lieu of transmission directly from the acquisition device. It is also important to note that the 12-lead Holter recorder, unlike the 12-lead electrocardiograph, does not produce a paper record output at the collection site. After acquisition of the continuous data, a complete Holter arrhythmia report can be generated and the appropriate 12-lead segments selected for review. Subsequent analysis of these 12-lead segments can be performed with onscreen caliper tools to generate the aECG XML files.

Telemetry

Alternate modes for 12-lead digital data collection also exist. In particular, 12-lead telemetry technology could be used for future data collection in clinical trials. The telemetry use model would be similar in to that of 12-lead Holter where a continuous record would be obtained.

Telemetry, much like Holter, is traditionally thought of as being limited to a few leads. However, with the X-12 digital transmitter it is possible to obtain continuous transmission of the 12-lead ECG. This technology, coupled with potential future developments, could be leveraged to the advantage of ECG data collection for clinical trials.

In lieu of recording the data to a removable memory card, the 12-lead digital data would be transmitted to a central monitoring station and stored. Subsequent analyses would follow a similar path as the Holter use model discussed previously.

12-LEAD ELECTROCARDIOGRAPH SIGNAL PROCESSING

With the acquisition of digital ECG data, digital signal processing follows naturally. Digital signal processing includes both ECG filters and the possible automatic processing of measurements utilizing ECG algorithms. Specific implementation of the signal processing depends upon a given device model, but some general observations are included in the following sections.

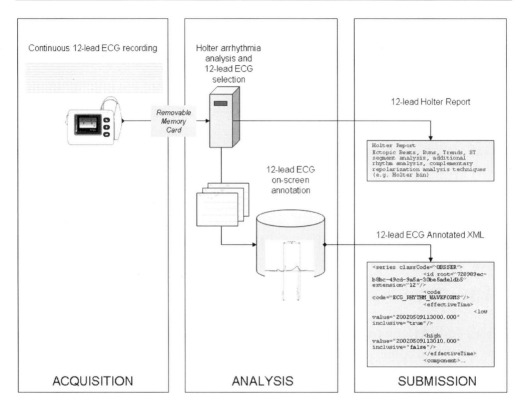

Fig. 6. Process flow for 12-lead Holter acquisition, analysis, and submission.

Digital ECG Filters

Digital ECG filters are applied to reduce noise associated with different sources. The three basic sources of noise that impact the ECG, include AC noise due to mains power, baseline wander due to high impedance between electrodes, and skin and muscle noise due to noncardiac muscle signals. In general, since digital filters can impact the underlying ECG signal, it is important to understand the nature of these filters in order to ensure the fidelity of the collected data.

AC Filters

AC filter technology is focused on elimination of noise arising from nearby or connected mains sources. AC filters are designed to operate at the appropriate line frequency that is either 50 Hz or 60 Hz. An example of an ECG with AC noise is illustrated in Fig. 7. AC noise is characterized by sharp, or fast rising, periodic noise most easily visible in the baseline of the ECG. The primary challenge for AC filters is to successfully dampen the periodic signal arising from line interference, while minimizing any impact on portions of the true ECG signal that have similar frequency content. This is particularly true in the QRS complex portion of the ECG.

Although the AC noise is present throughout the recording, it is most visible in the baseline of the ECG and difficult to *see* in the R wave itself. Distinguishing signal from noise in the QRS is both visually and hence computationally more challenging. Application of simple Fourier Transform techniques (FFT), which can easily identify power

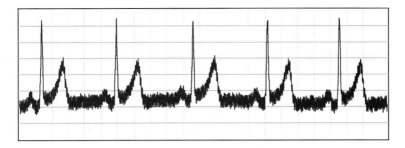

Fig. 7. ECG signal with typical AC noise.

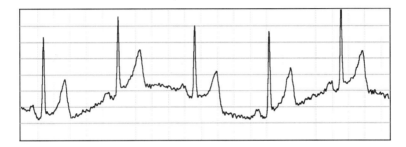

Fig. 8. ECG signal with typical baseline wander.

peaks at 50 or 60 Hz for removal, will inevitably diminish the amplitude of the true QRS signal that has nonzero power at those frequencies.

For this reason, robust AC filters for digital ECGs require an adaptive technique that takes into account the rapid change associated with the true ECG signal, and limits the magnitude of the sinusoidal AC cancellation in the presence of these rapid changes *(9)*. Implemented properly, AC filters can effectively remove line noise without compromising the true underlying ECG signal.

Baseline Filters

Baseline filters, also known as high pass filters, are used to reduce baseline wander as shown in Fig. 8. The basic challenge for baseline filters is to continuously properly estimate the isoelectric baseline of the ECG. There are several different implementations of these filters, some of which can have a potentially negative impact on the low-frequency component of the ECG.

Diagnostic electrocardiograph requirements state that the low frequency response of the ECG should range down to 0.05 Hz or meet the impulse response requirements outlined in the standard *(10)*. On some electrocardiograph devices it is possible to apply more aggressive filters that result in the reduction of this low frequency response. This is indicated on the ECG printout and is typically stated as a frequency response range, for example, 0.2 Hz to 150 Hz. Anytime an ECG states a low-frequency response range that does not extend down to 0.05 Hz, it is not to be considered a diagnostic ECG. Such nondiagnostic filters have a problematic effect in transition areas between low- and high-frequency components of the ECG. This is particularly true with the ST segment, where such filters can result in false episodes of ST segment depression (in the case of a positive QRS) or reduction of overall sensitivity to ST segment elevation.

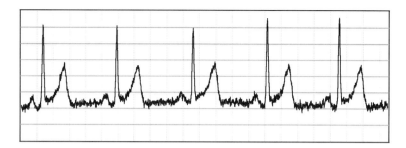

Fig. 9. ECG signal with typical muscle noise.

A particular class of baseline filters that are not easily characterized in terms of frequency response, utilize a "spline" technique to remove baseline wander. This approach relies on the proper identification of isoelectric points on the ECG waveform and the subsequent splining (cubic or otherwise) of these points to remove baseline wander. Such techniques should be avoided since they rely on the perfect identification of isoelectric points on the ECG, firstly in terms of algorithmic location and secondarily that these perfectly identified points are always physiologically isoelectric.[e] Failure in either sense can result in distortion of the isoelectric line that can significantly impact any analysis that depends upon absolute amplitude measurements or threshold crossing.

In lieu of a "spline" approach, it is preferable to use baseline filter approaches that are not built upon the assumptions discussed previously. More advanced digital filters that involve the use of a zero-phase FIR digital filter, can be designed to meet the normative standards for impulse response. Such a FIR filter results in substantially improved baseline stability compared with single pole filters without compromise of the underlying ECG signal response.

Muscle Filters

Muscle filters, also known as low pass filters, are used to remove noncardiac muscle noise from the ECG signal. These filters typically impact the upper range of the ECG frequency response. An example of muscle noise is shown in Fig. 9. Typical settings for muscle filters ranging from most sensitive to most aggressive include 300 Hz, 150 Hz, and 40 Hz. In some electrocardiographs these filters are applied to the printed output and not on the original digital signal that is saved and ultimately transmitted for further analysis. Thorough understanding of the device used to collect the data is required to understand what, if any, effect the muscle filter has on the underlying digital data.

Alternative approaches to muscle filters, based on the redundancy of information provided by the 12-lead ECG, have been developed (11). These approaches filter the ECG signal based on the notion of signal source consistency that can be established based on the redundancy of ECG leads. This type of filter has the advantage that it can achieve significant noise reduction in the 12-lead ECG without, as is the case with a standard 40 Hz filter, reducing true ECG signal components that are present above 40 Hz in the frequency spectrum.

---

[e]For example, a spline technique may assume that the segment preceding the QRS onset is isoelectric. In the presence of a premature QRS, this may not be the case.

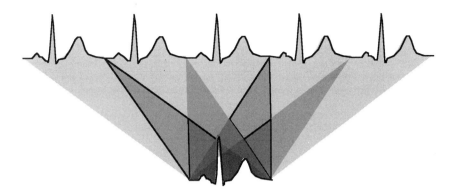

Fig. 10. Schematic illustration of formation of "median" beat.

Digital ECG Algorithms

ECG algorithms provide the capability to automatically analyze the ECG signal to provide a multitude of outputs, including morphology, interval duration measurements, and rhythm analyses. In the case of a resting ECG interpretation algorithm, automatic measurements are accompanied by diagnostic statements that can provide a silent second opinion for evaluation by a clinician.

Median Beats

Typically, interpretation algorithms perform their analyses on what are called "median" beats that are constructed from the acquired rhythm ECG data. Although the term "median" is often used, it would perhaps be better to use a more generic term such as "representative cycle." The construction of median beats for the ECG is not unambiguously defined, and in fact different algorithms utilize different techniques to do so. Hence, in the following text the term median beat is utilized, but it should be understood as a "median beat" with the previous caveats attached.

In ECG signal processing, median beats are utilized to minimize the impact of noise present in any given single beat. Multiple measurements can be determined utilizing the median beats including the P, QRS, and QT duration. Median beat formation involves the identification of a "primary" beat type within a sequence of beats. This categorization identifies beats that are to be included in the median or average beat formation. Beats that are not considered part of the "primary" class are not included in the formation of the median. In applying these criteria, beats such as occasional premature ventricular complexes are excluded from the median beat formation. Following selection of beats, the beats are aligned and combined to form the median beat. These remarks are generally true for established ECG algorithms and are illustrated in Fig. 10 for a single lead. Moving into discussions of specific measurement techniques requires reference to a specific platform. The comments that follow are therefore specifically relevant to the Mortara Instrument algorithm.

Global Measurements

With the median beats constructed, a series of "global" measurements can be obtained. These measurements are global in the sense that they are not lead specific, but rather span the 12-lead simultaneous data.

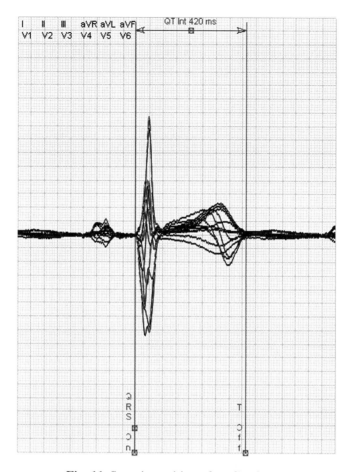

Fig. 11. Superimposition of *median* beats.

In the case of the P, QRS, and QT duration, the Mortara Instrument algorithm determines onsets and offsets by reference to a composite measure of electrical activity, reflecting the total activity across all leads formed from the independent median beats. In the particular case of the QT interval, this results in an interval defined by the earliest ventricular depolarization activity and the latest "end-of-T," considering all leads.

One way in which to visualize the earliest onset of ventricular depolarization and latest offset of repolarization concept is to display the digital medians overlaid upon each other. In Fig.11, the limb lead and precordial lead medians from Fig. 4 are shown superposed. The common moment of earliest depolarization and latest repolarization, as determined by the algorithm looking at all independent leads, is indicated by the vertical lines.

An alternate means to visualize this global activity is to utilize the digital medians to construct a single median reflective of the total electrical activity.^{f} This complex is constructed utilizing all independent leads to create an orthogonal basis and resulting

---

^{f}TEA is a trademark of Mortara Instrument.

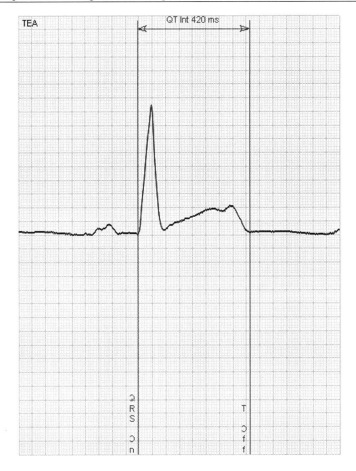

Fig. 12. TEA composite measure.

vector magnitude. An example of this complex is shown in Fig. 12 complete with the automatic algorithm onset and offset determinations.

Compared with Fig. 11, the total electrical activity visualization has the benefit that a single complex can be evaluated in lieu of the 12 superimposed complexes, and hence provides a more clear indication of global onset and offset of cardiac activity. However, it does have the disadvantage that it is constructed from all leads, and hence does not resemble a typical single lead that a reviewer may be accustomed to analyzing. Furthermore, when assessing the accuracy of automatic interval determination by algorithms that produce a global interval duration measurement, the use of the total electrical activity can often provide a clearer visualization of what the automatic algorithm evaluates. This, in turn, provides reviewers with an easier means to evaluate the accuracy of such automatic algorithm determinations.

QT Measurement: Automatic vs Manual

A complete discussion of the subject of automatic or algorithmic versus manual measurements of the QT interval is beyond the scope of this chapter. However, some important technical remarks regarding the expected differences between these techniques and the relevant applicability of both methodologies follows.

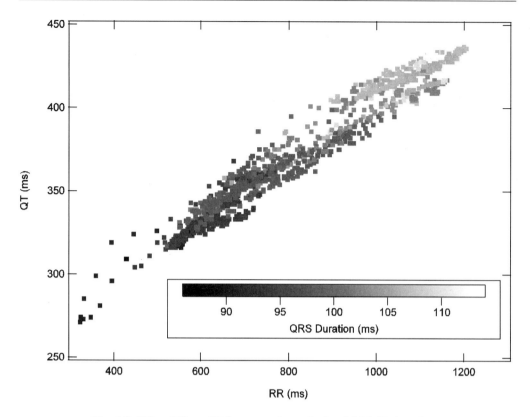

Fig. 13. QT vs RR vs QRS automatic analysis of 24-h Holter data.

Comparison of global automatic measurements with manual measurements performed in a single lead can result in the observation that global absolute QT measurements are longer than individual lead measurements. The "global QT" is naturally longer (statistically) than the QT measured in a single lead, due to the impact of isoelectric onsets/offsets in a single lead measurement. Moreover, in the presence of QT interval increases within a single individual's ECG, concomitant axis shifts of the T wave may cause the full extent of the QT increase to be more accurately recorded by the global QT measure. This could result in greater sensitivity to QT changes utilizing an algorithmically measured global QT versus that of a manual measurement in a single lead.

The applicability and appeal of automatic measurements are most evident in the analysis of large data sets that could include hundreds or thousands of measurement points for a single subject. Such analysis is especially true of data coming from continuous Holter studies. The automation provided by algorithmic approaches enables the analysis of such data in a practical sense. The results of such analysis can be used to investigate QT/RR relationships over 24 h which in turn can provide input into individualized correction factors, repolarization reserve, or utilization of the so called "Holter bin" method for QT analysis. Fig. 13 demonstrates the potential power of automatic measurements where Holter data from a 24-h recording has been automatically analyzed to reveal a multiparameter relationship of QT, RR, and QRS duration.

CONCLUSION

As the number of digital ECGs collected in clinical trials increases, it will become increasingly important that a broader audience within the clinical research community grasps the relevant issues surrounding high-fidelity ECG acquisition. The volume of digital data and subsequent analysis is fundamentally built upon the initial data acquisition and digital processing. Whether the ECGs are acquired by resting electrocardiograph, Holter, or other means, it is essential that the devices and the settings used are well understood by sponsors and core laboratories. This will enable the collection of a robust ECG data set that in turn can be analyzed with a host of tools based on manual, automatic, or combined methods.

REFERENCES

1. Einthoven W. Ueber die Form des menschlichen. Electrocardiogramms. Arch f d Ges Physiol 1895;60:101–123.
2. Fisch C. Centennial of the String Galvanometer and the Electrocardiogram. JACC 2000; 36:1737–1745.
3. Bjerregaard P, Gussak I. Naming of the waves in the ECG with a brief account of their genesis. Comments. Circulation 1998;98:1937–1942.
4. Wilson NF, Johnston FE, Macleod AG, Barker PS. Electrocardiograms that represent the potential variations of a single electrode. Am Heart J 1934;9:447–458.
5. Barnes AR, Pardee HEB, White PD, et al. Standardization of precordial leads. Am Heart J 1938;15: 235–239.
6. ANSI/AAMI EC-11-1991 Standard.
7. [Federal Register: October 24, 2001 (Volume 66, Number 206)], Department of Health and Human Services, Food and Drug Administration, [Docket No. 01N-0476], Electronic Interchange Standard for Digital ECG and Similar Data; Public Meeting
8. Sarapa N, Morganroth J, et. al. Electrocardiographic indentification of drug-induced QT prolongation: assessment by different recording and measurement methods. ANE 2004;9:48–57.
9. Mortara, D. AC filters for ECG, conference proceedings, Computers in Cardiology 1976.
10. ANSI/AAMI EC-11-1991 Standard, section 3.2.5.2.
11. Mortara D. Source consistency filtering, application to resting ECGs. J Elect 25:200–206.

8

Digital 12-Lead Holter vs Standard Resting Supine Electrocardiogram for the Assessment of Drug-Induced QTc Prolongation

Assessment by Different Recording and Measurement Methods

Nenad Sarapa, MD

CONTENTS

INTRODUCTION

Ever since it was introduced in routine clinical cardiology practice *(1)*, the continuous ambulatory electrocardiogram (Holter ECG) has been routinely used for diagnostic assessment of patients with different types of heart disease like cardiac arrhythmias, transient ischemic episodes and silent myocardial ischemia. The incidence of cardiac arrhythmia and myocardial ischemia, as well as the assessment of heart rate variability on Holter ECG acquired continuously over 24 h or longer have been useful for predicting clinical disease outcomes *(2–5)*. Likewise, Holter ECG is often used in clinical drug research for the monitoring of general cardiac safety of novel drugs under development, particularly during the early phase I trials. In contrast, Holter ECG has only rarely been used in drug development for the formal assessment of drug-induced effects on cardiac

From: *Cardiac Safety of Noncardiac Drugs:*
Practical Guidelines for Clinical Research and Drug Development
Edited by: J. Morganroth and I. Gussak © Humana Press Inc., Totowa, NJ

repolarization, and the experience of central ECG laboratories in measuring ECG intervals on Holter is limited. Pharmaceutical sponsors and patients alike would benefit if reliable QT/QTc assessment were possible by Holter ECG, whereby the continuous ambulatory digital 12-lead ECG would be used to substitute for standard resting supine 12-lead ECGs in the assessment of drug-induced QT/QTc prolongation.

DISCUSSION

The risk of drug-induced QT/QTc prolongation, potentially causing malignant polymorphic ventricular tachycardia Torsades de Pointes (TdP), has had significant implications for drug development in the last decade. Regulatory authorities require that the effect of novel drugs on cardiac repolarization be thoroughly investigated as early as practically possible in clinical trials (6). Regulatory actions consistently indicate that even small degrees of drug-induced QT prolongation relative to placebo will raise safety concerns, necessitating that favorable risk–benefit ratio be demonstrated before marketing approval is granted. Several efficacious non-antiarrhythmic drugs shown to cause QT prolongation have been removed from the market (e.g., terfenadine, astemizole, cisapride, grepafloxacin, and sertindole) (7–10). Using a reliable and fully effective method of ECG acquisition, as well as a precise method of QT and RR interval measurement, is therefore critical for detection of small but potentially clinically significant drug-induced QT prolongation. Inadequate acquisition or inaccurate measurement of ECG data may lead to approval of a drug with unacceptable risk–benefit ratio, or to inappropriate discontinuation of a promising drug during development (11–14).

In the seminal regulatory document on the assessment of the risk from QT interval prolongation induced by noncardiovascular drugs from 1997, the European Committee for Proprietary Medicinal Products (CPMP) has requested that ECGs be recorded frequently over extended periods of time at baseline and on drug treatment to determine the mean and maximum change from baseline, peak amplitude, and time course of drug-induced QTc prolongation (15). The timing of QT measurements should coincide with the maximum expected peak plasma concentration of the active substance and its most significant metabolites. In addition, the ECG measurements should be done before as well as after the occurrence of peak concentrations in plasma. All of these requirements are still present in the most recent regulatory concepts from 2004 (6). Drug regulatory bodies universally accept the use of discrete resting ECGs for the assessment of risk from cardiac arrhythmia, but it appears that this methodology has reached the limit of its information value for adequate and complete assessment of drug effects on cardiac repolarization. Serial discrete 10-s recordings of resting supine 12-lead ECGs at a limited number of times give only a static picture that does not reflect the dynamic changes in QT/QTc interval duration and its true relationship to heart rate. Even the improved precision and reproducibility of QT interval measurement on discrete resting ECG would only address the methodological variation, and would not alleviate the issues around the high biological variability of the QT/QTc interval. Cardiac repolarization involves a complex interplay between heart rate and the autonomic nervous system, so the relationship between the absolute values of QT and RR interval evaluated by linear regression analysis must be determined from many QT/RR data points obtained on long-term ECG tracings. If this approach is to correctly address the adaptation of the QT interval duration in response to the variations in heart rate, ECG tracings must be recorded continuously over long-term periods and not only as standard resting supine ECG (16,17). Moreover, frequent serial resting supine ECGs can only be recorded in subjects hospitalized in specially equipped phase I clinics for prolonged periods of time *(8,18)*. Such phase I trials invariably enroll only healthy volunteers and not patients with the target indication for the drug under development, phase I trials also include too few subjects to fulfill the regulatory requirements for thorough QT/QTc assessment. Another issue is using complex standard ECG schedules in patients with certain diseases associated with poor mobility of other disability (e.g., cancer, rheumatoid arthritis, osteoarthritis, Parkinson's and Alzheimer's disease). These patients would find it very difficult or even impossible to comply with lengthy hospitalizations or frequent outpatient visits. The continuous 12-lead digital Holter ECG allows collection of data continuously over extended periods of time to ensure detection of peak QT/QTc effects of the drug. Unlike resting supine ECGs that can only be collected at pre-scheduled time points, Holter ECG ensures availability of QT/QTc and RR interval data at times of potentially critical drug activity even if these are unknown beforehand (e.g., before pharmacokinetics or dose–concentration–response in humans are characterized). This ensures that drug effects on cardiac repolarization can be evaluated at the time of maximal concentration of the parent drug (or its active metabolite, if any) in plasma and/or at the time of maximal effect. Thus, continuous Holter ECG recording should prove useful for the assessment of cardiac repolarization at numerous discrete time points following drug administration in clinical drug trials. In addition, novel methods of data analysis applied on continuous Holter ECG may provide better insight into drug-induced effect on cardiac repolarization than the conventional measurement of QT interval duration.

Thus, the clinical trial sponsors and patients participating in them alike would benefit if reliable QTc assessment were possible by an ambulatory ECG acquisition that requires no hospitalization and a minimal number of outpatient visits. Despite intuitive notion that digital 12-lead Holter ECG could be used instead of standard resting supine ECGs in the assessment of drug-induced QTc prolongation, Holter is still very infrequently used for QT/QTc assessment in clinical trials. Drug regulators have only recently started reviewing Holter data in the context of the potential of a novel drug to cause QT/QTc prolongation. Most likely prompted by technical deficiency of the two- or three-channel Holter recorders available at the time, the CPMP stated in 1997 that Holter ECG do not sufficiently correlate with those from standard resting ECGs to be of value in QTc assessment *(15)*. Different commercially available Holter recorders may not be equally useful for the assessment of cardiac repolarization. Good quality recording at a sufficiently high sampling rate (preferably 500 Hz or above) with T-wave amplitude ideally above 0.25 mV in the lead chosen for QT measurement, as well as the availability of an interactive QT measurement software that allows verification and editing by an experienced human operator are the most important technical prerequisites for accurate QT analysis from continuous Holter ECG recordings. Since 1997, significant technological advances have enabled digital Holter devices to continuously capture 12-lead ECGs with greater precision and reproducibility. Modern digital Holter recorders that simultaneously capture 12-lead tracings are superior to two- or three-channel Holter recorders for a reliable assessment of cardiac repolarization *(19)*.

At their meeting on May 29, 2003, the FDA Cardiovascular and Renal Drugs Advisory Committee endorsed the study that utilized the digital 12-lead Holter WinAtrec *RR bin* approach for the definitive assessment of QT prolongation by alfuzosin (UroXatral®, Sanofi-Synthelabo); the drug was subsequently approved for marketing with the Holter-derived QTc data inserted into the label. At present, the draft ICH E14 guidance on the clinical evaluation of QT/QTc prolongation *(6)* does not yet include formal endorsement of Holter ECG for QT/QTc assessment in drug development. On the other hand, the reference to Holter ECG in Section 2.2.3 (p. 9) of the draft guidance *(6)* is encouraging by stating that "... newer systems that allow for the collection of multiple leads that more closely approximate a surface ECG have potential value to collect interval data. The use of Holter monitors might additionally allow detection of extreme QT/QTc interval events that occur infrequently during the day and asymptomatic arrhythmias. Data on the QT/RR from Holter monitoring can also prove useful in the calculation of individualized QT corrections." Somewhat disappointingly, this section of the guidance finished by stating that "However, as QT/QTc intervals measured by Holter methodology might not correspond quantitatively to those for standard surface ECGs, data obtained from the two methodologies might not be suitable for direct comparison or pooling."

It has been suggested that lengthening of the QT interval is not a sufficient criterion for the development of drug-induced TdP *(20)*. Not all drugs that have been linked with TdP cause significant QT prolongation and, in addition, accurate measurement of QT interval is confounded by a number of difficulties. The development of abnormal U waves, probably representing the summation of early afterdepolarizations, may be involved in the genesis of TdP. With the advent and wider adoption of digital ECGs, a spectrum of new electrocardiographic parameters will likely be added to the QT interval and heart rate in the assessment of cardiac repolarization. Quantitative computerized processing and analysis of digital ECGs will include QT/U intervals, QT/RR relationships, T-wave morphology, spatial heterogeneity of repolarization, and dynamic beat-to-beat T-wave changes (T-wave lability and microvolt T-wave alternans) *(11)*. These measurements are likely to supplement and some day possibly even replace the conventional QT and RR interval measurement of today. Such new digital techniques may identify drug-induced adverse repolarization effects more accurately and reliably than current methods, thus improving the safety screening of drug candidates in clinical development *(11)*. Clinical drug research aims to achieve high statistical power in the assessment of cardiac repolarization without the need to enroll unreasonably high number of subjects, so the collection and analysis of ECG data must be performed in a cost-effective manner. With digital 12-lead Holter, large number of ECG data can be collected over 24 h at a cost equal to recording five serial resting supine ECGs over the same time frame, and novel data analyses might increase the statistical power of detecting a drug effect on cardiac repolarization by means of averaging QT and RR data across defined time periods ("epochs" or "bins"). Beat-to-beat QT interval variability (QT dynamics) has been proposed as another novel and potentially useful noninvasive index of ventricular repolarization lability. Several reports have linked QT dynamics to cardiac disease outcome and sudden death *(2–5,21,22)*. Beat-to-beat QT variability is influenced by even the short transitory changes in sleep/wake state, posture, physical activity, or psychological stress *(23,24)*. In addition, QT interval exhibits a circadian rhythm with prolongation at nighttime that is mostly due to the lower heart rate. More recently, 24-h Holter monitoring has revealed a heart rate independent diurnal variation contributing to circadian QT/QTc oscillations *(25,26)*. It is well known that when the RR interval changes, the adaptation of the QT interval to such changes in heart rate is delayed (QT lag) for up to 2–3 min *(27)*. The QT adaptation is different whether the RR interval is accelerated or decelerated (QT hysteresis) *(28,29)*. Because QT dynamics is so sensitive to diverse changes in autonomic tone and heart rate, it is paramount for a meaningful interpretation that cardiac repolarization is assessed on ECG tracings acquired continuously over longer periods of time.

Modern digital Holter ECG equipment has made it possible to perform beat-to-beat QT/RR interval measurements on long-term ECG recordings by automated software, usually preceded by human review of the tracings (17,30,31). Acceptable short-term reproducibility of the automated Holter QT analysis has been demonstrated, albeit thus far only with two- or three-channel Holter recorders (17,31–34). The QT measurements in narrow heart rate windows ("bins") showed the best reproducibility (34).

ELECTROCARDIOGRAPHIC IDENTIFICATION OF DRUG-INDUCED QT PROLONGATION: ASSESSMENT BY DIFFERENT RECORDING AND MEASUREMENT METHODS

The current strict regulatory requirements for thorough pre-approval characterization of the proarrhythmic potential of drug candidates warrant search for new better methods of ECG acquisition and measurement. It is critically important in this context that the comparative value of different ECG acquisition and interval measurement methods be determined. To this end, Pfizer and its academic collaborators have compared the precision of QT and RR interval measurement by manual digitized methods (digitizing board and digital onscreen calipers) when applied on paper and onscreen digital 12-lead ECGs recorded by standard resting or continuous ambulatory Holter method.

To our knowledge, this was the first study to compare the standard 12-lead ECGs to discrete ECGs derived from continuous digital 12-lead Holter recorder for their utility in the assessment of drug-induced changes in QT/QTc and RR intervals, measured on a very large number of serial ECGs (1600 simultaneously recorded pairs). It is also the first study to compare the precision of QT/QTc and RR interval measurement by the two most relevant manual digitized methods (digipad and onscreen calipers). The results from this study were published elsewhere (35) and are reiterated here to illustrate the valuable potential of using digital 12-lead Holter in the assessment of drug-induced cardiac repolarization.

METHODS

Study Design

This open-label, nonrandomized study included a fixed treatment sequence administered on three successive days: 24-h baseline (d –1), a single 160 mg dose of sotalol (Betapace® 80 mg tablets, Berlex Laboratories, Montville, NY) (d 1) and a single 320 mg dose of sotalol (d 2). The study was conducted in Pfizer's Phase I clinic in Kalamazoo, MI. All subjects gave written informed consent to the study protocol approved by an independent institutional review board.

Electrocardiogram Recordings

Standard digital 12-lead ECGs were recorded for 10 s after 5 min supine rest (ELI-200 from Mortara Instrument, Milwaukee, WI; 10-by-2 rhythm strip format, paper speed 25 mm/s, amplitude 1 mV/10 mm). The recordings were acquired with a sampling frequency of 500 Hz (2 ms resolution) and with a 16-bit amplitude (2.5 μV) resolution. Sixteen standard ECGs were recorded at identical times on d 1 and 2 (immediately pre-dose and at 1, 1.5, 2, 2.5, 3, 3.5, 4, 4.5, 5, 6, 8, 10, 13, 16, and 22.5 h after dosing) and at corresponding clock times at baseline (d –1). Digital 12-lead Holter ECGs were recorded continuously for

22.5 h on d –1, 1, and 2 (H12 Recorder from Mortara Instrument). Holter recordings were sampled at 180 Hz (5.6 ms resolution) and with a 16-bit amplitude (2.5 μV) resolution. They were time-stamped simultaneously with the start of each standard ECG. Sixteen discrete 12-lead ECG digital files per study day were derived from Holter to the H-Scribe analysis system and printed out (10-s rhythm strip, paper speed 25mm/s, amplitude 1 mV/10 mm) at the time points coinciding with standard ECGs. Holter and standard ECGs were recorded from the same location on each subject by dual snap electrodes (Nikomed U.S.A., Inc. #4500, Doylestown, PA) utilized for precordial leads. Single snap electrodes (Nikomed U.S.A. Inc. #4520) were utilized for limb leads. All study equipment was validated and recently serviced and calibrated.

QT and RR Interval Measurement Systems

Two manual ECG interval measurement systems were used: first, a digitizing board (*digipad*, eResearchTechnology Inc., Philadelphia, PA) with magnification of the paper ECG coupled with digitization software, whereby point-to-point determination of onset and offset points was made by two trained analysts *(36);* second, an electronic caliper system (CalECG Software v1.0, AMPS, LLC, New York, NY) applied on a computer screen to digital ECG files from the standard ECG recorder by the same trained analysts. At the time of the study, the onscreen calipers could not be directly applied to the source digital ECG files from H12 Holter recorder, so the 16 Holter-derived paper ECG print-outs were scanned into a portable network graphics file at 300 dpi and calipers were applied to the scanned image. The RR and QT interval measurements by both manual methods were an average of three consecutive sinus rhythm beats. QT intervals were corrected for heart rate using Fridericia's (cube root) correction (QTcF).

The repeatability of the digipad method was examined to support its use as a standard for pairwise comparisons between measurement methods. The inter- and intra-observer variability in digipad measurements was tested by repeating the initial digipad analysis (ED-1) twice within 5 and 6 mo (ED-2 and ED-3, respectively) on all standard ECGs by the same two analysts. In ED-2, all ECGs were randomized between the two analysts. In ED-3, all ECGs from the same subject were read by one analyst (50% by the same analyst from ED-1 and 50% by the other).

Statistical Analysis

Primary statistical comparisons were made for manual measurements of QT, QTcF, and RR intervals in limb lead II of the standard and Holter-derived 12-lead ECGs. Statistical comparisons measurements made in precordial lead V5 produced similar results and are not presented. Measurement methods were compared in a pairwise fashion, whereby digipad was the reference for all comparisons. Descriptive statistics and Bland-Altman plots *(37)* were used to compare methods, incorporating results for absolute QT/QTcF interval values and QT/QTcF changes from baseline from all subjects. Baseline was the average of all 16 ECGs obtained on d –1. It is recognized that these do not represent independent data points, but support the primary objective of comparing ECG acquisition and measurement methods across a wide range of QT intervals.

RESULTS

Subject Disposition and Electrocardiogram Acquisition

Thirty-nine healthy adult volunteers (11 females) aged 18–45 yr (mean: 27 yr), weighing 47–108 kg (mean: 74 kg) with a body mass index of 18.2–30.8 kg/m^2 (mean: 24.4 kg/m^2)

were evaluated. There were 33 Caucasians, 2 African-Americans, and 4 with unspecified race. All subjects received the 160 mg dose of sotalol and 22 of them (all males) also received the 320 mg dose.

A total of 3200 ECG tracings were obtained from standard ELI200 and H12 Holter recorders (22 subjects × 48 ECGs + 17 subjects × 32 ECGs = 1600 per acquisition method). ECG results based on digipad measurements on standard ECGs are presented in Table 1.

Reproducibility of the Digipad Measurement Method

Table 2 presents the agreement between the for QT, QTcF, and RR intervals produced by the initial digipad measurement, and the two repeated measurements performed by the same two analysts in limb lead II of all 1600 standard ECGs, 5 and 6 mo apart.

Comparability of Electrocardiogram Recording and Measurement Methods

Table 3 presents the pairwise comparisons between QT, QTcF, and RR interval measurement methods on simultaneously recorded standard and Holter-derived 12-lead ECGs. Agreement between selected pairwise comparisons is depicted by Bland–Altman plots in Fig. 1. The mean difference indicates the lack of agreement between the compared methods *(37)*, whereas the degree of variation about the mean difference is described by the range of ±2 standard deviations, expected to include 95% of differences in individual pairwise comparisons.

Outlier Analysis for QT Change From Baseline

Table 4 presents the outlier analysis, i.e., the classification of individual QTcF changes from baseline determined by each measurement method on standard and Holter-derived ECGs. Considering the initial digipad QT measurements on 1600 standard ECGs obtained on d −1 to 2 (ED-1), the absolute QTcF change from baseline of 30–60, 61–90, and >90 ms was observed in 36.3, 9.1, and 0.2% of all ECGs, respectively. Considering the initial digipad measurements on day 1 ECGs, a change from baseline in QTc interval corrected by Fridericia's formula of 30–60, 61–90, and > 90 ms was observed in 41.0, 12.4, and 0% of ECGs in women, and in 35.3, 8.4, and 0.3% of ECGs in men.

Comparability of Methods for Detecting QT and RR Change From Baseline Over Time

Figure 2 presents the mean changes from baseline in QT, QTcF, and RR intervals after dosing with sotalol on d 1 and 2, as detected by each measurement method on standard and Holter-derived ECGs.

DISCUSSION

The high-resolution digitizing board is the standard approach for manual QT interval measurement on paper ECG *(36,38)*, although automated measurements by the standard ECG recorder's computer algorithm are also commonly used. The U.S. Food and Drug Administration and Health Canada jointly proposed that for new drug approvals, digital ECGs should be obtained with annotation of the onset and offset of the prolonged QT intervals *(39)*. Digital onscreen calipers would be the method of choice for manual QT interval measurement on digital ECGs.

Table 1
ECG Results by Study Day Based on Digipad Measurements (ED-1) in Limb Lead II of Standard ECG

	Day −1 mean (range)			Day 1 mean (range)			Day 2 mean (range)
	All subjects (n = 39)	Males (n = 28)	Females (n = 11)	All subjects (n = 39)	Males (n = 28)	Females (n = 11)	All subjects* (n = 22)
RR (ms)	910.7 (737 to 1088)	934.2 (744 to 1088)	850.8 (737 to 1004)	1030.6 (843 to 1176)	1055.8 (876 to 1176)	966.4 (843 to 1103)	1090.1 (945 to 1233)
HR (bpm)	67.2 (56 to 82)	65.4 (56 to 81)	71.7 (60 to 82)	59.5 (51 to 72)	57.9 (51 to 69)	63.4 (55 to 72)	55.8 (49 to 64)
QT (ms)	355.9 (318 to 395)	354.7 (318 to 395)	359.0 (337 to 386)	393.6 (357 to 432)	388.3 (357 to 424)	407.3 (378 to 432)	412.9 (379 to 446)
QTcF (ms)	368.1 (343 to 402)	363.6 (343 to 293)	379.7 (358 to 402)	390.8 (362 to 431)	382.1 (362 to 407)	412.9 (386 to 431)	401.9 (374 to 430)
ΔRR (ms)	N/A	N/A	N/A	119.9 (6 to 229)	121.6 (25 to 203)	115.6 (6 to 229)	164.5 (61 to 254)
ΔHR (bpm)	N/A	N/A	N/A	−7.7 (−15 to 0)	−7.5 (−15 to −2)	−8.3 (−15 to 0)	−10.1 (−18 to 4)
ΔQT (ms)	N/A	N/A	N/A	37.8 (20 to 66)	33.6 (20 to 51)	48.3 (34 to 66)	60.9 (41 to 84)
ΔQTcF (ms)	N/A	N/A	N/A	22.7 (5 to 45)	18.6 (5 to 32)	33.2 (22 to 46)	40.3 (23 to 57)

*Subjects evaluated on d 2 were males only.

ED-1, first measurement by digipad on standard ECG; QT; absolute QT interval; QTcF, absolute QT interval corrected for heart rate by Fridericia's formula; RR, absolute RR interval; HR, heart rate; Δ, change from baseline, where the baseline constitutes an average of all 16 measurements on d −1; N/A, not applicable.

Table 2

Agreement Between Repeated QT, QTcF, and RR Interval Measurements by Digipad in Limb Lead II of Standard ECG

Pairwise comparisons	QT Interval				QTcF Interval				RR Interval			
	Absolute		Change from baseline		Absolute		Change from baseline		Absolute		Change from baseline	
	Mean difference (ms)	SD	Mean difference (ms)	SD	Mean difference (ms)	SD	Mean difference (ms)	SD	Mean difference (ms)	SD	Mean difference (ms)	SD
ED-1 vs ED-2	−11.6	9.8	1.0	8.7	−11.5	9.8	1.6	8.6	−1.0	6.3	−0.1	6.5
ED-1 vs ED-3	−6.4	9.7	0.2	8.2	−6.3	9.7	0.4	8.2	−1.0	5.6	−0.1	5.5

ED-1, first digipad measurement; ED-2, ED-3, digipad measurements repeated within 5 and 6 mo after ED-1 by the same two analysts; SD, standard deviation of difference; QTcF, QT interval corrected for heart rate by Fridericia's formula.

155

Table 3

Agreement Between Manual Methods for the QT, QTcF, and RR Interval Measurement in Limb Lead II of Standard and Holter-Derived Digital 12-Lead ECGs

Pairwise comparisons	QT Interval				QTcF Interval				RR Interval			
	Absolute		Change from baseline		Absolute		Change from baseline		Absolute		Change from baseline	
	Mean difference (ms)	SD	Mean difference (ms)	SD	Mean difference (ms)	SD	Mean difference (ms)	SD	Mean difference (ms)	SD	Mean difference (ms)	SD
ED-1 vs HD	-3.3	10.5	0.5	10.4	-2.7	12.5	-0.3	12.6	-3.5	67.3	7.3	72.9
EX vs HX	5.2	19.1	2.4	18.2	6.0	20.1	1.4	19.8	-5.0	70.3	6.8	74.0
ED-1 vs EX	-14.8	13.2	-1.2	14.0	-16.0	13.3	-0.7	13.9	9.0	8.6	2.2	8.2
HD vs HX	-6.1	15.6	0.9	12.8	-7.2	15.2	1.1	12.0	7.6	19.0	1.7	18.6

ED-1, first measurement by digipad on standard ECG; EA, measurement by the standard ECG recorder's automated algorithm; EX, measurement by digital on-screen calipers on standard ECG; HD, measurement by digipad on Holter-derived ECG; HX, measurement by digital on-screen caliper on Holter-derived ECG; SD, standard deviation of difference; QTcF, QT interval corrected for heart rate by Fridericia's formula.

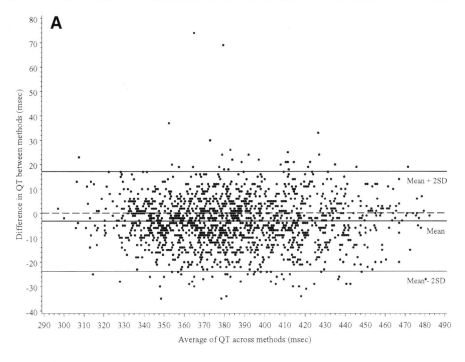

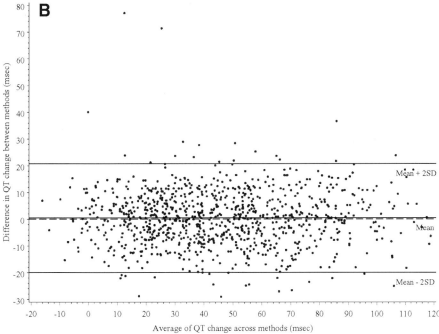

Fig. 1. Bland-Altman plots of agreement between digipad and onscreen measurements on standard and Holter-derived ECGs. abbreviations as in Table 3. Part 1a. QT Interval by digipad on standard and Holter-derived ECG (ED-1 vs HD). Part 1b. QT change from baseline by digipad on standard and Holter-derived ECG (ED-1 vs HD). Part 2a. QTcF interval by digipad on standard and Holter-derived ECG (ED-1 vs HD). Part 2b. QTcF change from baseline by digipad on Standard and Holter-derived ECG (ED-1 vs HD). Part 3a. RR interval by digipad on Standard and Holter-derived ECG (ED-1 vs HD). Part 3b. RR change from baseline by digipad on atandard and Holter-derived ECG (ED-1 vs HD).

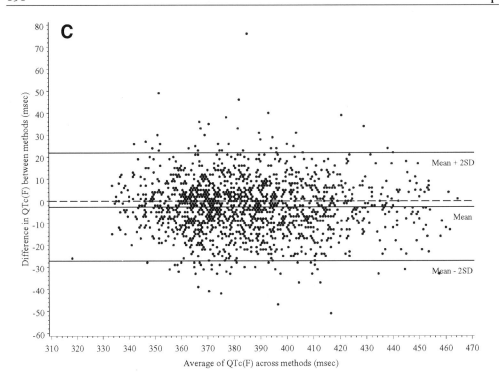

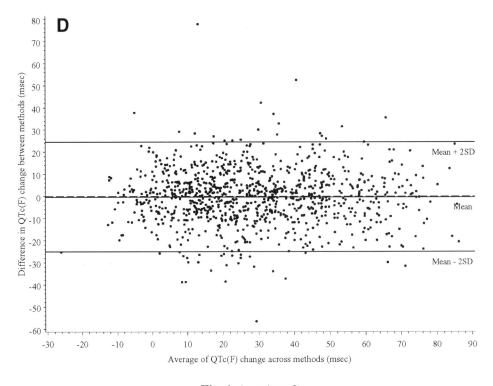

Fig. 1. (*continued*)

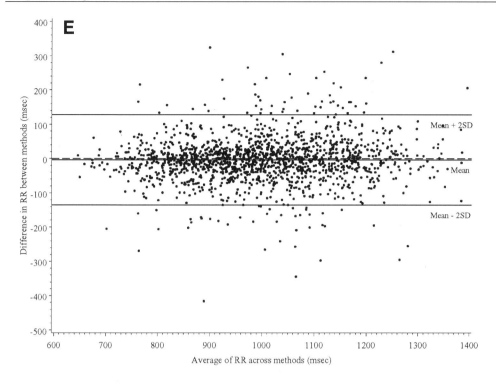

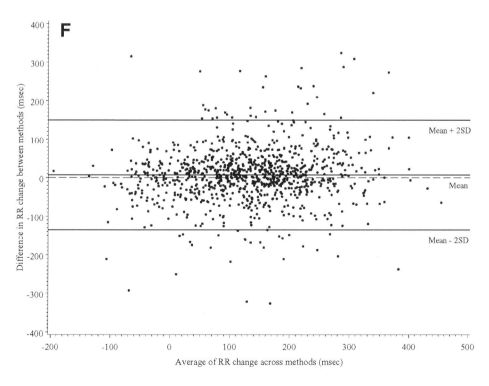

Fig. 1. (*continued*)

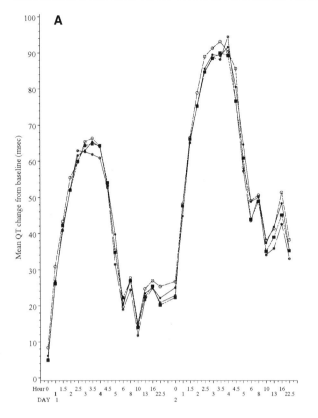

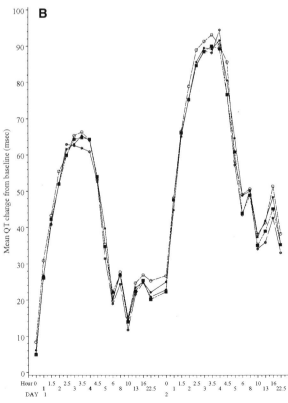

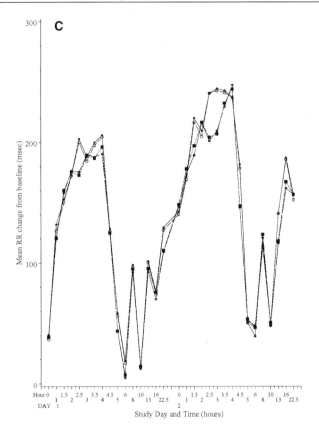

Fig. 2. Pairwise method comparisons by mean QT, QTcF, and RR change from baseline over time after oral administration of 160 mg and 320 mg of sotalol Part 1. Mean QT change from baseline. Part 2. Mean QTcF change from baseline. Part 3. Mean RR change from baseline. Legend: •-•-• ED-1; ■-■-■ HD; ○-○-○ EX; ⌊-⌊-⌊ HX. Abbreviations as in Table 3.

Whereas substantial error was observed in repeated digitizing board measurement by untrained volunteers *(38)*, other studies reported low relative inter-observer error in QT interval measurement when this method was used by trained observers *(39,40)*. A small mean QTc change from baseline of only 6 ms caused by terfenadine was detected by digipad *(18)*. We performed two repeated measurements by digipad on 1600 standard ECGs to examine the reproducibility of this method in our study. The repeated absolute QT interval measurements were on average 11.5 and 6.4 ms longer than the initial values of 5 and 6 mo earlier, indicating a small but systematic inter-run bias in the method for measurement of the absolute QT interval. We did not find differences between readers, or when ECGs were grouped by subject vs being read at random, and we were unable to account for the drift in the repeated digipad measurements of the absolute QT interval over time. This implies that for any manual method, the variability of QT interval measurement over time on different prospectively obtained ECGs should be taken into account. If the shorter duration of the trial makes it feasible, it would be prudent to ensure that all ECGs from the same subject are manually read within a reasonably short time frame (e.g., 1 wk). In this study both repeated digipad analyses showed only a negligible bias from the initial analysis for the mean differences in the change from baseline in QT (1.0 and 0.2 ms) and QTcF (1.6 and 0.4 ms). The mean differences between repeated and the initial digipad analyses were very small for the absolute RR interval (–1.0 ms) and virtually nonexistent for the RR change from baseline (–0.1 ms). Such results indicate very good reproducibility of digipad for detection of sotalol-induced QT/QTc, and RR changes from baseline in this trial and justify the use of digipad as a reference method for QT interval measurement to which other methods were compared.

Numerous serial ECGs recorded at baseline and upon repeated dosing with novel drugs and placebo are necessary for conclusive characterization of the potential of a new drug to prolong the QT interval (*see* Chapter 4 for details) *(12,42)*. Such intensive evaluation is generally performed in healthy volunteers hospitalized in well-equipped phase I units, and not in patients with the target disease indication enrolled in large multicentric phase II/III clinical trials where the vast majority of QT and RR data come from infrequently obtained standard ECGs, with often a single baseline recording. If QT and RR intervals could be reliably obtained from ambulatory digital 12-lead Holter recordings, this technology may become the method of choice for more intensive QT assessment in clinical trials *(42)*. In our study, QT, QTcF, and RR data produced by digipad on standard ECGs were essentially equivalent to those from digital 12-lead Holter ECGs (Table 3). We have observed a very small mean difference in the absolute QT and QTcF intervals (–3.3 and –2.7 ms) and a negligible mean difference in the QT and QTcF change from baseline (0.5 and –0.3 ms) when digipad was applied to standard ECGs and Holter-derived paper ECG copies, respectively. There were only two ECGs where the individual QTcF changes by digipad differed from those by onscreen by 60 ms or more *(*Fig. 1, part 2b*)*. Upon re-inspection of these ECGs, we found that both had a flat T wave in limb lead II, making it technically difficult to identify the same end point of T wave by both manual methods. Digipad RR data from standard ECGs were very similar to those from Holter-derived ECGs (mean differences, –3.5 ms for absolute RR and 7.3 ms for RR change from baseline), although with a considerably large standard deviation of difference. The mean difference of 7 ms between the RR changes from baseline produced by digipad on standard and Holter ECGs is so small relative to the total duration of RR interval that it would not affect the QT/RR relationship. The mean differences between the absolute QT, QTcF, and RR data produced by onscreen calipers applied to standard ECGs imported as digital files and to Holter ECGs scanned from paper were also small, although with greater standard deviation than digipad (Table 3).

Overall, despite somewhat different lead positions (12 lead Holter ECG has electrodes only on the torso, whereas the standard ECG uses also the limb leads) and differences in the sampling frequency of ECG recordings, our results validate the utility of digital 12-lead Holter for the assessment of QT prolongation in clinical drug research. With its inherent ease of capturing ECG continuously over long periods of time, digital 12-lead Holter would facilitate more intensive QT risk assessment in clinical trial patients who cannot comply with complex standard ECG schedules at baseline and on treatment. Holter will also make digital 12-lead ECG recordings available for retrospective analysis at critical time points after dosing that are difficult or impossible to capture by advance scheduling (maximum plasma concentration of the parent drug and active metabolites, clinical adverse events possibly related to QT prolongation). Numerous QT and RR intervals derived from continuous Holter ECGs will allow for employment of subject-specific QT correction formulae that might be more accurate than the Bazett's or Fridericia's in evaluating the true drug-induced QT effect at different heart rates *(42,43)*.

We observed negligible bias between the digipad and onscreen methods for QT, QTcF, and RR changes from baseline produced on standard and Holter-derived ECGs (mean

Table 4
Classification of Individual QTcF Changes From Baseline Determined by
Manual Measurement Methods in Limb Lead II of Standard and Holter-Derived ECGs

QTcF change from baseline (ms)	ED-1 N = 975		HD N = 961		EX N = 979		HX N = 960	
	n	%	n	%	n	%	n	%
0 to 30	530	54.4	527	54.8	529	54.5	547	57.0
31 to 60	354	36.3	346	36.1	338	34.5	311	32.4
61 to 90	89	9.1	86	8.9	93	9.5	96	10.0
> 90	2	0.2	2	0.2	15	1.5	6	0.6

ED-1, first measurement by digipad on standard ECG; EA, measurement by the standard ECG recorder's automated algorithm; EX, measurement by digital on-screen calipers on standard ECG; HD, measurement by digipad on Holter-derived ECG; HX, measurement by digital on-screen caliper on Holter-derived ECG; SD, standard deviation of difference; QTcF, QT interval corrected for heart rate by Fridericia's formula. N, the total number of ECGs (d 1 and d 2) evaluated; n, the total number of ECGs (d 1 and d 2) where a given QTcF change was detected.

differences: −1.2 vs 0.9 ms for QT change, −0.7 vs 1.1 for QTcF change, and 2.2 vs 1.7 ms for RR change on standard and Holter ECGs, respectively), although the standard deviations of difference between RR interval measurements on standard and Holter ECGs were quite high for both digipad and onscreen methods. The absolute QT, QTcF, and RR intervals by onscreen were on average longer than those by digipad (Table 3). As the only manual method currently available for true digital ECG files, onscreen calipers are likely to replace the digitizing board as the standard manual measurement method in the digital ECG era. The absolute duration of QT/QTcF intervals up to 16 ms longer by onscreen than by digipad might be an issue in drug trials utilizing the onscreen method. However, the negligible mean differences between onscreen and digipad in detection of sotalol-induced QT or QTcF change from baseline (−0.7 to 1.2 ms) indicate that digital onscreen calipers are a reliable method for the assessment of drug-induced QT/QTc interval prolongation. Both manual methods applied to standard or Holter-derived ECGs produced a similar proportion of QTcF changes from baseline between 0–30 ms, 31–60 ms and 61–90 ms (Table 4). The incidence of extreme outliers for QTcF change (> 90 ms) was higher with the onscreen method than digipad on both standard and Holter-derived ECGs. Lower resolution on a computer screen after paper ECGs are scanned into portable network graphics image files, in contrast to digipad's high power image magnification, might explain the greater variability of onscreen method than digipad on Holter-derived ECGs. Importing true digital ECG files directly from the Holter recorder into the measurement system (available now but not during our study) would be a more appropriate way to perform manual onscreen measurements than scanning the paper ECG copies. The sotalol-induced changes in T wave morphology or amplitude by potassium channel blockade (44) could increase the variability of QT measurement by any manual method, and pure human measurement errors can also occur.

Exposure to single 160 mg and 320 mg doses of sotalol had no adverse effects while causing a wide range of QT, QTcF, and RR changes from baseline in all study subjects (Table 1), which makes our results representative of a variety of clinical situations. All measurement methods, whether applied to standard and Holter-derived ECGs, were comparable in describing the magnitude as well as the temporal dynamics of changes in

QT, QTcF and RR interval induced by 160 mg and 320 mg of sotalol (Fig. 2). Although the sotalol-induced QT/QTc prolongation was larger in this study than those likely to be encountered in the assessment of non-antiarrhythmic drugs' effect on cardiac repolarization, the Bland–Altman plots (Fig. 1) show uniform variability of pairwise comparisons over a wide range of QT/QTcF prolongation, including the smaller degrees of < 30 ms. Given this, our results would be applicable to the detection of smaller degrees of QT/QTc prolongation that must be ruled out during drug development.

CONCLUSIONS

ECGs derived at discrete time points from a digital 12-lead Holter recorder provide QT/QTc and RR data of equal value to those from a standard resting 12-lead ECG for the assessment of drug-induced change from baseline in QT/QTc and RR intervals. Digital 12-lead Holter may allow for a more comprehensive assessment of drug effects on cardiac repolarization. Manual digitized QT/QTc and RR interval measurement systems, whether on paper using a digitizing pad or by digital onscreen calipers, produce comparable mean sotalol-induced changes from baseline in QT/QTc and RR interval. The variability of QT/QTc and RR measurement by the onscreen method in this study was greater than digipad.

Our results appear to validate the utility of digital 12-lead Holter for the assessment of QT prolongation in clinical drug research. With its inherent ease of capturing ECG continuously over long periods of time, digital 12-lead Holter would facilitate more intensive QT risk assessment in clinical trial patients. Numerous QT and RR intervals derived from continuous Holter ECGs will allow for employment of individual QT correction formulae or the analysis of the *data clouds*, which might be more accurate in evaluating the true drug-induced effect on cardiac repolarization than the conventional endpoints (change from baseline in QT interval corrected by Bazett's or Fridericia's methods). This would ultimately ensure that safer drugs are brought to market to the significant benefit of patients and clinicians.

REFERENCES

1. Holter NJ. New methods for heart studies. Science 1961;134:1214.
2. Atiga WL, Calkins H, Lawrence JH, et al. Beat-to-beat repolarization lability identifies patients at risk for sudden cardiac death. J Cardiovasc Electrophysiol 1998;9:899–908.
3. Atiga WL, Fananapazir L, McAreavey D, Calkins H, Berger RD. Temporal repolarization lability in hypertrophic cardiomyopathy caused by beta-myosin heavy-chain gene mutations. Circulation 2000;101:1224–1226.
4. Berger RD, Kasper EK, Baughman KL, et al. beat-to-beat QT interval variability; novel evidence for repolarization lability in ischemic and nonischemic dilated cardiomyopathy. Circulation 1997;96: 1557–1565.
5. Vrtovec B, Starc V, Starc R. Beat-to-beat QT interval variability in coronary patients. J Electrocardiol 2000;33119–33125.
6. International Conference on Harmonization. The clinical evaluation of QT/QTc interval prolongation and proarrhythmic potential for non-antiarrhythmic drugs. Preliminary Concept Paper, Step 1 Draft 4, June 10, 2004.
7. Yap YG, Camm AJ. Arrhythmogenic mechanisms of non-sedating antihistamines. Clin Exp Allergy 1999;29(Suppl. 3):174–181.
8. van Haarst AD, van't Klooster GA, van Gerven JM et al. The influence of cisapride and clarithromycin on QT intervals in healthy volunteers. Clin Pharmacol Ther 1998;64:542–546.
9. Morganroth J, Talbot GH, Dorr MB, et al. Effect of single, ascending, supratherapeutic doses of sparfloxacin on cardiac repolarization (QTc interval). Clin Therapeutics 1999;21:818–828.

10. Darpö B. Spectrum of drugs prolonging the QT interval and the incidence of torsades de pointes. Eur Heart J 2001;3(Suppl. K):K70–K80.
11. Haverkamp W, Breithardt G, Camm AJ, et al. The potential for QT prolongation and proarrhythmia by non-antiarrhythmic drugs: clinical and regulatory implications. Report on a Policy Conference of the European Society of Cardiology. Cardiovascular Research 2000;47:219–233.
12. Morganroth J. Focus on issues in measuring and interpreting changes in the QTc interval duration. Eur Heart J Supplements 2001;3(Suppl. K):K105–K111.
13. Malik M, Camm AJ. Evaluation of drug-induced QT interval prolongation. Implications for drug approval and labeling. Drug Safety 2001;24:323–351.
14. Shah RR. The significance of QT interval in drug development. Brit J Clin Pharmacol, 2002;54: 188–202.
15. Committee for Proprietary Medicinal Products (CPMP). Points to Consider: The assessment of the potential for QT interval prolongation by non-cardiovascular medicinal products. The European Agency for the Evaluation of Medicinal Products, 17 December 1997.
16. Merri M, Moss AJ, Benhorin J, et al. Relation between ventricular repolarization duration and cardiac cycle length during 24-hour Holter recordings.
17. Jensen BT, Larroude CE, Rasmussen LP, et al. beat-to-beat QT dynamics in healthy subjects. Ann Noninvasive Electrocardiol 2004;9:3–11.
18. Pratt CM, Ruberg S, Morganroth J, et al. Dose-response relation between terfenadine (Seldane) and the QTc interval on the scalar electrocardiogram: distinguishing a drug effect from spontaneous variability. Am Heart J 1996;131:472–480.
19. Lee K-T, Chu C-S, SU H-M,et al. Circadian variation of QT dispersion determined by twelve-lead Holter Electrocardiography. Cardiology 2003;100:101–102.
20. Morganroth J. Relations of QTc prolongation on the electrocardiogram to torsades de pointes: definitions and mechanisms. Am J Cardiol 1993;72:10B–13B.
21. Extramiana F, Neyroud N, Huikuri HV, et al. QT interval and arrhythmic risk assessment after myocardial infarction. Am J Cardiol 1999;83:266–269.
22. Bonnemeier H, Hartmann F, Wiegand UK, et al. Course and prognostic implications of QT interval and QT interval variability after primary coronary angioplasty in acute myocardial infarction. J Am Coll Cardiol 2001;37:44–50.
23. Pohl R, Yeragani VK. QT variability in panic disorder patients after isoproterenol infusion. Int J Neuropsychopharmacol 2001;4:17–20.
24. Yeragani VK, Pohk R, Jampala VC, et al. Effect of posture and isoproterenol on beat-to-beat HR and QT variability. Neuropsychobiology 2000;41:113–123.
25. Extramiana F, Maison-Blanche P, Badilini F, et al. Circadian modulation of QT rate dependence in healthy volunteers: Gender and age differences. J Electrocardiol 1999;32:33–43.
26. Lande G, Funck-Brentano C, Ghadanfar M, et al. Steady-state vs. non-steady-state QT-RR relationships in 24-hour Holter recordings. Pacing Clin Electrophysiol 2000;23:293–302.
27. Lang CC, Flapan AD, Neilson JM. The impact of QT lag compensation on dynamic measurement of ventricular repolarization: Reproducibility and the impact of lead selection. Pacing Clin Electrophysiol 2001;24:366–373.
28. Sarma JS, Venkataraman SK, Samant DR, et al. Hysteresis in the human RR-QT relationship during exercise and recovery. Pacing Clin Electrophysiol 1987;10:485–491.
29. Yamada A, Hayano J, Horie K, et al. Regulation of QT interval during postural transitory changes in heart rate in normal subjects. Am J Cardiol 1993;71:996–998.
30. Bosner MS, Kleiger RE. Heart rate variability and risk stratification after myocardial infarction. In Malik M, Camm AJ (eds). Heart rate variability. Futura, Armonk, NY, 1995, pp. 331–340.
31. Atildsen H, Christiansen EH, Pedersen AK, et al. Reproducibility of QT parameters derived from 24-hour ambulatory ECG recordings in healthy subjects. Ann Noninvasive Electrocardiol 2001;6:24–31.
32. Copie X, Alonso C, Lavergne T, et al. Reproducibility of Qt interval measurements obtained from 24-hour digitized ambulatory three-lead electrocardiograms in patients with acute myocardial infarction and healthy volunteers. Ann Noninvasive Electrocardiol 1998;3:38–45.
33. Savelieva I, Yap YG, Yi G, et al. Comparative reproducibility of QT, QT peak, and T peak – T end intervals and dispersion in normal subjects, patients with myocardial infarction and patients with hypertrophic cardiomyopathy. Pacing Clin Electrophysiol 1998;21:2376–2381.
34. Baranowski R, Poplawska W, Buchner T, et al. day-to-day reproducibility of Holter beat-by-beat analysis of repolarization. Acta Cardiol 2003;58:185–189.

35. Sarapa N, Morganroth J, Couderc JP, et al. Electrocardiographic Identification of Drug-Induced QT Prolongation: Assessment by Different Recording and Measurement Methods. Ann Noninvasive Electrocardiol 2004;9:48–57.
36. Morganroth J, Silber SS. How to obtain and analyze electrocardiograms in clinical trials: Focus on issues in measuring and interpreting changes in the QTc interval duration. A N E 1999;4:425–433.
37. Bland JM, Altman DG. Measuring agreement in method comparison studies. Stat Methods Med Res.1999;8:135–160.
38. Malik M, Bradford A. Human precision of operating a digitizing board: implications for electrocardiogram measurements. PACE 1998;21:1656–1662.
39. Food and Drug Administration and Health Canada. The clinical evaluation of QT/QTc interval prolongation and proarrhythmic potential for non-antiarrhythmic drugs. Preliminary Concept paper, November 15, 2002 http//www.fda.gov/cder/workshop.htm#upcoming.
40. Kautzner J, Gang Y, Camm AJ, et al. Short- and long-term reproducibility of QT, QTc, and QT dispersion measurement in healthy subjects. PACE 1994;17:928–937.
41. Kautzner J, Gang Y, Kishore AGR, et al. Interobserver reproducibility of QT interval measurement and QT dispersion in patient after acute myocardial infarction. Ann Noninvas Electrocardiol 1996;1: 363–374.
42. Malik M, Camm AJ. Evaluation of drug-induced QT interval prolongation. Implications for drug approval and labeling. Drug Safety 2001;24:323–351.
43. Malik M, Färbom P, Batchvarov V, et al. Relation between QT and RR intervals is highly individual among healthy subjects: implications for heart rate correction of the QT interval. Heart 2002;87: 220–228.
44. Darpö B, Almgren O, Bergstrand R, et al. Assessment of frequency-dependency of the class III effects of almokalant. A study using programmed stimulation and recordings of monophasic action potentials and ventricular paced QT-intervals. Cardiovasc Drug Therapy 1996;10:539–554.

9

Holter Monitoring for QT

The RR Bin Method in Depth

Fabio Badilini, PhD
and Pierre Maison-Blanche, MD

CONTENTS

BACKGROUND

Many noncardiovascular drugs have the adverse effect to delay cardiac repolarization, a phenomenon that can be quantified in humans on the surface electrocardiogram (ECG) by the QT interval *(1,2)*. Despite a number of limitations associated with its assessment, the drug-induced prolongation of QT interval is considered an important marker for the risk of life-threatening arrhythmias (torsades de pointes [TdP]) *(3,4)*.

An additional challenge associated with the measurement of the QT interval is its intrinsic property of being inversely related to heart rate (QT interval shortens as heart rate increases) *(5,6)*, a characteristic that justifies the need for a way to normalize QT interval changes whenever the heart rate also changes. This normalization is more commonly known as QT correction and the never-ending debate on which regression formula should be used to define the best model (or formula) to normalize the QT interval is far from being resolved.

While waiting for more reliable and more reproducible markers of drug-induced delayed repolarization, we need to define methodologies capable to reliably capture changes in the QT intervals while minimizing the risks associated with correction formula or regression models.

From: *Cardiac Safety of Noncardiac Drugs:*
Practical Guidelines for Clinical Research and Drug Development
Edited by: J. Morganroth and I. Gussak © Humana Press Inc., Totowa, NJ

The so-called Holter bin approach (also known as the RR bin method) is one of the methods that have been proposed in the pharmaceutical arena.

In this chapter, the technical characteristics of the Holter bin method used to assess drug-related changes in both the QRS and the QT intervals *(7,8)* will be described in detail. The method presented is part of a larger research package called WinAtrec designed to cover various aspects in continuous ECG monitoring analysis.

THE HOLTER BIN METHOD

General Concepts

INTERFACING WITH COMMERCIAL SYSTEMS

WinAtrec entry point is validated Holter data. This means that all beat validation and editing (positioning and labeling) is assumed to be correctly performed beforehand, on the commercial system environment. In general, commercial systems store ECG waveform and the validated annotation information on disk files with proprietary (and sometimes compressed) data formats.

The interface between WinAtrec and these commercial systems depends on data organization; some systems include tools for the export of ECG and annotations information into public domain formats (such as ISHNE or MIT) that are directly supported by WinAtrec. Others simply provide the format description of their internal file structures and authorize the usage. In general, the first step is to perform a reformatting from the original formats of ECGs and annotation files (different for each separate vendor) to a unique internal format used by WinAtrec which, for the ECG waveforms, is that proposed by the International Society for Holter and Noninvasive Electrocardiology (ISHNE) *(9)*.

SMOOTHING OF ANNOTATION FILES

Proper implementation of the RR Holter bin approach requires a correct computation of the continuous (beat-to-beat) averaged heart rate needed to compensate for nonsinus events, noise, intermittent data, and similar conditions typical of Holter recordings. To handle these situations, WinAtrec computes a so-called smoothed annotation file, where the original (raw) sequence of beat labels is replaced by a new interpolated sequence. The portions of the raw annotation file where interpolation is applied can be based on one or more user-selectable set of events (e.g, sequences of ventricular and/or supraventricular beats, pauses, and short RR intervals). The position of beat labels to be inserted is then computed using a cubic-spline interpolation technique by considering the last and first three valid RR intervals, before and after the portion to be smoothed.

The result of this procedure is to obtain an interpolated annotation sequence characterized by inserted beat labels not associated with real beats (and, thus not used for analysis) but only used for the computation of the correct rate beat-to-beat averaged heart rate. Figure 1 is an example of the interpolation of an isolated ventricular beat (PVC). Please note that an L (interpolation) label has been placed on the normal beat after the PVC. This is to avoid the post-PVC beat to be subsequently used by the Holter bin method, but only for the computation of the beat-to-beat averaged RR interval.

SELECTIVE BEAT AVERAGING: THE SUBSTRATE OF HOLTER BIN

The RR Holter bin is a beat averaging approach. In general, beat averaging is applied to *consecutive* sinus beats within a time window, and it is used to obtain low noise level templates (the noise content decreases by a factor of $\frac{1}{\sqrt{n}}$ when we average n beats). The

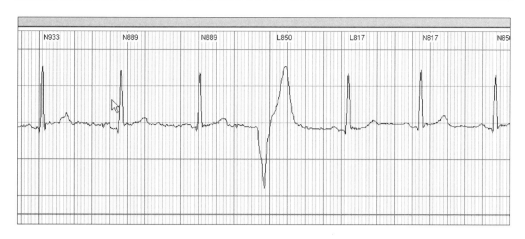

Fig. 1. Example of interpolation: The two L-labeled beats will not be used by the RR bin method but only for the computation of the beat-to-beat averaged heart rate.

averaging technique used in the Holter bin approach employs a more complex selection model to group the individual beats to be average that is called selective beat averaging.

The concept of selective beat averaging is not new, as it was applied to study arrhythmia events. Sequences of RR intervals preceding frequent ventricular extrasystoles have been investigated to assess the electrophysiological mechanisms associated with ventricular excitability *(10,11)*. Dynamic behavior of high resolution body surface ECG recordings was also analyzed with a selective beat approach, either using short–long RR sequence generated by ventricular extrasystole *(12)*, or at different values of cardiac cycle length *(13)*. Modes of onset of TdP were also identified with a selective beat averaging model that identified the presence of oscillatory patterns preceding the arrhythmia onset *(14)*.

In WinAtrec, selective beat averaging is used to group (average) individual P–QRS–T complexes preceded by the same stable heart rate as computed over an "observation period" preceding each of the beats to be averaged. The observation period can be reduced to a single beat (the "RR-1 only" model) where all the beats will be considered for analysis, regardless of the stability conditions preceding them. The philosophy behind the concept of imposing stability aims to respect the restitution curve of ventricular repolarization that demonstrates how full adaptation of QT interval to changes in heart rate is only achieved after a time period that can be longer than a minute *(15)*. Thus, despite an identical RR interval, beats occurring "in the middle of heart rate changes" may have a different repolarization shape than those occurring at stable heart rate. Most of all, they will have a different QT duration. This phenomenon, known as hytesresis, will be covered in details in a later section.

One simple way to define stability is to impose the averaged RR interval computed over the observation period (RR_{Per}) to match with the immediately preceding RR interval (RR_{-1}):

$$RR_{-1} = RR_{Per} \pm th1 \qquad (1)$$

where th1 is a user-selectable threshold set by default to 15 ms. Alternatively, stability may require the equivalence of RR intervals calculated over more subperiods, or imply the usage of other variables such for example heart rate variability parameters *(16)*. Recently, more sophisticated definitions based on the usage of the best fit model applied on a per case basis have been proposed *(17)*.

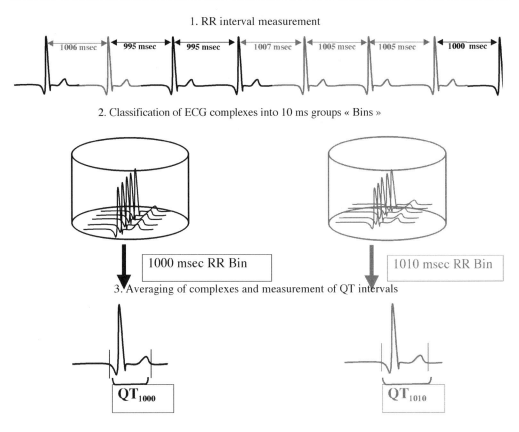

1. RR interval measurement

2. Classification of ECG complexes into 10 ms groups « Bins »

1000 msec RR Bin

1010 msec RR Bin

3. Averaging of complexes and measurement of QT intervals

QT_{1000}

QT_{1010}

Fig. 2. Flowchart of RR Holter bin method.

Given a rule of selection and the time period where to apply it (e.g., a circadian period or a the peak concentration of a compound), the algorithm used in the Holter bin determines a family of averaged templates, one per class of RR intervals (from here the terminology RR bins). The stratification (bin) resolution is user selectable and can be as small as 10 ms that is appropriate for systems with high sampling rate. The total number of templates obtained within a family depends on bin resolution and on the effective range of heart rates available in the time period analyzed. Figure 2 summarizes the process of beat selection/allocation of Holter bin method: starting from the RR interval measurements, individual beats are allocated (averaged) in the bin whenever they meet the selection criterion imposed. At the end of the process, a single QT interval (or other quantitative parameter) is measured on the averaged waveform. Figure 3 shows a cascade display of a family of templates together with the associated histograms of RR bins.

CORRECTING THE TRIGGER JITTER OF ANNOTATION FILES

Commercial Holter systems implement proprietary algorithms and mathematical definitions for QRS fiducial markers (e.g., the center of mass or maximum velocity in the QRS). Because of these differences, consistency in the positioning of QRS fiducials cannot be assumed *a priori*. Even worse, a so-called trigger jitter effect, which can be defined as an inconsistent positioning of the fiducial QRS markers (even between a beat and the next) is known to affect many systems. When averaging, trigger jitter would typically produce larger (longer) and smaller (less amplitude) QRS complexes. In addi-

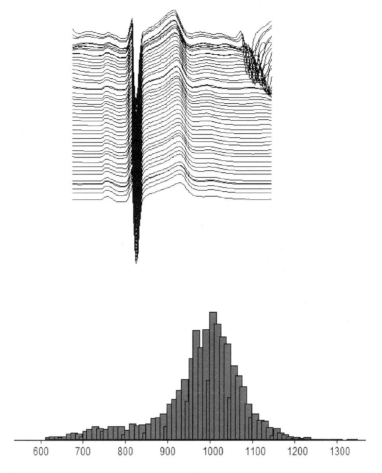

Fig. 3. Cascade display of a family of RR bin templates with the associated histogram.

tion, even the RR bin assignment would be effected as the sequence of RR intervals would also be modified by a wrongly positioned fiducial point.

All methods that implement some form of beat averaging, including Holter bin, should include proper signal pre-processing to avoid (or to correct for) trigger jittering. In WinAtrec, the correction algorithm is based on a complete re-analysis of the QRSs positions and on the application of a parabolic interpolation to reliably define the apex of the QRS complex of each beat *(16,18)*. Figure 4 is a real-case example where trigger jitter is overtly seen within a few seconds of data; the strip in the upper part is extracted before the correction and the lower strip after the correction. Figure 5 shows the effect of trigger jittering in an extreme case: the two overlaid templates are the averages of QRS complexes from the same time window before (light pen) and after (black pan) trigger jitter correction (from the same ECG subject of Fig. 4). The before correction template is clearly affected by *both* a distorted QRS (smaller amplitude plus an artifact S wave) and even a T wave alteration. The importance of applying proper trigger jitter correction is apparent.

PROPER BEAT ALIGNMENT

Most commercial systems produce digital ECGs at a relatively low sampling rate (in the range of 200 Hz). When performing beat averaging, single beats need to be aligned

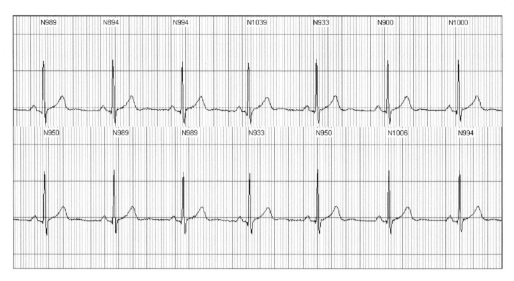

Fig. 4. ECG strip shown before (upper panel) and after (lower panel) jitter correction. Before correction, the positioning of beat labels fluctuates form one beat to another whereas after correction they are stabilized. Even the RR interval sequence is seriously affected with changes up to 100 ms long.

(superimposed) on the top of each other. This process, even when the effect of trigger jitter has been compensated, can still determine small distortions in the averaged complexes as a result of the random positioning of the alignment (fiducial) markers associated with sampling rate.

To cope with this problem all individual beats to be averaged are oversampled (at 400 Hz) and resynchronized with respect to the apex of the R wave as estimated by the peak of the fitted parabola *(16,18)*. More details on the mathematical model used to perform this realignment can be found in the original article that introduced selective beat averaging *(16)*.

Of note, this resampling procedure is not applied with the aim to increase or to add information (a purely utopian goal), but only with the intent to produce better alignment of individual beats before averaging. To give a quantitative ballpark, on a commercial system with a sampling rate in the range of 200 Hz (i.e., digital samples 5 ms apart) an averaged complex obtained without realignment can produce QRS complexes from 3 to 8 ms longer than that of the individual beats used for the averaging (data extrapolated from WinAtrec validation documentation).

MEASUREMENTS ON AVERAGED WAVEFORMS VS BEAT-TO-BEAT MEASUREMENTS

Even after reducing the variability linked with heart rate variations (using bin stratification), hysteresis (imposing stability), or autonomic factors (focusing on well-defined circadian periods), some residual variability related to other factors (on for all the short-term respiratory related variations) will still characterize the individual beats used for averaging. Thus, it is legitimate to question how representative a measurement performed on an averaged waveform can be with respect to the population of measurements from the individual beats used to obtain the averaged waveform.

WinAtrec validation addressed this specific issue on both real and on simulated data, and we will report three significant examples. In Fig. 6A, results from a real case example are reported: the distribution of beat-to-beat QT measurements is displayed together with the single-value QT measurement (vertical line) obtained on the waveform derived av-

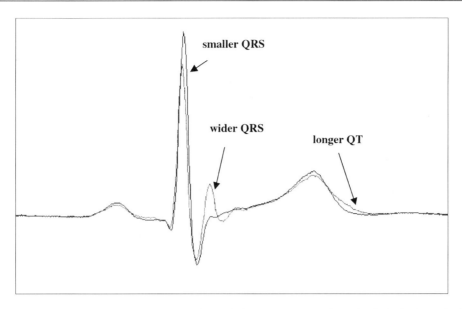

Fig. 5. Averaged complexes from the ECG of Fig. 4. The waveform in light is that obtained averaging beats before jitter correction; the bold waveform is that obtained averaging the same beats after correction. The distortions (resulting is a smaller and wider QRS and in a longer QT intervals) are apparent.

eraging all the individual beats from a 8-h time window (12:00–20:00; RR interval range: 610–1230). In both cases (i.e., on beat-to-beat and on the averaged waveform) the QT interval was measured by the same algorithm implemented in WinAtrec used in fully automatic (no user overreading) mode. In this algorithm, the T wave offset definition is based on first derivative adaptive threshold *(16)*.

Of note, the averaged waveform of this experiment was intentionally derived without using any selection criteria (no RR bin stratification, no stability imposed), and thus maximizing all sources of variability. Indeed, the range of QT intervals is fairly large and also contains the algorithm "mistakes" (in the small tail of the left hand of the distribution, and above 500 ms on the right hand). The range of beat-to-beat QT intervals typically seen with RR bin is, of course, much smaller and reduced to only few milliseconds, particularly when a stable model is imposed.

The beat-to-beat distribution of Fig. 6A is not symmetric and it has a faster descend at QT intervals higher than then mean value (423 ms) and with a small tail centered around 300 ms. The median and the mode (most frequent) values were 420 and 411 ms, respectively. The measurement derived from the averaged waveform was 410 ms, thus reflecting the mode (most frequent value) of the distribution.

The same behavior is confirmed on simulated data. In Fig. 6B and 6C, the distribution of individual QT intervals was predetermined to have respectively a rectangular and a triangular shape centered at 400 ms and covering the 350–450 ms range. As in the real case example, the QT interval measured on the averaged template matched with the mode of the distribution (which for these two simulations also correspond the mean and median values).

These results indicate that from a pure mathematical standpoint, and at least with respect to the measurement algorithm implemented in WinAtrec, measurements performed

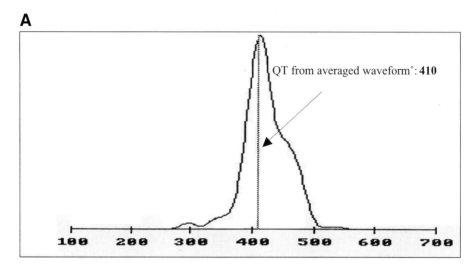

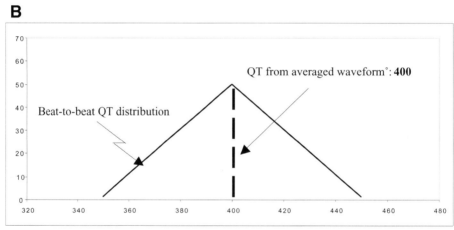

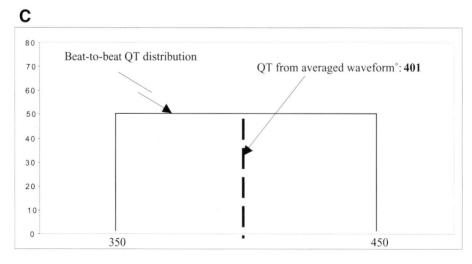

Fig. 6. Comparison between beat-to-beat distributions and single-value (from the averaged waveform) of QT intervals from a real case example (**A**) and from two simulation experiments based on triangular (**B**) and rectangular (**C**) beat-to-beat distributions.

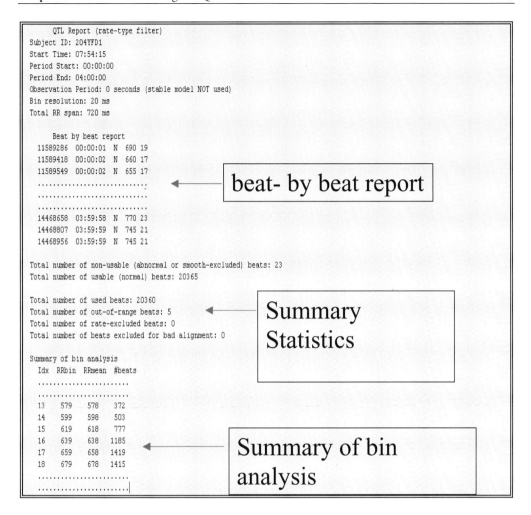

Fig. 7. Extract of Holter bin beat-to-beat report.

on the averaged waveform reflect the most frequent values of the measurements from the individual beats used for the averaging, and thus are not biased by extremes values from the individual beat population.

Audit Trail of RR Holter Bin

One of the big concerns with the implementation of Holter bin approach in clinical trials is that of a proper audit trail on the individual beats used (averaged). For each period analyzed, WinAtrec automatically generates a log file where a beat-to-beat report is stored. The log file includes a header where user selectable options chosen are reported (e.g., the length of the observation period, bin resolution, span of RR interval considered). The header is followed by a beat-to-beat table where time of occurrence, beat label, RR interval, and bin allocation of each individual beat in the analyzed period is reported. This table allows *a posteriori* verification of proper bin allocation and verification of proper beat exclusion (based on either beat labeling or on stability criteria). The table is followed by a summary where basic statistics (total number of included/excluded beats) and number of individual beats averaged in each bin are reported. Figure 7 is an extract of the Holter bin beat-to-beat report from a real case.

THE HYSTERESIS DILEMMA

Repolarization duration does not respond instantaneously to sudden heart rate changes and the QT interval takes time to adapt to heart rate changes. This phenomenon is well-known and has been observed and described for many years *(15)*. During exercise, hysteresis is very easily seen in the QT/RR plane as the state map curves follow two completely separate patterns during the exercise and the recovery phases *(19)*. The most critical consequences of this phenomenon is that using the preceding RR interval, either for correcting or even, as in our case, to decide bin allocation, may be quite dangerous. In Fig. 8, an ideal model for hysteresis is shown on the QT/RR plane (each circle identifying a singe beat): in the center we have a steady-state (QT_1, RR_1) pair. If we imagine an ideal step increase in heart rate (i.e., a sudden acceleration) the RR interval will jump from RR_1 to RR_3 $(RR_3 < RR_1)$, whereas the QT interval will take time to reach the new steady-state value QT_3. During the adaptation phase QT intervals are "longer" than at steady-state value QT_3.

Conversely, an ideal step decrease in heart rate (a sudden deceleration), will trigger a jump increase in RR $(RR_2 > RR_1)$, and an adaptation phase with observed QT intervals shorter that the new steady-state QT interval (QT_2). These shorter/longer QT intervals during adaptation times will have two major consequences:

1. During adaptation, for a fixed RR interval we would observe several different values of QT with a consequent altered correction mechanism (if we correct the QT interval). In the context of an averaging approach such as the Holter bin, individual beats with different QT intervals would be included in the same RR bin.
2. *Any* QT/RR regression model fitted to all observed data would produce altered results with weaker (less steep) slopes observed when keeping all (stable and unstable) observations.

The model of Fig. 8 is purely ideal, as we do not have sudden step changes in a daily standard scenario (the closest we can get would be using pacemakers or running an exercise test protocol). On the other hand, the hypotheses derived can be verified on real data. Figure 9 has been obtained from a normal subject with substantial physical activity during the recording. The averaged RR interval in the period analyzed in the example was 700 ms (see the histogram in upper right corner of Fig. 8). The superimposed waveforms shown in Fig. 9 were obtained averaging all the beats with a preceding RR interval of 630 ms (dark pen waveform), and only averaging the beats preceded by a stable heart rate (light pen waveform). Thus, the RR bin shown (RR = 630), corresponds to a heart rate faster than the mean heart rate of the explored period, and potentially includes both steady-state values (for the RR = 630 level) and adapting periods that we could assume to be acceleration sequences. The *ALL* beat (unstable) waveform overtly shows a longer QT interval than the stable waveform, confirming the hypotheses of the model. Of note, the number of averaged beats in the stable waveform is significantly smaller than that in the unstable waveform (70 vs 151).

The example shown in Fig. 9 was taken intentionally as an extreme case with *a lot* of hysteresis (a normal subject who was active during the period analyzed). However, the same type of results (observing shorter QT intervals whenever the heart rate is below the averaged heart rate, and longer QT intervals in heart rate ranges above the mean heart rate), can be confirmed in general, although in many cases (particularly when the subject analyzed was forced to keep resting condition by the clinical protocol) the differences between the stable and unstable model were minimal.

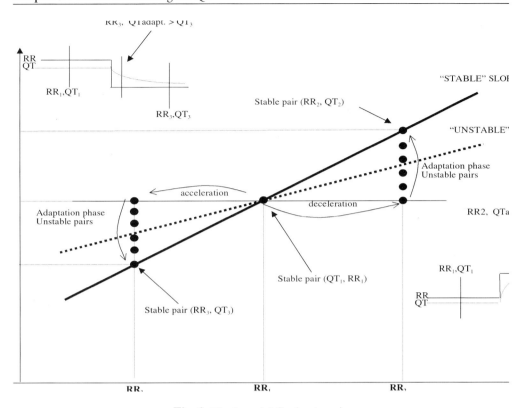

Fig. 8. Ideal model for hysteresis.

Ideally, the amount of hysteresis should be quantified on a case-by-case basis and a stable model should be imposed anytime the hysteresis would cross a certain threshold. Certainly, a good way to minimize the problem would be to carefully define protocols aimed to minimize *a priori* the presence of hysteresis (e.g., limiting physical activity and making sure the ECGs analyzed would be taken only after stable heart rate conditions).

What needs to be clear is that hysteresis is not a methodological pitfall of an approach more than another, but rather a physiologic phenomenon that can affect the data on a case-by-case magnitude. We strongly believe that the Holter bin method, through the intrinsic concept of selective beat averaging, is actually one of the existing methods that better control the presence of hysteresis. Clearly, the price paid to take this into account can be that of excluding a significant amount of beats that, depending on the definition of stability imposed, can become a big percentage of total available data.

Table 1 reports the results from a real case example that helped us understand the price of hysteresis. Data from the table are taken from a normal subject and are based on a 2-h time period (16:00–18:00), with an averaged heart rate of 60 beats per minute (RR = 1000). The RR Holter bin algorithm was run using a "RR-1 only" model (i.e., no control of hysteresis, or all beats included) and using the stability criteria defined in Equation 1 with a progressively increasing observation period (10, 20, 30, and 60 s). In the second column of Table 1, the QT interval from the RR bin at the averaged RR of the considered period (RR_{1000}) is reported with (in parentheses) the number of individual beats averaged. The last columns also reports the QT interval associated with two RR bins away from the averaged RR, respectively RR_{1050} and RR_{950}.

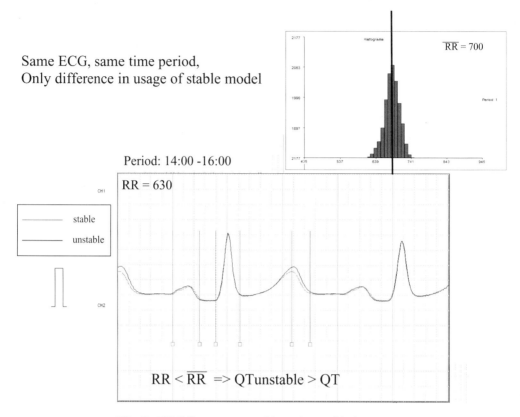

Fig. 9. QT differences at stable and unstable heart rate.

The price *paid* to impose stability is apparent. Even with a short observation period (10 s), the *loss* of beats is already significant, although more important (in percent) away from the averaged RR (in the RR_{1000} bin the number of included beats changed from 1406 to 1048, a 25% loss; in the RR_{1050} bin it changed from 318 to 152 beats, a 52% loss). This loss of beats progressively augmented by increasing the length of the observation, although it was less pronounced in the central RR bin. With a 60 s observation period, the loss was 31, 75, and 77%, respectively for the RR_{1000}, RR_{950}, and RR_{1050} bins, with an overall total loss of 842 beats out of 1937 initially available (43%). In the central (averaged RR) bin, the QT interval did not change with the imposed stability, whereas it progressively increased and decreased in the RR_{1050} and RR_{950} bins. This observation is perfectly in line with the ideal model previously described, i.e., without hysteresis control the QT interval is longer at faster heart rates (shorter RR intervals) and shorter at lower heart rates (longer RR intervals).

In the Alfusozin study, the study that gave the visibility of this technology to the pharmaceutical world, the Holter bin method was applied using the "only RR-1" model, i.e., without using the stable model and hysteresis was intentionally minimized at the protocol level *(8)*. This decision (whose discussion is beyond the scope of this chapter) led to some confusion and criticisms that created the misconception that the Holter bin approach cannot correct hysteresis, or (even worse) that hysteresis is a problem specific to this method. All the arguments reported should have clarified that this is definitely not the case.

Table 1
The Price of Hysteresis

Model	QT_{RR1000} (n)	QT_{1050} (n)	QT_{950} (n)
RR-1 only	345 (1406)	358 (318)	345 (213)
10 s	345 (1048)	360 (152)	345 (124)
20 s	345 (988)	360 (122)	343 (87)
30 s	345 (982)	362 (105)	343 (84)
60 s	345 (967)	362 (79)	340 (49)

QT/RR RELATION WITH THE HOLTER BIN METHOD

An intrinsic feature of the Holter bin method is that only a single QT interval will be derived from a given RR interval. In the QT/RR plane this characteristic leads to a plot with a limited number of QT/RR pairs (one per each bin). A thorough discussion on the advantages and problems of this is beyond the scope of this chapter and has been exhaustively covered in literature. Actually, the method itself was initially developed with the purpose of better assessing QT dynamicity, and in particular the QT/RR relationship. The most important and well-accepted findings can be summarized as follows:

• When the inspected period (i.e., the period where the method is applied) is well defined from an autonomic nervous system perspective (e.g., avoiding to mix day and night) the QT/RR relationship is strongly linear with high correlation coefficients *(16,20–22)*.
• The relationship is stronger (i.e., steeper) if we focus on stable heart rate conditions. In other words, mixing stable heart rate and hysteresis periods lead to a different QT/RR relationship *(18)*. Figure 10 show the QT/RR plot from a real case example and are extracted from a 4-h period. In Figure 10a all the beats (n = 19846) were included, whereas in Fig. 10B a 60 s stability period was imposed (n = 7412, i.e., almost two-thirds of total beats were excluded). While remaining in both cases highly linear (r = 0.96), the slope of the stable model was significantly steeper (again in perfect line with the model of Fig. 8).

Assessment of QT dynamicity has been one of the initial focuses of WinAtrec and several works confirming the above statements have been published on the matter, both on healthy subjects *(20,23)* and in pathological populations *(21,22)*.

WORKING WITH RR BIN TEMPLATES: THE SERIAL APPROACH

One of the strongest and most practical opportunities offered by the Holter bin approach is certainly its intrinsic orientation toward serial analysis, i.e., toward the comparison of records taken at different time points.

Indeed, the fact of sorting all the analyzed periods by heart rate and to obtain a single reference waveform for each RR interval bin facilitates the superimposition and quantitative comparison of templates obtained under different conditions during the same recording (e.g., day vs night or comparison between periods with different drug concentrations), or across recordings taken at separate time-matched periods (e.g., baseline vs drug). Thus, it is possible to compare parameters and measurements from ECG waveforms from different periods (the so-called comparison at identical heart rate), without the need to normalize or correct the observations (e.g., the QT intervals) for heart rate changes.

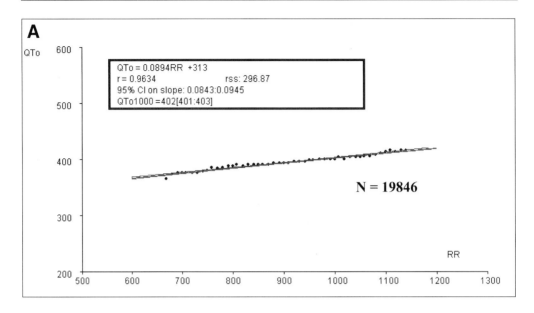

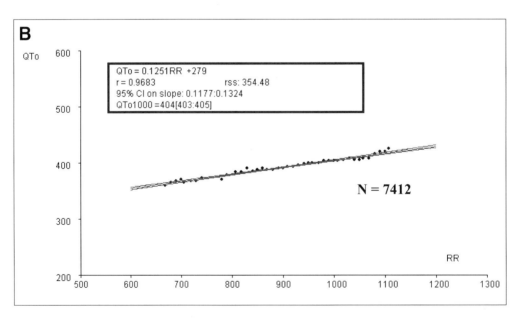

Fig. 10. QT/RR plots using the "RR-1 only" model with all beats included (**A**), and using 60 s stable model (**B**).

An example of this serial analysis comparison at identical heart rate is shown in Fig. 11 where all the templates (i.e., from all the families) of a given RR bin are overlaid. The user can make direct assessment of the QT changes throughout the periods at the same heart rate.

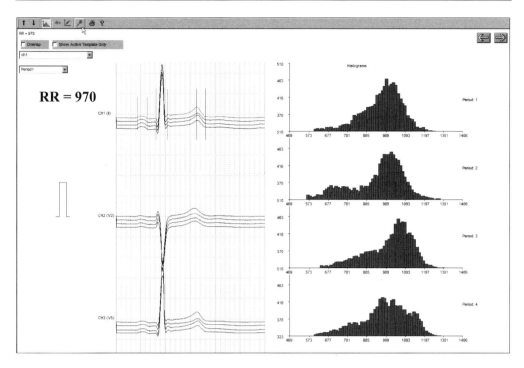

Fig. 11. Example of serial analysis: the five templates overlaid are from five different Holter systems and come from time-matched 4-h periods (12:00–16:00).

In Fig. 11, there are four separate time-matched periods and the overlapped templates are those associated to the bin RR = 970 (which is common to all four periods). A user can jump to the next or previous RR bin by using the arrow buttons in the upper right part of the screen.

The output of this comparison at identical heart rate is a serial table where each measurement variable chosen for the analysis is repeated (columns) over each RR bin (rows). This worksheet organization enables easy derivation of statistics (e.g., delta of variables when comparing).

LIMITATIONS OF HOLTER BIN METHOD AND POSSIBLE EVOLUTION

From a pharmacological point of view, the most relevant limitation of the Holter bin approach is that long enough period of stable conditions (in particular, plasma concentrations) are required to populate an acceptable number of bins. This may become a problem with compounds characterized by a fast response where important periods to be captured (such as the peak concentration period) would be just too short to apply the method. Under these circumstances, a more standard beat-to-beat approach, or even a time-based averaging applied over short durations may be more suitable. WinAtrec can already generate time-based templates and apply the same type of comparative analysis (in particular the serial approach described in the previous section) available from the Holter RR bin method.

The architecture of the method facilitates the extension toward other selection criterion models. For example, the selection of bins could be based on different physical activity periods with the use of an activity status index, considering different sleep conditions *(25)* or focusing over awakening periods *(26)*. The support for these more sophisticated stratification criteria would require additional biomedical sensors that could become available with continuous ECG recording. Alternatively, selection could be driven by the occurrence of specific events, such as arrhythmias or ischemia. As a future direction it may also be interesting to take into account, in addition to the dependence of the actual QT value on a certain number of previous RR intervals, the action of inputs capable to modify QT interval independently of RR interval changes *(27)*.

Lastly, the Holter bin approach should not be seen as a method limited to the analysis of repolarization, but rather as a technique suited for the quantitative analysis of ECGs in the broad sense. Interestingly, the first application of the method in a pharmaceutical clinical trial was for the analysis of QRS intervals.

HOLTER BIN METHOD USAGE IN PHARMACEUTICAL TRIALS

Usage of Holter Bin Method for Assessment of Drug-Induced QT Prolongation in Class III Antiarrhytmic Agent

The objective of this study was to study the influence of heart rate on dofetilide-induced QT prolongation among healthy volunteers *(24)*. Ten healthy volunteers underwent two 24-h ECG recordings, one in the absence of dofetilide and the other after a single oral dose of 0.5 mg dofetilide. Two 4-h periods were defined during the second recording: Dh, which corresponded to stable high concentration of the drug, and D1, which corresponded to low concentration of the drug. Corresponding baseline recording periods, Ch and C1, matched by time with Dh and D1 were selected from the control ECG recording in the absence of dofetilide. Rate-independent changes in QT duration were analyzed using the Holter bin method with a 60 s stable model. The serial comparison approach described in the section entitled Working With RR Bin Templates: The Serial Approach was used both to compare in-between recordings (comparison between different concentration periods) and across recordings (baseline vs drug).

During Dh, dofetilide induced a mean 12% lengthening of ventricular repolarization. Dynamic ECG analysis showed that this prolongation increased as RR intervals became longer, a phenomenon known as reverse-rate dependence. However, QT prolongation persisted at the shortest (600 ms) RR intervals that could be analyzed. More interestingly, during D1 dynamic ECG analysis showed a persistent, although small, effect of dofetilide on both QT prolongation (3%) and reverse-rate dependence of this effect. The study concluded that dofetilide prolongs QT duration, and this class III effect is influenced by heart rate. The Holter bin method was shown to be sensitive to detect small changes during low concentration periods.

Usage of Holter Bin Method for QRS Interval Changes Assessment: The Flecainide Extended Release Study

This study was conducted in the Lariboisiere Hospital between 1999 and 2002 *(7,28)*. The goal of this trial was to inspect pharmacodynamic equivalence of flecainide acetate immediate-release (IR) and controlled-release (CR) formulations as assessed from QRS duration in patients previously treated with the IR formulation. Patients were blindly

Table 2
Results for the Flecainide Extended Release Study

	Flecainide IR (N = 25)	Flecainide CR (N = 23)
Baseline (ms)		
Median (ms)	102.00	100.10
Q1; Q3 (ms)	98.00; 110.38	95.43; 109.92
Week 8		
Median (ms)	103.15	99.00
Q1; Q3 (ms)	98.00; 109.00	94.24; 105.36
% change between baseline and Week 8		
Median	0.04	–0.5
Q1; Q3	–0.88; 2.74	–2.33; 0.92
Hodges–Lehman estimate [95% CI]	0.9 [–0.4; 2.2]	–0.7 [–2.7; 0.2]
Hodges-Lehman estimate of IR–CR [95% CI]	1.6 [–0.1; 3.7]	

Q1, Q3, First and third quartiles; IR, immediate-release formulation; CR, controlled-release formulation; 95% CI, 95% confidence interval.

randomized to the IR group (100 mg b.i.d, n = 25) and to the CR group (200 mg o.d, n = 23), and ECG parameters were measured at baseline and at wk 8 from 24-h Holter.

The Holter bin approach was used to derive QRS interval durations at different classes of constant RR intervals (bin resolution: 10 ms; stability period: 1 min) over the entire 24 h. Using Hodges–Lehmann estimates of the difference between IR and CR groups for percent change in QRS duration between baseline and wk 8 was 1.6% [–0.1; 3.7], indicating that both formulations were pharmacodynamically equivalent. Median QRS values (102 ms vs 100.1 ms at baseline; 103.15 ms vs 99 ms at wk 8) as well as first and third quartiles were very similar in both groups (Table 2). The correlation between QRS duration and RR classes at baseline was highly significant ($p < 0.0001$). The study conclusion was in favor of pharmacologic equivalence between the two different concentration formulations.

Usage of Holter Bin Method for QT Interval Changes Assessment: The Alfusozin Study

This crossover study included two single doses of the α_1-adrenergic receptor blocker alfuzosin, placebo, and a QT-positive control arm (moxifloxacin 400 mg) in 48 healthy subjects (8). Bazett, Fridericia, population-specific (QTcN), and subject-specific (QTcNi) correction formulae were applied to 12-lead ECG recording data. QT1000 intervals (QT at RR = 1000 ms) were obtained from Holter recordings using custom software to perform time-matched, subject-specific, rate-independent QT analysis.

The Holter bin approached was applied to analyze a 4-h period centered around the peak concentration of alfusozin. At the therapeutic dose (10 mg), alfuzosin did not induce any significant change in the QT1000 (+0.1 ms 95%CI[-2.5;2.6]), QTcN (+0.5 ms 95%CI[-2.0;3.0]) or QTcNi intervals (+0.5 ms 95%CI[-2.0;2.9]). Alfuzosin at a supra maximal dose 40 mg induced a small but significant QT1000 increase of 2.9 ms 95%CI[0.3;5.5]. This increase was lower than that induced by moxifloxacin at the therapeutic dose (+ 7.0 ms 95%CI[4.4;9.6]). Alfuzosin 40 mg increased heart rate by 3.7 bpm, concordant with the greater increase observed with the Bazett formula. The direct Holter-based QT interval measurement method is sensitive to detect small drug-induced QT changes. Alfuzosin produced a slight nonsignificative increase in heart rate and did not significantly prolong QT interval at the therapeutic dose. Alfuzosin's effect on QT interval at four times the therapeutic dose was less than 5 ms.

REFERENCES

1. Viskin S. Long QT syndromes and torsade de pointes. Lancet. 1999;354:1625–1633.
2. Crouch MA, Limon L, Cassano AT. Clinical relevance and management of drug-related QT interval prolongation. Pharmacotherapy 2003;23:881–908.
3. Redfern WS, Carlsson L, Davis AS, Lynch WG, MacKenzie I, Palethorpe S, et al. Relationships between preclinical cardiac electrophysiology, clinical QT interval prolongation and torsade de pointes for a broad range of drugs: evidence for a provisional safety margin in drug development. Cardiovasc Res. 2003;58:32–45.
4. Vos MA, van Opstal JM, Leunissen JD, Verduyn SC. Electrophysiologic parameters and predisposing factors in the generation of drug-induced Torsade de Pointes arrhythmias. Pharmacol Ther. 2001;92:109–122.
5. Franz MR, Swerdlow CD, Liem LB, Schaefer J. Cycle length dependence of human action potential duration in vivo: effects of single extrastimuli, sudden sustained rate acceleration and deceleration, and different steady state frequency. J Clin Invest 1988;82:972–979.
6. Viitasalo M, Karjalainen J. QT Intervals at heart rates from 50 to 120 beats per minutes during 24-hour electrocardiographic recordings in 100 healthy men. Circulation 1992;86:1439–1442.
7. Coumel P, Maison-Blanche P, Tarral E, Perier A, Milliez P, Leenhardt A. Pharmacodynamic equivalence of two flecainide acetate formulations in patients with paroxysmal atrial fibrillation by QRS analysis of ambulatory electrocardiogram. J Cardiovasc Pharmacol. 2003;41:771–779.
8. http://www.fda.gov/cder/foi/nda/2003/021287_uroxatral_toc.htm.
9. Badilini F, "The ISHNE Holter Sandard Output File Format", A.N.E., 1998; 3(3):263–266.
10. Zimmermann M, Maison Blanche P, Cauchemez B, Leclercq JF, Coumel P. Determinants of the spontaneous ectopic activity in repetitive monomorphic idiopathic ventricular tachycardias. J Am Coll Cardiol 1986; 7: 1219–1927.
11. Albrecht P, Cohen RJ, Mark RG. A stochastic characterization of chronic ventricular ectopic activity. IEEE Trans Biomed Eng 1988; 35:539–550.
12. Narayanaswamy S, Berbari EJ, Lander P, Lazzara R. Selective beat averaging and spectral analysis of beat intervals to determine the mechanisms of premature ventricular contractions. In Comp in Cardiology Proceedings 1993: 81–84.
13. Romberg D, Patterson H, Theres H, Lander P, Berbari R, Baumann G. Analysis of alternans in late potentials. J Electrocardiol 1995; 28 (suppl): 198–201.
14. Locati E, Maison Blanche P, Dejode P, Cauchemez B, Coumel P. Spontaneous Sequences of onset of Torsade de Pointes in patients with acquired prolonged ventricular repolarization: quantitative analysis of Holter recordings. J Am Coll Cardiol 1995; 25: 1564–1575.
15. Franz MR, Swerdlow CD, Liem LB, Schaefer J. Cycle length dependence of human action potential duration in vivo: effects of single extrastimuli, sudden sustained rate acceleration and deceleration, and different steady-state frequency. J Clin Invest 1988; 82: 972–979.
16. Badilini F, Maison-Blanche P, Childers R, Coumel P. QT interval analysis on ambulatory electrocardiogram recordings: a selective beat averaging approach. Med Biol Eng Comput 1998;36:1–10.
17. Pueyo E, Smetana P, Hnatkova K, Laguna P, Malik M. Time for QT adaptation to RR changes and relation to arrhythmic mortality reduction in amiodarone-treated patients. Proc in Computers in Cardiology 2002; 565–568.
18 Merri M, Farden D, Mottely JG, Titlebaum EL. Sampling frequency of the electrocardiogram for the spectral analysis of heart rate variability. IEEE Trans Biomed Eng 1990; 37: 99–106.
19. Sarma JSM, Venkataraman K, Samant DR, Cadgil U. Hysteresis in the human RR-QT relationship during exercise and recovery. Pace 1987; 10: 485–491
20. Extramiana F, Maison-Blanche P, Badilini F, Pinoteau J, Deseo T, Coumel P. Circadian modulation of QT rate dependence in healthy volunteers. J Electrocardiol 1999;32:33–43.
21. Extramiana F, Neyroud N, Huikuri HV, Koistinen MJ, Coumel P, Maison-Blanche P. QT interval and arrhythmic risk assessment after myocardial infarction. Am J Cardiol 1999;83:266–269.

22. Extramiana F, Maison-Blanche P, Tavernier R, Jordaens L, Leenhardt A, Coumel P. Cardiac effects of chronic oral beta-blockade: lack of agreement between heart rate and QT interval changes. Ann Noninvasive Electrocardiol. 2002;7:379–388.

23. Lande G, Funck-Brentano C, Ghadanfar M, Escande D. Steady-state versus non-steady-state QT-RR relationships in 24-hour Holter recordings. Pacing Clin Electrophysiol. 2000;23:293–302.

24. Lande G, Maison-Blanche P, Fayn J, Ghadanfar M, Coumel P, Funck-Brentano C. Dynamic analysis of dofetilide-induced changes in ventricular repolarization. Clin Pharmacol Ther. 1998;64:312–321.

25. Verrier RL, Stone PH, Pace-Schott EF, Hobson A. Sleep related cardiovascular risk: new home-based monitoring technology for improved diagnosis and therapy. A.N.A. 1997; 2:158–175.

26. Toivonen L, Helenious K, Vitasalo M. Electrocardiographic replarization durino stress from awakening on alarm call. J Am Coll Cardiol 1997;30:774–779.

27. Porta A, Baselli G, Caiani E, Malliani A, Lombardi F, Cerutti S, Quantifying electrocardiogram RT-RR variability interactions, Med. Biol. Eng. Comput., 1998;36: 27–34.

28. Badilini F, Maison-Blanche PM, Ngo P, Coumel P, Leenhardt A. Computerized QRS analysis from 24 hour ambulatory monitoring to assess pharmacodynamic changes. J Electrocardiol. 2003;36 Suppl:109–110.

IV

APPLICATION OF ELECTROCARDIOLOGY IN CLINICAL RESEARCH

10 Fundamentals of ECG Interpretation in Clinical Research and Cardiac Safety Assessment

Ihor Gussak, MD, PhD, Robert Kleiman, MD, and Jeffrey S. Litwin, MD

CONTENTS

INTRODUCTION

The interpretation of ECGs recorded during clinical drug trials shares many similarities with the clinical interpretation of ECGs, but also differs in several significant ways. The fundamental rules for measurement of ECG intervals and overall ECG interpretation (cardiac rhythm, conduction, etc.) are identical whether an ECG is recorded from a patient having chest pain in an emergency room, or from a healthy subject involved in a clinical drug trial. But, the overall purpose of the evaluation of two such ECGs differs greatly.

There are four major areas of clinical utility of electrocardiology in clinical trials:

1. Screening, selection, and enrollment of study participants
2. Assessment and monitoring of cardiac safety of the investigational drug through evaluation of changes in ECG morphology and interval duration measurements (with emphasis on changes in QTc)
3. Assessment of efficacy of the investigational drug or intervention in cardiovascular trials.
4. Indirect benefits to the subject and subject's physician in diagnosing undetected structural or electrical cardiac diseases, as well as detecting progression of cardiac disease (unrelated to the investigational agent) during the course of the clinical trial

From: *Cardiac Safety of Noncardiac Drugs:*
Practical Guidelines for Clinical Research and Drug Development
Edited by: J. Morganroth and I. Gussak © Humana Press Inc., Totowa, NJ

Evaluation of the "safety" of the investigational drug via clinical and electrocardiographic evaluations is the most pivotal part of the global safety strategy during Clinical Research and Drug Development (R&D). High among the concerns during the development and testing of any new drug is the fear of cardiac toxicity, and particularly of lethal cardiac arrhythmias. Many new pharmaceutical agents have been withdrawn from the market, or their use severely restricted to very specific indications as a result of unexpected adverse events, including fatalities. Life-threatening arrhythmias and sudden cardiac death are the most severe clinical manifestations of cardiac toxicity. Of lesser, but still significant concern, are the potential of a medication producing significant bradyarrhythmias caused by sinus node suppression or heart block, or producing new or worsening of pre-existent congestive heart failure.

Recent regulatory developments have thrust cardiac safety to the forefront of clinical development. The effect of new drugs on ventricular repolarization—specifically the prolongation of ventricular repolarization as demonstrated by a prolongation of QTc—is now the most common cause of drug withdrawal from the market and delays in regulatory approval for marketing. This explains why the "safety and tolerability" studies in R&D commonly precede the studies on clinical efficacy of the investigational drug.

The "primary goal" of electrocardiology in R&D is to evaluate the effect of the investigational drugs on the electrical functions of the heart, beginning with early phase clinical studies in healthy volunteers and continuing through to later phase studies that further define drug effects in the target population (where subjects are most susceptible to the cardiac effects of agents and where effect modifiers exist, which may enhance cardiac actions). The "primary objectives" of the cardiac safety assessment in R&D are to determine the drug-associated ECG changes (and their magnitude), and their relationship to the pharmacokinetic/pharmacodynamic peculiarities of the investigational drug. This can only be ascertained based on a statistical analysis of a large ECG database comprising the study and control (placebo) groups (see Chapter 14). The "secondary objectives" of the cardiac safety assessment in R&D are the detection and monitoring of ECG abnormalities identified in any subject who has been exposed to the investigational drug, including placebo. As the result of the very low incidence of life-threatening arrhythmias and/or sudden cardiac death, the detection of lethal ventricular arrhythmias is generally limited to post-marketing surveillance and not a main focus in earlier phases of R&D.

In addition, through the use of inclusion or exclusion criteria, the ECG is widely utilized in the screening/selection/enrollment process of many cardiac and noncardiac clinical trials in order to ensure a homogenous target population. The utility of the ECG as a screening tool in the enrollment of study participants, as well as the specifics of the ECG interpretation in the efficacy assessment of the cardiovascular drugs are not the subjects of this chapter, therefore, will not be discussed.

The main focus of this chapter is to outline the scope of the clinical aspects of ECG interpretation that are pertinent to clinical research, the similarities and dissimilarities compared with those in clinical practice, and to address the utility of the ECG in defining cardiac toxicity of noncardiac investigational drugs.

DRUG-INDUCED CARDIAC TOXICITY AND ITS ECG INDICES

Cardiac Channelopathies

In the assessment of cardiac safety, abnormal drug reactions ("adverse effects") that are related to an investigational drug are usually viewed in the context of toxicity, associated with the potential for development of cardiac electrical instability and sudden cardiac death. In general, the majority of adverse effects are caused by inappropriate drug formulations and excessive exposure to the agent. However, adverse effects may occur even at normal doses ("idiosyncratic drug reactions") and are extremely difficult to predict. An idiosyncratic drug reaction is most commonly due to unexpected differences in drug absorption, distribution, metabolism, excretion, or metabolic drug–drug interaction in genetically predisposed individuals. Individual "pharmacokinetic/pharmacodynamic" peculiarities in metabolic pathways and/or drug targets may explain some of the idiosyncratic drug reactions.

Even with a normal genotype, "drug interactions," with co-administration of an agent that is a potent inhibitor of the enzyme system that normally degrades the drug modulating ion channel function can result in life-threatening arrhythmias (1,2). Because of the narrow therapeutic index, these pharmacokinetic interactions are of extreme importance and are a major safety concern in any drug development.

Advances in basic electrophysiology and genetics have greatly facilitated identification of "cardiac channelopathies," defined as abnormal alteration of ion channel function (3) that can occur due to:

- Primary alteration in ion channels
- Signaling or Ca^{2+} handling proteins
- Structural changes in the myocytes or extracellular matrix
- Changes in activity of the neurohumoral system

In addition to "inherited cardiac channelopathies," caused by genetic mutations or polymorphisms of various ion channels responsible for the normal ventricular repolarization, progression of the underlying disease and cardiac adaptation that occurs with disease ("ionic remodeling") can also modify the electrophysiologic drug actions (including "acquired cardiac channelopathies") (4), as can acquired conduction system disease and acquired intra-atrial or intraventricular conduction inhomogeneities. Depending on the underlying disease and its stage, the electrophysiologic and ionic changes in the heart may vary, resulting in differences in the pathophysiology of arrhythmias and their variability in response to treatments (5).

Commonly, ionic remodeling leads to a "silent" reduction in naturally redundant K^+ channels and reduced levels of expression ("cardiac repolarization reserve"), and therefore, increased sensitivity of the channel to inhibition. This may become manifest only after exposure to a K^+ channel blocker which prolongs repolarization (6,7), (e.g., increased sensitivity to I_{Kr} blockade in patients with congestive heart failure, where a reduction in I_{Ks} occurs in the ventricles) (8), with increased dependence of repolarization on I_{Kr}. Recently, a missense mutation in the KCNE2 subunit of the I_{Kr} channel was identified as the basis for clarithromycin-induced torsades de pointes (TdP) (9). This mutation decreases activation of the K^+ channel, resulting in a threefold increased sensitivity to drug inhibition compared to the wild-type channel (9).

A diminished repolarization reserve that by itself does not cause symptoms (10), may potentially lead to fatal arrhythmias in the presence of various drugs (11). For instance, otherwise innocent polymorphisms in ion channel genes may enhance drug binding and magnify the channel block (12). The prototype for such polymorphisms may be a mutation in KCNE2 that has been reported to be responsible for arrhythmias triggered by an antibiotic (9). Thus, reduction in the repolarizing K^+ current of any cause tends to prolong the QT interval and can set the background for the development of malignant ventricular tachyarrhythmias such as TdP.

A variety of electrophysiological factors determine and modulate the electrocardiographic contour and the duration of ventricular repolarization. Among "intrinsic" cardiac factors, the most important are:

- Shape and duration of the action potentials and their transmural heterogeneity
- Numbers of depolarizing cells participating in generation of the repolarizing currents
- Degree of electrotonic transmission and cell-to-cell coupling conductance
- Primary asynchrony of the repolarization
- Secondary asynchrony of the repolarization due to asynchrony of depolarization.

"Extracardiac" factors include:

- Neurotransmitters
- Electrolytes
- Temperature
- Hormones
- Age
- Gender

One of the most challenging questions in the ECG assessment of the cardiac safety of the investigational drug is differentiation of the drug's effects on the ECG parameters from numerous physiologic as well as pathologic factors, conditions, or diseases (e.g., diurnal variability, gender, aging, ventricular hypertrophy, congestive heart failure, electrolytes imbalance, dehydration). Therefore, planning the requirements for ECGs in global Clinical Development Plan (CDP) can vary significantly between different CDPs as well as from one clinical study to another within the same CDP. The "ECG design" is more universal for the early phases (e.g., thorough Phase 1 QT definitive study, *see* Chapter 11) and less generic in the late phase clinical trials (*see* Chapters 12 and 13). Nevertheless, in addition to clinical and statistical considerations, there are regulatory aspects that are mandatory in designing the unique ECG "support" for global CDPs and specific clinical studies (*see* Chapters 16, 17, 18).

Since both the sensitivity and specificity of the resting surface 12-lead ECG for detecting and quantifying changes in ventricular repolarization are limited, the potential for false-negative and false-positive ECG findings is always of concern. There is no unique or universal ECG marker of abnormal cardiac repolarization that can detect an arrhythmogenic substrate created by an investigational drug. Therefore, "any ECG changes" that are induced by an investigational drug—"even minimal changes" that still fall within the normal range—should be considered as potential surrogate markers of drug-induced cardiac toxicity unless proven otherwise. This is especially relevant for a drug not intended to affect electrophysiological properties of the heart, especially ventricular repolarization. The key concern, of course, is to determine if ECG changes noted during the course of a study are drug related or are coincidental, and due to development or progression of underlying cardiac disease not related to the study medication.

It has been postulated that abnormal cardiac repolarization is potentially arrhythmogenic. Furthermore, the most common electrophysiological mechanisms underlying drug-induced malignant ventricular arrhythmias, such as TdP, are those produced by abnormal cardiac repolarization in general, and specifically by delayed ventricular repolarization.

Among ECG indices of the ventricular repolarization that could be detected on the surface ECG are those that are associated with the "duration" of the QT interval and the "contour" of the ST–T (U) segment. They include:

- Duration of the QT interval and its correction for heart rate effects
- Displacement of the ST segment (e.g., elevation, depression, slope)
- Morphological pattern of T waves (normal, inverted, biphasic, isoelectric) and U waves (normal, abnormal)
- Their combination.

So far, only "QT interval duration corrected for the heart rate (QTc)" is accepted as a surrogate marker of abnormal (delayed) ventricular repolarization, and the only clinically proven ECG index to link to life-threatening ventricular tachyarrhythmias, such as TdP. Furthermore, the standard resting ECG remains the most utilized diagnostic tool in the evaluation of cardiac safety in clinical trials. It should be noted that not all QT-prolonging drugs are proarrhythmic, yet "a majority of proarrhythmic drugs that were removed from the market did demonstrate QT prolongation." The search for other more sensitive and more specific ECG indices to detect a potential arrhythmogenic "signal" of the investigational drug in human are in active progress (see Chapters 3 and 6).

It has been estimated that drug-induced TdP degenerates into ventricular fibrillation in approx 20% of cases and may account for 10–17% of drug-related cardiac fatalities (13). Some individuals are more prone to drug-induced QT prolongation and are at higher risk for TdP than others. In other words, how "acquired" is the drug-induced QT prolongation, or what is the true incidence of latent long QT carriers? It is currently estimated that long QT syndrome (LQTS) mutation carriers are present in 1 of 1000 to 3000 individuals (14). It is noteworthy that 10–15% of patients with drug-associated TdP have been demonstrated to have one of the currently understood variants of congenital long QT disease (14).

BASIC PRINCIPLES OF ECG INTERPRETATION IN CLINICAL RESEARCH AND CARDIAC SAFETY ASSESSMENT

The main principles of ECG interpretation in clinical research and cardiac safety assessment, in particular, are similar to ECG interpretation in clinical practice since they both are based on the same basic electrophysiologic fundamentals underlying clinical electrocardiography. Nevertheless, ECG processing in clinical research that includes (a) obtaining, (b) measuring, (c) interpreting, (d) analyzing, (e) storage, and (f) reporting of the ECG data, has distinct features compared with that in clinical practice. The cornerstone requisites for the ECG processing in R&D are:

- Accuracy, precision, and reproducibility of the interval duration measurements (IDMs). Unlike clinical ECG reading, where small errors in measurement of the RR or QT intervals are not likely to be of any significance at all, precise and accurate measurement of IDMs is absolutely critical to accurately assessing a drug's risk of cardiac toxicity.
- Consistent, uniform, blinded, bias-free, and reproducible ECG interpretation. Whereas these are important in clinical ECG reading, they reach critical importance in ECG interpretation for clinical cardiac safety assessment. Consistent interpretation of ECGs, ideally by a core lab with very small number of highly capable expert electrocardiographers, is necessary to avoid the introduction of "changes" in ECG findings during a study

that are not a result of drug- or disease-induced cardiac abnormalitics, but which arc instead caused by inconsistencies in the ECG interpreter's style. A perfect example is the interpretation of old myocardial infarction. In clinical ECG interpretation, it is common for different ECG readers to differ in calling an old myocardial infarction (MI), a septal MI, an anteroseptal MI, an anterior MI, a possible MI, or other variation. This completely unacceptable when discussing clinical cardiac safety assessment, as it would wreak havoc on the study database. Similarly, the appearance of serial ECGs may vary, and Q wave myocardial infarctions may seem more or less evident on serial ECGs due to subtle changes in lead position, subject positioning or heart rate. When interpreting clinical ECGs, the "appearance," "disappearance," and changes in size of Q waves may lead to inconsistent ECG interpretations, but will generally have no clinical effect. In contrast, the report of a "new" MI that is in fact a result of a slight change in ECG axis or lead positioning can have tremendous consequences during a clinical trial. It is absolutely critical that ECG interpretation in clinical trials be done with unerring consistency and adherence to strict guidelines in order to allow the detection of true drug related effects. We believe that the use of a core ECG laboratory for ECG interpretation is the only mechanism to insure such consistency.

- Full compliance with regulatory guidelines. This is not an issue in clinical ECG interpretation, but is of utmost importance in clinical trials that will lead to submission to governmental agencies.
- Active interaction with clinical sites and sponsor. When interpreting ECGs for clinical purposes, a life threatening new finding may need to be reported to a physician just a few feet or rooms away. In contrast, clinical trials may enroll sites in dozens of countries and time zones. Because many of these sites will be outpatient clinics in specialties other than cardiology, the finding of a new, potentially serious ECG abnormality must prompt notification of the site and possibly the sponsor, even though this may involve multiple continents, time zones, and languages.

Similar to the ECG evaluation in a clinic, "qualitative" interpretation of the rest single 12-lead ECG in clinical research is based on evaluation of: (a) interval ranges, (b) heart rate/rhythm and its irregularities, and (c) pattern/shape of the waveforms. Since the primary goal of cardiac safety in R&D is to detect drug-induced ECG changes on the heart and to differentiate the "cardiotoxic signal" from the effects of all other modifying factors, both the "individual spontaneous ECG variability" (e.g., QTc variability, *see* Chapter 9) and the "quantitative ECG analysis" (assessment of the magnitude of ECG changes in their serial comparison) are subjects of great scrutiny. In most clinical trials, IDM-based ECG abnormalities (e.g., atrio-ventricular delay, QT prolongation, bradycardia, tachycardia) and abnormal ECG changes (e.g., progressive deterioration of conduction within the left bundle branch) are determined by the study protocol and defined as those that are above or below predefined normal limits. ECG exclusion criteria and protocol alerts are also predefined by the study protocol and often "adjusted" to the clinical characteristics of the target population (e.g., age, gender, underlying diseases) and modified by nonclinical factors (e.g., statistical power to detect ECG "signal").

Although the main focus in ECG interpretation in clinical research is to detect true drug-induced ECG changes, there are indirect benefits to the individual subject participating in a clinical trial. They benefits include:

- Diagnosis of previously undetected structural heart disease, conduction system diseases, and channelopathies (e.g., LQTS, WPW syndrome, Brugada syndrome)

- Detection of ECG changes during the course of the study that may have clinical benefits for the subject (though completely unrelated to the study medication)
- Notification to the clinical site and sponsor's safety authorities about worrisome findings

ECG interpretation in clinical research has always been challenged by various dilemmas, such as a lack of consensus on:

- Strictly defined criteria for "normal" ECG and their normal ranges under various physiologic factors/conditions (e.g., age, gender, temperature)
- Clinical relevance of different ECG abnormalities/changes (e.g., progressive prolongation of the abnormally wide QRS complex in either the left or right bundle branch block, and the clinical relevance in healthy volunteers versus a population with coronary artery disease)
- ECG changes in serial ECG comparisons that are minimal but yet sufficient enough to "cross" an arbitrary chosen threshold (e.g., a normal ECG with a PR interval duration of 199 ms "becomes" abnormal if the PR interval measures 201 ms on the next ECG, resulting in the report of "deterioration").

In R&D, the definitions of interval related ECG abnormalities (such as the definitions of sinus bradycardia and sinus tachycardia, or of first-degree heart block) are often modified and "tailored" to the specific needs of the CDP or particular clinical trial in order to satisfy the requirements of sensitivity and the specificity of the ECG "signal" in the particular study or CDP (e.g., heart rate ranges in pediatric studies). Consequently, ECG "criteria for abnormal" could vary from one study to another, from one CDP to another, and from one sponsor to another. Thus, it is very unlikely that those additional ECG "standards" would become "universal" ECG standards and, therefore, positively impact "uniformity" of ECG interpretation. At the same time, minimizing inconsistencies and maximizing uniformity in ECG interpretation in clinical trials is a primary task in the clinical research community, and an active search for the *gold* ECG standards is warranted.

Normal ECG vs Abnormal ECG

Since the majority of participants in the early phases of R&D are healthy volunteers, the definition of both the "normal" ECG and its "normal" ranges has always been of paramount importance and an area of great debate in clinical electrocardiology. Traditionally, "normal" ECG in clinical practice has been defined on the basis of "normal is . . . anything that is not abnormal." Such a simplistic and somewhat dubious "strategy" in identification and classification of the abnormal ECG findings is often based on arbitrary chosen limits of normal and does not fully satisfy scientific standards in clinical research. Different approaches and procedures for deriving upper and lower normal limits for different ECG parameters and characteristics stratified by gender and age have been proposed in clinical research, based on a large ECG database of normal population.

In the normal heart, individual morphological patterns of the ECG waves and their durations are determined by basic intrinsic electrophysiological properties of the heart. The magnitude of changes varies between individuals ("inter-individual normal ranges") and within the same individual ("intra-individual normal ranges") dependent upon his/her health conditions, yet within predictable ranges. Age, gender, physical and emotional activities, temperature, and different circadian rhythms (e.g., diurnal, annual) are among the major modifying factors of ECG measurements. As an example, Figs. 1, 2, and 3 provide

A

Age and Gender Differences in J-Point Measurements in Leads V1-V2 (measurements are mean μV ± 1 SD)

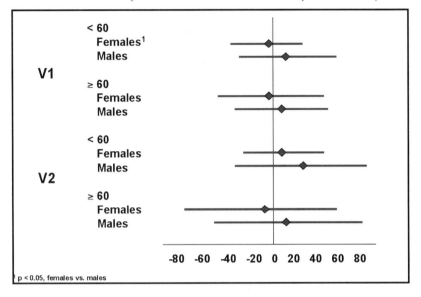

Age and Gender Differences in J-Point Measurements in Leads V3-V4 (measurements are mean μV ± 1 SD)

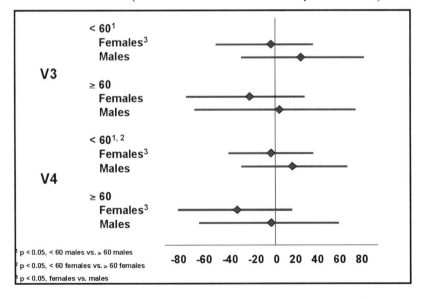

Fig. 1. Differences in ST-segment displacements (J point and J_{80} in leads V1–V4) between men and women in two age groups. Of note: (**A**) the elevations of the J and J_{80} points were most pronounced in younger males with a tendency toward decreasing their magnitude with age, (**B**) in

B

Age and Gender Differences in J_{80}-Point Measurements in Leads V1-V2 (measurements are mean μV ± 1 SD)

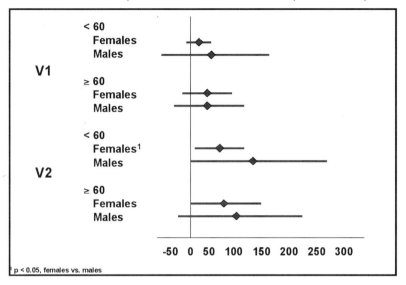

Age and Gender Differences in J_{80}-Point Measurements in Leads V3-V4 (measurements are mean μV ± 1 SD)

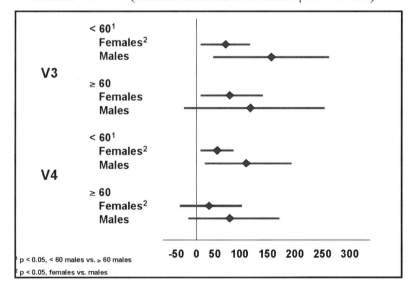

contrast, the J points in females were predominantly negative, with a significantly faster positive ST-segment slope compared with men (the latter decreased with age).

Age and Gender Differences in T-Wave Amplitudes
(measurements are mean μV ± 1 SD)

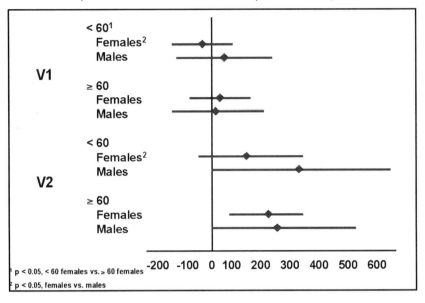

Age and Gender Differences in T-Wave Amplitudes
(measurements are mean μV ± 1 SD)

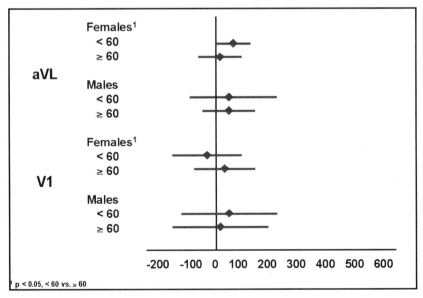

Fig. 2. Differences in T wave amplitude between men and women in two age groups. Of note: (A) in patients under age 60, T wave amplitudes in leads V1–V2 were smaller in females under 60 than in males, (B) the overall T wave amplitudes decreased in leads I, II, aVL, and V1 in females over age 60, (C) no statistically significant differences were noted in T wave area (in different leads) between men and women in different age groups (not shown).

Age and Gender Differences in QT Interval Duration
(msec ± 1 SD)

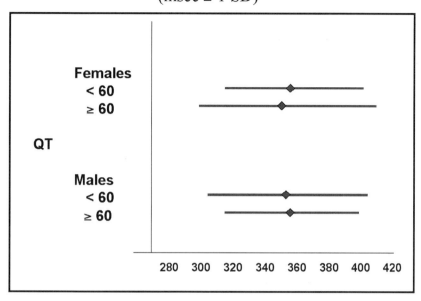

Age and Gender Differences in QTc Interval Duration
(msec ± 1 SD)

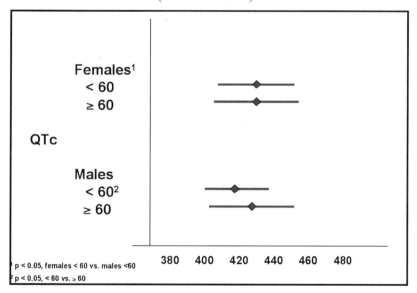

Fig. 3. Differences in QT and QTc between men and women in two age groups. Of note: (A) no statistically significant differences were found between any group with respect to the ventricular rate and QT interval, (B) QTc, however, was found to be shorter in young men than in young women, and increase with aging in men.

data on the age and the gender-determined changes of the different ECG indices of ventricular repolarization in the normal population. Of note, (a) all measurements were extracted from computerized ECG (12SL, GE-Marquette) and include J, J_{80} points (mV), T wave amplitude (mV), ventricular heart rate (bpm), QT and QTc (by Bazett), and (b) the patient population consists of 450 otherwise healthy subjects (34 women and 61 men younger than 60 yr, and 55 women and 300 men older than 60 yr) with clinically excluded cardiovascular abnormalities or diseases. In brief, these data demonstrate (a) significant physiological age- and gender-related ST–T and QTc differences in an otherwise healthy population, and (b) significant longitudinal age trends in ECG intervals (especially in men). This demonstrates that the recognition of baseline ECG changes independent of cardiac disease but associated with aging and gender is pivotal in serial rest ECG evaluation.

"Clinical relevance" of abnormal ECG findings is another area of great confusion, inconsistency, and debate. First, it is very difficult or even impossible to determine the clinical relevance of various ECG abnormalities or ECG changes, solely based on a single rest ECG tracing or even serial ECG comparisons. Clinical relevance is just that—a "clinical" decision, not a decision made in the vacuum or based interpreting a solitary piece of evidence. The clinical relevance of a particular finding must be judged in the context of the patient's prior history, current symptoms, and physical findings. Second, the clinical significance of different ECG abnormalities/changes is different in diverse populations. For instance,

- Right bundle branch block (RBBB) in an otherwise healthy individual could be considered a relatively "benign" ECG finding, whereas the same ECG abnormality in patients with an acute myocardial infarction is considered an independent mortality factor.
- A change in the heart rate from 60 bpm to 90 bpm (both within the normal range) may be clinically more important than a change in the heart rate from 99 bpm to 101 bpm ("crossing" the arbitrary limit from normal sinus rhythm to sinus tachycardia).
- Flat T waves are generally not felt to be clinically significant, but if the patient is experiencing chest pain at the time the T waves become flat that would be clinically significant. The core lab would be blinded to any patient symptoms and site reliance on a core laboratory determination that this finding was not significant could have an adverse effect on patient care.

Therefore, it is not appropriate for an ECG core laboratory to determine clinical relevance, as the core laboratory is blinded to all clinical information. If a determination of the clinical relevance of any particular ECG abnormality is desired, the investigator at the study site should determine this, as "clinical" information is needed to perform this assessment.

In most cases, "clinically relevant or noteworthy ECG abnormalities or ECG changes" in R&D are defined as those that require medical attention as to prognosis or treatment (e.g., new onset atrial fibrillation or flutter). Clinically noteworthy ECG abnormalities or ECG changes that are significant enough to initiate an active medical monitoring/follow-up and/or required changes in the subject's management are classified as "medical *(ECG)* alerts" (e.g., acute myocardial infarction). Such findings warrant expedited notification of all appropriate medical authorities (including both on site investigators and safety officers) identified by each study protocol. When faced with these "alerts" sites should follow normal and prudent procedures to ensure patient safety, and they should not delay appropriate care due to the fact that the patient is in a clinical trial.

"Comparison" between serial ECGs recorded during a trial is another area of contention and inconsistency. There is little agreement on which (or how many) ECGs should serve as the baseline comparator for a study, or whether comparisons should be made to baseline ECGs or to subsequent ECGs recorded during a trial. In addition, when multiple baselines are collected it is possible that some may have different morphology determinations. This prompts the question as to which of the baseline ECGs is the true comparator since morphologies, unlike interval duration measurements, cannot be combined.

Slight changes in a measurement can result in an ECG crossing an arbitrarily defined boundary and, as in the preceding example, a "deterioration" from normal sinus rhythm to sinus tachycardia. A slight increase in the QRS duration may result in a "deterioration" from incomplete Left bundle branch block (LBBB) to complete LBBB, and a slight increase in the PR interval may result in the appearance of first degree AV block and a "deterioration" in conduction. These rule related "deteriorations" or "improvements" do not aid the clinical site, the subject or the collection of the study data, and may simply result in confusion, added expense and delays.

Another major difficulty arises when ECGs are delivered to the ECG core laboratory out of sequence. If the comparator ECG is not available when later ECGs are evaluated, a comparison cannot be made. If the comparator ECG subsequently becomes available, the interpretation of all subsequent ECGs will need to be revised, resulting in added expense, delay and potential for errors.

For these reasons we do not recommend to include clinical relevance and comparisons in ECG interpretations during clinical trials. Instead, we prefer to rely upon the use of clinical alert criteria, which allow for notification of site and sponsor whenever a concern for subject safety arises.

Regulatory Electrocardiograph Guidance and Role of Physician Interpreter in Core ECG Laboratory

The Regulatory ECG Guidance is designed to provide comprehensive, balanced, and consistent cardiac safety evaluation to further improve early identification of drugs that might have pro-arrhythmic properties (*see* Chapters 17 and 18 for details). To a greater degree than ever before, the Regulatory ECG Imperative presents very specific guidance to the pharmaceutical industry on cardiac safety data collection, analysis, and distribution.

These guidelines rely on a combination of "manual/visual" evaluation of QT duration and increasingly on digital ECG signal-processing. ECGs performed in a definitive QT study are to be recorded and stored "digitally;" however, interpretation of digital waveforms or printed-paper records produced by the digital storage system are both permitted. The Regulatory ECG Imperative also includes technical standards referenced in the guidance (more detailed information can be find on the FDA official website, http://www.fda.gov/cder/guidance/index.htm). These standards apply to the manner in which digital ECG waveforms and the associated annotations created during the manual measurement process using onscreen calipers are to be submitted for regulatory review. Submission of annotated waveforms is required for all definitive QT trials, and other trials in a program as specified through collaboration with the appropriate therapeutic group within the target regulatory agency.

There are several benefits to digital ECG data acquisition for cardiac safety assessment using either standard resting ECG recordings or 24-h digital 12-lead Holter ECG recordings (that allow access to multiple ECG waveforms) *(15)*, Specifically, digital Holter recordings offer continuous access to monitor digital ECG data allows for the analysis of:

- Dose-dependent effects of a tested drug (and possible arrhythmias)
- Assessment of adaptation of QT interval to a wide spectrum of changing heart rates, including night hours
- Analysis of dynamic features of repolarization, including QT–RR relationship (regression analysis, slope), QT interval or repolarization morphology variability, or T wave alternans
- Application of novel algorithms for repolarization analyses including automatic area-based approaches or T wave loop morphology

Holter-derived digital ECG data acquisition provides the ability to reassess data and acquire ECGs at additional time points if necessary (e.g., to reassess pharmacokinetic issues related to metabolites or to increase statistical power). Holter digital ECG acquisition also provides the opportunity to improve "quality control" and "quality assurance" of ECG analysis (*see* Chapter 17), and allows for more comprehensive auditing (review) of ECG interpretation. In particular, regulatory authorities are interested in reviewing ECG recordings acquired during drug testing with additional access to interpreter's annotation. Access to digital ECG recordings will provide a better opportunity to perform direct comparisons of repolarization duration and morphology when recorded off and on tested drug.

The majority of currently used ECG machines record the ECG signal in digital format, though the format of data acquisition and storage is proprietary and varies among manufacturers. Similarly, digital acquisition of long-term digital 12-lead Holter recordings may replace analog recordings, but again, the format of digital ECG data files varies among manufacturers of digital Holter systems. For the above reasons, there is a need to develop a uniform standard for ECG/Holter output files allowing universal access to acquired data.

FUTURE DIRECTIONS

In conclusion, the following areas of the clinical and experimental sciences are identified as subjects of intensifying efforts in clinical research:

1. Basic cellular, molecular, and pharmacologic mechanisms underlying the drug-induced electrical instability of the heart
2. Clinical validity and prognostic value of various ECG indices of the drug-induced proarrhythmic toxicity
3. Risk factors and pre-existing cardiac abnormalities influencing the likelihood of the fatal iatrogenic arrhythmias

REFERENCES

1. Legebrve RA, Van Peer A, Woestenborghs R. Influence of itraconazole on the pharmacokinetics and electrocardiographic effect of astemizole. Br J Clin Pharmacol 1997;43:319–322.
2. Neuvonen PJ, Kantola T, Kivisto KT. Simvastatin but not pravastatin is very susceptible to interaction with the CYP3A4 inhibitor itraconazole. Clin Pharmacol Ther 1998.63:332–341.
3. Jahangir A, Terzic A, Shen W-K. Antiarrhythmic Drugs, Repolarization, and Future Direction. In Cardiac Repolarization: Bridging Basic and Clinical Science. Gussak I, Antzelevitch C, Hammil SC, Shen W-K, Bjerregaard P, eds. Humana Press: Totowa, NJ 2003.

4. Nattel S. Effects of ionic remodeling on cardiac antiarrhythmic drug actions. J Cardiovasc Pharmacol 2001;38:809–811.

5. Nattel S. New ideas about atrial fibrillation 50 years on. Nature 2002;415:219–26.

6. Roden DM. Pharmacogenetics and drug-induced arrhythmias. Cardiovasc Res 2001;50, 224–231.

7. Roden DM, Spooner PM. Inherited long QT syndromes: a paradigm for understanding arrhythmogenesis. J Cardiovasc Electrophysiol 1999;10:1664–1683.

8. Nattel S, Li DS. Ionic remodeling in the heart—Pathophysiological significance and new therapeutic opportunities for atrial fibrillation. Circ Res 2000;87:440–447.

9. Abbott GW, Sesti F, Splawski I, Buck ME, Lehmann MH, Timothy KW, Keating MT, Goldstein SA. MiRP1 forms IKr potassium channels with HERG and is associated with cardiac arrhythmia. Cell 1999;97:175–187.

10. Marban E. Cardiac channelopathies. Nature 10;415:213–218, 2002

11. Roden DM, Spooner PM. Inherited long QT syndromes: a paradigm for understanding arrhythmogenesis. J Cardiovasc Electrophysiol 1999;10:1664–1683.

12. Roden DM. Pharmacogenetics and drug-induced arrhythmias. Cardiovasc Res 50, 224–231.

13. Shah RR. Drug-induced prolongation of the QT interval: why the regulatory concern? Fundam Clin Pharmacol 2002;16:119–124.

14. Yang P, Kanki H, Drolet B, Yang T, Wei J, Viswanathan PC, Hohnloser SH, et al. Allelic variants in long-QT disease genes in patients with drug-associated torsades de pointes. Circulation 2002;105:1943–1948.

15. Morganroth J. Focus on issues in measuring and interpreting changes in the QTc interval duration. Eur Heart J 2001;3 (Suppl K): K105–K111.

11

Design and Conduct of the Thorough Phase I ECG Trial for New Bioactive Drugs

Joel Morganroth, MD

CONTENTS

BACKGROUND

Drug-induced prolongation of the QTc interval, when excessive and in conjunction with the right risk factors, can degenerate into torsades de pointes (TdP), a frequently fatal form of polymorphic ventricular tachycardia. While it is clear that the QT interval on the electrocardiogram (ECG) may not be highly correlated with the risk of TdP, change in the QTc duration is the one relied upon by drug developers and regulatory authorities as the best predictor of a new drug's cardiac safety. As commented on by Dr. Robert Temple from the Food and Drug Administration (FDA) in an FDA co-sponsored public meeting in Shady Grove, MD, in January 2003, if a drug prolongs the QT interval this effect is the commonest cause of new drug development delays, disapprovals, or removal from the market. Such drugs have come from many different therapeutic groups and from many different, related, and unrelated chemical structures. Some examples include the antihistamine terfenadine; the antibiotic grepafloxacin; the antispasmodic terodiline; the

From: *Cardiac Safety of Noncardiac Drugs:*
Practical Guidelines for Clinical Research and Drug Development
Edited by: J. Morganroth and I. Gussak © Humana Press Inc., Totowa, NJ

calcium channel blocker lidoflazine; the atypical antipsychotic sertindole; the opioid levomethadyl; and the gastric prokinetic agent cisapride.

In March 2002, the Cardio-Renal Division of the FDA developed the concept of defining a drug's effect on the standard ECG from a single clinical research trial in a robust, intense, or thorough manner so that the results would be "definitive." The author believes that the motivation for this new concept was to prevent the public's exposure to drugs with uncertain or unknown effects on the ECG (with particular focus on cardiac repolarization as determined by the QTc interval duration from the standard scalar ECG). Specific details of this "intensive or definitive ECG Trial" first appeared in the November 2002 FDA–Health Canada ECG concept paper (1) entitled, "The Clinical Evaluation Of QT/QTc Interval Prolongation And Proarrhythmic Potential For Non-Antiarrhythmic Drugs." The adjectives that have been used to characterize this trial, intensive, definitive, and thorough are comparable, but since no single trial should be viewed as 100% definitive the best descriptor for now is "Thorough ECG Trial" as used by the International Committee on Harmonization (ICH) in their current discussions on this topic. The emphasis of this chapter does not include any changes under consideration since these deliberations are still ongoing and not in the public domain, and final international guidance is likely to still respect local regulatory concepts.

The FDA Concept paper is one in a series of regulatory guidances for cardiac safety determination starting first with the Committee for Proprietary Medicinal Products (CPMP) from Europe in 1997. As these ECG guidances have evolved, they have become more detailed or "recipe-like" on how clinical research should be conducted to determine cardiac safety as defined from drug induced changes in the surface ECG (2,3). Obviously, it is important in defining the cardiac safety of drugs to also understand their agent's effect on cardiac conduction (PR and QRS interval duration) and morphology (especially the T–U complex) as well as non-ECG derived effects on cardiac function and arrhythmogenic or proarrhythmic potential from adverse cardiac event reports.

Lack of observing TdP or its other manifestations such as syncope in a typically sized 5000 patient marketing application, is not reassuring that a drug has no cardiac liability since the 95% confidence interval for TdP would range from 0 to 1 in 1600, and 1/1600 is a very high event rate for this life threatening adverse event when millions of patients may be exposed in the market following its approval and routine clinical use. Post-marketing surveillance can help in detecting TdP but underreporting and ascribing TdP solely to underlying risks, such as heart disease limits this approach. Thus, the QTc interval duration in clinical development is the best, albeit flawed, surrogate marker available today.

The rational for the selection of which drugs when in development and how to conduct the Thorough ECG Trial is the purpose of this chapter. The principles involved in the analysis of the resultant data from the trial and their interpretation for regulatory decisions will also be addressed. Since this is a new type of trial in drug development, it is likely that many of the recommendations suggested herein will be modified as further experience is gained.

WHICH DRUGS SHOULD HAVE A DEFINITIVE ELECTROCARDIOGRAPH TRIAL? WHEN IN DEVELOPMENT SHOULD THE TRIAL BE CONDUCTED?

The FDA–Health Canada Concept paper (1) states that the need to understand precisely the ECG effects of drugs applies to all new bioactive agents, as well as any marketed drugs that are brought back to the agency for approval of new formulations, dosage regimens, indications, or target populations, especially relevant when there is higher exposure to the agent or a broader market application or inclusion of higher medical risk subjects. The author has personally seen requests from the FDA for a Thorough ECG Trial for biologics, orphan drugs, and drugs derived from naturally occurring vitamins or hormones. It seems likely that there will be cases when drugs are from a therapeutic class without a history of TdP or QTc effects, or when stereoisomers of known drugs are evaluated when a Thorough ECG Trial may not be required. This is likely to be on a case-by-case basis as defined by individual therapeutic divisions and the general policy may change with time.

The Concept paper *(1)* further points out the recommendation to record, process, and store ECGs digitally. The use of a central or core analysis laboratory, as has been the standard for hematology and chemistry analyses, will reduce the great variability of methods of analyzing ECGs reducing noise in the ECG data. Paper ECGs are acceptable only when digital ECGs are not practical. Paper ECGs can be digitized and processed similarly to digitally recorded tracings if desired to harmonize an ECG database. It is also clear from all the three ECG regulatory guidance documents that ECG interval durations should be measured by a manual method using either a digitizing board, or with electronic calipers applied manually to electronic digital ECG wave forms on screen *(4)*. Employing automated ECG interval duration measurements may provide lower variability even though the measurements may be less accurate, and further comparisons between these two methods in Thorough ECG Trial's will be illuminating.

When in the course of drug development should a sponsor conduct a Thorough ECG Trial depends on many scientific, regulatory, and sometimes drug development process issues. Scientifically, one should not conduct this trial until there is a clear understanding of the drug's pharmacokinetic profile, metabolism, nature of metabolites (if any), and a good estimate of a clinically effective dose. Thus, the earliest time to conduct such a trial would be usually at the end of phase I or early phase II. Sponsors may want to be certain of the ECG effects or cardiac safety liability of their new drug before launching a very costly phase III set of trials in which large numbers of patients will be exposed, and thus potentially be placed at risk if the ECG effects of the drug are not fully delineated. For some compounds, however, the clinically useful dose(s) may not be known until a phase III trial, and thus the Thorough ECG Trial will not be conducted until phase III. Of course, recently many Thorough ECG Trial are being conducted late in phase III (since the policy and concept for such a trial is new) or in some cases after the NDA has been filed (examples include Vardenafil, [Bayer, and GSK] and Alfusozin [Sanofi], which were publicly addressed at a joint Genitourinary and Cardio-Renal Advisory Committee Meeting at the FDA on May 29, 2003).

Certain new agents cannot be investigated in a Thorough ECG Trial. The primary example is drugs that are cytotoxic, such as in the oncology therapeutic area where their administration to normal volunteers (see later) is neither ethical nor can control groups be employed.

Another example of drugs not suited for a Thorough ECG Trial would be the antipsychotic agents that produce intolerable side effects at a far lower dose in healthy volunteers than the dose that will be employed in the target patient population. In such cases, the Thorough ECG Trial should be undertaken in the patient population if its value can be bolstered by using higher than usual clinical doses when feasible, and additional treatment arms employing therapeutic agents within the same class that have at least market experience or known ECG effects.

DESIGNING THE TRIAL: PHARMACOLOGICAL PRINCIPLES

Single vs Multiple Dosing Designs

Since the objective of the Thorough ECG Trial is to define the effect of a treatment on ECG parameters, that treatment must be given in a manner that reflects the extent of exposure of parent compound and its metabolites in the target population when the drug is in clinical use. If the pharmacokinetics of a drug following a single dose and at steady-state following multiple doses is essentially identical, then a single dose trial can be conducted. If there is any evidence of accumulation of parent or if the metabolites are not well characterized and the drug is to be used in a multiple dose manner for therapy, it seems logical that only a multiple dose study design to steady-state would be appropriate. Generally, any drug that is used for chronic therapy or at least for multiple days is likely to need a multiple dose trial design unless the sponsor has definitive data to show that there is no difference in exposure of parent/metabolites after such multiple dosing vs a single dose. The only advantage of a single dose in the Thorough ECG Trial is to reduce the duration of the trial (decreases also any time effects on ECG intervals) and the cost of conducting the trial, and therefore when in doubt a multiple dose design should be employed.

Rationale for and Selection of the Supratherapeutic Dose Treatment Arm and the Study Population

From a clinical point of view, it seems more meaningful to conduct the Thorough ECG Trial in the population that is the target of the drug's use; however, selecting patients with clinical diseases or older apparently healthy people will make the ECG results in the Thorough ECG Trial nondefinitive. This is because patients who have multiple degrees of disease intensity often have multiple comorbidities and take different concomitant medications, the balancing of all these factors that can effect the duration of the QTc interval, would require too large a sample size and too difficult a recruitment to make the ECG trial thorough. Because the effect of drugs on cardiac intervals will occur in healthy as well as abnormal hearts or other clinical conditions, it is more effective to select as the study population a homogeneous disease and drug-free group of healthy volunteer men and women from age 18–45 yr. Above this age range, the concern for subclinical heart and other disease and use of concomitant medications increases greatly. The individuals in a Thorough ECG Trial Trial should have no variables that will influence the ECG parameters, and thus the study population for the Thorough ECG Trial should be healthy young volunteers. However, to mimic the new drug's interaction with any effect modifiers that might be present in the target population (e.g., heart disease, metabolic abnormalities, concomitant drug metabolic inhibitors, or abnormal metabolism) a supratherapeutic dose treatment arm in the healthy volunteers must be employed. It is anticipated that this supratherapeutic dose given to healthy volunteers will mimic the worst-case effects (save for a frank overdose) of the drug in the target population, allowing the Thorough ECG Trial study to be conducted in healthy volunteers rather than in the target population.

The selection of the supratherapeutic dose is one of the most critical features in defining whether the Thorough ECG Trial was adequately designed. The use of a combination of metabolic inhibitors with the new agent to achieve a supratherapeutic dose equivalent: should usually be avoided since such inhibitors (particularly drugs like ketoconazole) may affect ECG intervals (QTc duration) themselves, making study design and data analysis issues quite complex. Many times the sponsor is reluctant to try a higher dose than has been used before in the development program, but without a properly selected supratherapeutic dose the Thorough ECG Trial loses its objective to define "definitively" the ECG effects of the new agent. The selection of the supratherapeutic dose should be modeled based on the known pharmacologic properties of the drug and how the extent of exposure will change when it is taken by a patient who has effect modifiers, with special attention to a higher than anticipated dose (patient becomes confused and takes more pills then prescribed), metabolic inhibitors that magnify the extent of exposure as often defined from interaction trials, organ dysfunction that results in drug accumulation, presence of heart disease (mean QTc duration in this population is longer by about 10–20 ms) (5), and metabolic conditions such as hypokalemia. Once this modeling has identified the maximum extent of exposure then the dose that provides the equivalent exposure is the best definition of the supratherapeutic dose. Alternatively, the magnitude of this supratherapeutic dose can be just below the maximum tolerated dose that has been defined in the typical multiple ascending phase I dose trial, if, in fact, the intolerability was clinically significant and that a maximum toleration was properly obtained. As a rough guideline, the minimal clinical dose compared to the supratherapeutic dose is at least 3–5× apart and for certain agents such as antihistamines or antibiotics may be over 10× apart.

Need for and Timing of Pharmacokinetic Samples

Generally, to adequately characterize a new drug its dose–response or concentration response relationship for QTc prolongation should be provided using a sufficient number of ECGs, paired with the highest levels of drug concentration that may occur in the target population under the potential maximum extent of exposure. For all clinical trial phases, collection of plasma samples around the time of the ECG measurement is encouraged so as to permit an exploration of these relationships. In phase I and II clinical trials, a range of dose groups are studied allowing the collection of this data. The Thorough ECG Trial provides an opportunity to further characterize this relationship because the use of the supratherapeutic dose will at least add to or often provide the highest concentration of drug by which to evaluate ECG interval changes. Important considerations in characterizing the dose– or concentration–response relationship include:

- the maximal degree of the QTc prolongation
- the steepness of the slope between QTc prolongation and dose–concentration
- the relationship between the threshold dose for QTc prolongation and the therapeutic dose range, linearity or nonlinearity of the dose–concentration-effect dependency, and the time course of QTc prolongation in relation to plasma levels

To be certain that all treatment arms in the Thorough ECG Trial are subjected to the same experimental conditions, all subjects in the trial should have pharmacokinetic blood samples obtained. Usually only the blood samples in the supratherapeutic new drug arm are actually analyzed for this analysis, because the concentrations of the lower dose of the new drug or the positive control are not of much value in defining the concentration response relationship for ECG effects of the new agent. If a QTc effect of the agent is identified, then analyzing all paired ECG-plasma samples of drug can be used to identify perhaps the lowest drug concentration associated with a QTc effect.

CLINICAL TRIAL DESIGN ISSUES: ELECTROCARDIOGRAPHIC DATA ISSUES

Value of HR, PR, QRS, and Morphological Considerations

While the primary focus of most concern with regard to cardiac safety is the effect on cardiac repolarization (QTc interval), it is important not to forget that the standard ECG provides additional information that must also be analyzed and considered. Drugs that affect heart rate (HR) have potential implications whether the slow the rate (e.g., dizziness or syncope) or increase the rate (e.g., inducing cardiac ischemia). Cardiac conduction as manifested by the PR interval (atrio-ventricular [AV] conduction) and QRS interval (intraventricular conduction) should be carefully considered, because drugs that affect calcium and sodium channels may show such effects by prolonging these intervals. Induction of bradyarrhythmias from effects on AV conduction and increases in proarrhythmic responses from sodium channel blockade (established for example for class IC antiarrhythmic drugs) has important safety implications. Morphological changes in the ECG waveforms may be signals of myocardial cell integrity disturbance by a new drug, and the effects on T–U wave complexes may be an important determinant of an affect on cardiac repolarization.

ELIMINATION OF SOURCES OF VARIABILITY

The basic tenet of the Thorough ECG Trial is that it is as "definitive" as possible, meaning that all sources of variability in ECG intervals (especially the QTc duration) have been controlled so that any ECG effects observed in the trial will solely (or almost so) be as a result of the new agent under study. The sources of variability in QTc duration are important to identify. First, it has been well established that the QTc duration is subjected to a large degree of spontaneous variability averaging 75 ms over a day *(6)*. This fact alone emphasizes why it is difficult in routine phase I or II-III trials to be confident about QTc or ECG drug effects, especially when there are limitations in sample size, frequency of ECGs, and/or use of control groups. Hence, the need for a targeted phase I Thorough ECG Trial. To reduce the spontaneous variability, attention must be given to basic clinical trial design issues such as sample size, frequency of measurements taken (number of ECGs at baseline and on therapy), accuracy of the ECG interval durations (centrally validated and consistent manual determinations), homogeneity of the study population (healthy volunteers, half of whom should be females), controls for environmental stresses (activity, food, diurnal effects, time effects, etc.), and especially the effect of heart rate on QT duration (*see also* Chapter 14.)

QT vs QTc and How to Derive a QTc

The QT interval duration varies inversely with the magnitude of the heart rate (as the heart rate slows, the QT increases), and therefore it is very important to correct the measured QT interval duration for heart to derive the ECG interval of interest—the corrected QT interval or QTc. The Bazett correction formula (QTcB = QT/square root of the RR interval in seconds), used almost exclusively in clinical practice, overcorrects at elevated heart rates and under corrects at rates below 60. Since 1999, in drug development the Fridericia formula (QTcF = QT/cube root of the RR interval in seconds) has been used widely because this correction tends to be more resistant to the effects of heart rate changes. In the experience of this author, there is no advantage of linear regression QTc correction formulae over the exponent approach. ECG analyses in individuals will generally provide these two fixed exponent QTc durations, and for individual clinical trials data analysis using the Fridericia correction which is preferred (Bazett data are often provided for historic interest, but their analysis should be considered secondary). However, at the time of integrating all ECG data across all studies at the end of phase III (an integrated summary of safety) using the QTc corrected by defining a population-based exponent is recommended. A population-based QTc formula is determined by taking the QT and heart rate paired data in the population studied at baseline or on placebo and defining the best correction exponent that provides as flat a slope as possible between heart rate and the resultant QTc (population). For example, for atypical antipsychotic agents that are used to treat schizophrenia, the population exponent for the correction formula was defined by the Neuro-Pharm Division of the FDA as 0.37 rather than 0.5 (square root) for Bazett, or 0.33 (cube root) for Fridericia. This exponent, of course, should not be applied in general to all neurologic drugs or even to other atypical antipsychotic agents but should be determined for each study population used in the trials.

Subject specific or individual defined correction formulae are by design the most accurate method in correcting for the heart rate effect on the QT duration. The individual corrected QT (QTcI) is determined by taking each individual in a trial and calculating that individual's exponent that best eliminates the influence of heart rate on QT duration. This requires at least 35 to 50 or more ECGs on placebo/baseline in which these ECGs encompass a range (usually 50–80 beats per minute) of spontaneous heart rate changes to have enough power to accomplish this task. The individual QTc has been routinely employed in the Thorough ECG Trial and should be considered the primary endpoint for this trial's determination of the effect of the new drug on cardiac repolarization in such cases. QTcF is a secondary endpoint and the QTcB data are provided for historical reasons *(7)*.

What Should Be the Baseline Set of Electrocardiograms?
How Many Electrocardiograms Should Be Obtained on Treatment?

The accuracy of obtaining the best point estimate of an individual's ECG interval at baseline (pre-treatment) is another factor that critically influences the observed variability in the QTc interval effects in a trial. Even for typical research trials in which the primary focus is not on ECG effects, the FDA–Health Canada Concept paper *(1)* notes that the "use of baseline values from single ECGs is a practice to be discouraged." The recommendation is that baseline ECGs should be computed as the mean of multiple ECGs to enhance the precision of the measurement in light of the large degree of spontaneous variability in QTc duration. Regulatory guidance is to collect drug-free ECGs on two or three different days to help document inter-day variability in the baseline. Baseline ECGs should be collected at similar times of the day to minimize the possible effects of diurnal fluctuation and food. In addition, posture and activity levels at the time of the ECGs should be standardized to the extent possible for all recording periods. It is the author's opinion that in routine clinical trials that at least three baseline ECGs should be obtained even if only a few minutes apart to reduce the QTc variance, thus providing that the change from baseline in the treatment and control groups will be more likely not as a result of chance (spontaneous variability). When these concepts are applied to the Thorough ECG Trial, especially with the desirability to define individual correction formulae for QT to QTc, careful attention to the number of ECGs used to define the baseline and the treatment effects is critical.

It is critical that the ECG sampling frequency covers the entire period of exposure to the drug and its metabolites and also accounts for diurnal variation, food effects, and differences in posture and activity. Therefore, the author recommends that the best time points for ECG selection to best characterize the *baseline* is constructed to be very similar to a standard set of time points used to define the pharmacokinetic profile of the new drug. For most drugs, this set is usually at least 10 to 20 time points over a day when blood samples are taken. To construct these time points the pharmacokinetics of the new drug must be known so that adequate time point selection will encompass the Cmax-Tmax of parent and metabolites, as well as time to penetrate cardiac tissue and affect protein ion channels. Even if the pharmacokinetic profile of parent and metabolites extend for only 12 h, it may be of some value to select a few time points during the last 12 h of a day to account for some late effects of metabolites or tissue penetration and also diurnal variability (or effects of additional dosing if not a once a day therapy). In total for most drugs, the time points to be selected will encompass about 12–16 points, and at each of these time points the author recommends at least three ECGs be taken about 1 min apart (high degree of variability makes these three ECGs almost always different in terms of QTc duration). Thus, the baseline with this approach will have 12–16 time points with three ECGs per point or 36–48 separate ECGs. This number of ECGs should be enough to compute under most circumstances an individual correction for QTc, and overall provide sufficient power to adequately characterize the QTc duration (and other ECG parameters).

For thorough ECG trials in which the new drug can be used as a single dose when parent and metabolites (if present) are all dissipated by 24 h, a crossover design is frequently employed. This design allows for the collection of baselines before each treatment arm of the crossover, and therefore the baseline time points may be taken for just a few hours before each single dose. Adding all the ECGs together from the baseline periods before each treatment arm should provide sufficient numbers of ECGs off-treatment to calculate an individual correction for QTc. On-treatment time points should extend until there is no evidence of parent or metabolite being present. With careful attention to meals and activity during the baseline and time points on treatment, this design is effective in defining the ECG effects of the treatments. An example of this design is the Vardenafil ECG Trial ([Bayer and GSK] joint Genitourinary and Cardio-Renal Advisory Committee Meeting at the FDA on May 29, 2003).

How Many Treatment Groups? At Least Four and Often Six

In a Thorough ECG Trial it is important, in my opinion, to study at least two doses of the new agent to define if there are any dose-related ECG effects:

- One of the doses should be close to the standard clinical dose.
- The other is the supratherapeutic dose, which must cover the expected or theoretical maximum concentration that might occur under the worst circumstance in clinical care (excluding an intentional overdose).

If a QTc effect is observed then information regarding the steepness of that dose-QTc effect will be critical in defining the cardiac risk. Having only the supratherapeutic dose in a trial eliminates the ability to define dose-effect (if present), and internal consistency checks for the resultant ECG data. For example, if the standard clinical dose has a 6 ms placebo-corrected QTc change from baseline but the supratherapeutic dose group displays a further 2 ms QTc change, then the agent is likely showing a nonclinically relevant effect on cardiac repolarization on the lower dose (assuming that the positive control and placebo groups data results are appropriate).

Furthermore, to interpret the results of a Thorough ECG Trial adequate control groups are required. Without a placebo treatment arm it is difficult to determine the effects of QTc spontaneous variability. Thus, the primary purpose of the placebo group is to be certain that the spontaneous variability of QTc durations have been adequately handled in the trial, and thus the placebo change from baseline for QTc duration must be close to 0 ms (it is probable that a placebo induced change of over 10 ms means that the trial was not adequately controlled). Reasons for inadequate control may be too few ECGs, too few subjects, poor quality in ECG duration measurements, poor control of activity and food, poorly defined timing for ECG time points, etc.

The most significant new regulatory proposal is the requirement for inclusion of a positive control group. The positive control group is required to demonstrate precisely a placebo-corrected 5–10 ms change from baseline in the QTc duration. Thus, the drug used to define this response must be carefully selected for if too potent (e.g., sotalol) or too weak and a 5–10 ms effect is not demonstrated, then the positive control arm and thus the trial's thoroughness would have failed. This magnitude of a 5–10 ms QTc effect (placebo corrected change from baseline) is considered to be the threshold where risk of TdP begins. Thus, if one claims the trial shows no difference between the new agent and placebo, it is critical to be certain the trial had sensitivity to rule out a 5 ms effect by showing that a positive control arm demonstrated just that magnitude of an effect in the same trial under the same experimental conditions. Hence, it is advisable that all treatment arms in the trial be conducted under the same experimental conditions to insure that the positive and placebo control groups are demonstrating the effects under the same conditions as the new agent. Some have tried to reduce costs by using a single dose of the positive control drug in a sample of or in all the subjects, and then going on to randomize the study population to the placebo and new drug doses in a multiple-dose design. This approach should be discouraged because it does not allow the positive control group to experience the same study conditions as the other treatment arms.

At least these four treatment groups are necessary for a Thorough ECG Trial in the author's opinion:

- placebo group
- positive control group
- clinical dose group, and
- supratherapeutic dose group.

The fifth and sixth arms are optional and are relegated to the use of two doses of a therapeutic agent in the same class as the new drug under study. The use of a therapeutic agent from the same class is often very beneficial, especially when that drug is marketed and ECG data of a thorough nature previously have not been obtained. The best example is again from the Vardenafil ECG Trial referred to earlier. Besides placebo and moxifloxacin (positive control), the sponsors employed a clinical and supratherapeutic dose of vardenafil (Levitra) and also sildenafil (Viagra). Viagra is a drug from the same therapeutic category available on the market worldwide for several years without thorough ECG data, but without evidence of clinical TdP. In the Thorough ECG Trial, vardenafil and sildenafil showed comparable QTc effect durations (about 6–8 ms), and thus the argument was made and accepted for approvability of vardenafil that the dose effect was very flat (about 8–10× exposure but only an additional 2 ms change in QTc from clinical to supratherapeutic dose) and with the benign marketing experience of sildenafil the risk of a QTc effect on vardenafil was acceptable. The use of a drug from the same therapeutic category (the fifth and sixth treatment arms) in this trial was very informative in understanding the clinical importance of the ECG effects observed on vardenafil. Similar beneficial information is likely to be obtained with other compounds, so the use of a comparator drug in the same therapeutic category should be considered when appropriate in a Thorough ECG Trial. In fact, the Concept paper (1) states that if "an investigational drug belongs to a therapeutic class that has been associated with QT/QTc interval prolongation, active controls should be selected from other members of the same class to permit a comparison of effect sizes, preferably at equipotent therapeutic doses." In the author's opinion, one selects such drugs to compare to the new drug for clinical interpretation and *not* as a substitute for the use of a standard positive control arm as defined later, because such therapeutic class agents are usually not well characterized and their effect size may not be 5–10 ms raising assay sensitivity issues for the trial.

The Positive Control: Feasibility, Choice, and Implementation

The important design requirement for a Thorough ECG Trial is the need to define the trial's *assay sensitivity* using a positive control arm that is conducted under exactly the same trial conditions as the other treatment arms and produces a 5 to 10 ms change in QTc duration from baseline (placebo-corrected). The antibiotic, moxifloxacin given intravenously or orally either as a single or multiple doses, reliably produces an effect of this magnitude as detailed in its product labeling. Moxifloxacin appears to be the best agent to employ at present as the positive control in the Thorough ECG Trial. Initially, there was great concern that inducing a QTc effect in a healthy volunteer would be unethical because it poses a theoretical health risk. Because any new agent when used in man for the first time poses a health risk because toxicity has not been defined in man phase I trials, research is conducted only after appropriate preclinical data has been obtained, proper informed consent is obtained from the volunteer, and the study conditions are designed to detect and minimize risks. The use of an antibiotic like moxifloxacin that has been widely used in the market (over twenty million patient exposures) in critically ill subjects with rare reports of TdP (usually associated with other drugs or conditions that could cause TdP) speaks to the relative benign nature of this drug. Its use in a healthy volunteer under clinical research conditions with an induced change of 5 to 10 ms in QTc duration should prove to be of no risk, because an increase in QTc duration only translates into a clinical arrhythmia if co-factors are present such as hypokalemia, heart failure ischemia, atrial fibrillation, excessive bradycardia, and the like. These conditions by definition should not be present in the healthy volunteer population. The duration of the induced small QTc effect (time on study) is generally very short since usually only one to five doses will be used. Thus, in the author's opinion, the use of a marketed antibiotic like moxifloxacin under these conditions does not raise any ethical issues. The inclusion of a positive control to assure assay sensitivity when that assay is judging the cardiac liability or lack thereof of a new agent under consideration for widespread market use is obviously well justified.

Alternately, if one is concerned about the antibiotic effects of moxifloxacin, a single dose can be employed in a multiple dose regimen by providing placebo tablets on the interim days from baseline to steady-state, because the single dose of moxifloxacin should be as remote from the baseline as is the study drug.

Choice of a Parallel vs a Crossover Design

The FDA–Health Canada Concept paper *(1)* notes that a "Crossover or parallel group study designs may be suitable for trials addressing the potential of a drug to cause QT/QTc interval prolongation." The choice of which of these two designs is employed depends on the pharmacokinetic facts about the new drug and the clinical use. Crossover studies can use smaller numbers of subjects than parallel group studies, as the subjects serve as their own controls when the endpoint is to define the differences between the treatment groups effect on a variable. In the Thorough ECG Trial the primary analysis is the change from baseline in the placebo group to evaluate the control of spontaneous variability, the moxifloxacin (positive control) group to be sure that a 5–10 ms change from baseline placebo corrected response is obtained, and then the analysis of the two different doses of the test agent. With the analysis being descriptive change from baseline in each treatment group, the crossover or parallel design does not affect sample size in a critical way. In either case, the sample size is defined by the power and alpha needed to be certain that one can detect a 5 ms (± 5 ms) drug effect assuming a certain QTc variance (which is defined by the number of ECGs obtained—which when enough to do an individual correction is usually <10 ms). Crossover designs also facilitate heart rate correction approaches based on individual subject data when there is no carry over effects, and the baselines before each arm can legitimately be used to enhance the number of ECGs employed in the analysis. Parallel designed studies are needed, in my opinion, for drugs with multiple dosing with half-lives long enough that it takes several days to reach steady-state. When metabolites are not well characterized and likely present, a parallel study is best because carryover effects in the crossover trial cannot be assured. With a parallel design there is no issue about carryover or period effects to invalidate the trial, and the number of baseline ECGs to provide for an individual correction for QT can easily be recorded as a result of new technology (*see* later). Of course, with a parallel design you cannot test for period effects and to some this is considered a limitation of a parallel design choice; to others it may be considered an advantage.

Blinding

The FDA–Health Canada Concept paper *(1)* states that "Clinical studies assessing QT/QTc interval prolongation should be randomized and double-blinded, with concurrent placebo control groups." However, the standard use of moxifloxacin as an ideal positive control has complicated this general principle because placebo matching for moxifloxacin is not available. Over encapsulation is possible, but that requires further equivalence testing and the risk of not matching the known 5–10 ms effect. Because the endpoint data are all based on blinded digital ECG information that is analyzed in a blinded manner by a central ECG laboratory, the need for strict blinding of all treatment arms (specifically the moxifloxacin arm) is not apparent. Clearly, when feasible the placebo and new drug arms under evaluation should be "double-blinded." At a public meeting in Washington, D.C., FDA officials agreed with this viewpoint that double-blinding of the moxifloxacin arm was not a requirement for the Thorough ECG Trial. Of course, the central ECG laboratory should be completely blinded, and generally it is advisable to have the central ECG analyzer review all ECGs for a given subject to reduce variability.

ELECTROCARDIOGRAPHIC TECHNICAL ISSUES

Role of a Centralized Electrocardiograph Laboratory

Inadequate acquisition or measurement of ECG data may lead to an incorrect assessment of the drug's ECG effects and lead to approval of a drug with unacceptable risk–benefit ratio or to inappropriate discontinuation of a promising drug during development *(4,8,9)*.

To provide for a more standardized approach to ECG acquisition and measurement, the FDA–Health Canada Concept paper *(1)* notes that:

- The clinical ECG database should be derived primarily from the collection of standard 12-lead ECGs.
- The ECGs should be recorded and stored as a digital signal, but the assessment of intervals and the overall interpretation may be made from the digital record or from a printed record. If the analysis will be based on a paper record and the resolution for QT/QTc interval verification is within the desired range of < 5.0 ms, a paper speed of 25 ms is preferred, as higher speeds (e.g., 50 ms) may lead to distortion of low amplitude waves such as U waves.
- The QT/QTc interval should be determined as a mean value derived from at least three to five cardiac cycles (heart beats), preferably—from lead II.

"Historically, lead II has been preferred for QT/QTc interval measurements, as the end of the T wave is usually most clearly discerned in this lead. . . . While a description of morphological changes in the T–U complex is important, a discrete U wave of small amplitude should be excluded from the QT/QTc interval measurement. If the size of the U wave and the extent of T–U overlap are such that the end of the T wave cannot be determined, inclusion of the U wave in the QT/QTc interval measurement may be necessary and should be discussed with the regulatory authority. . . Pending improvements in automated technologies, the ECG readings should be performed manually. Although automated ECG recorders can be programmed to calculate many ECG intervals (RR, QRS, QT, QTc, and PR) from digital data signals, automated measurements of low amplitude wave forms, such as the P, T, and U waves, can result in inaccurate PR and QT interval measurements. While these automated recordings have a useful role in the rapid assessment of ECGs for safety, manual recalculation of the intervals ("over-read") is needed for the clinical trial database. Inconsistency between manufacturers in terms of the algorithms used for calculation of the intervals is another problem in the interpretation of computerized readings. Manual ECG readings are performed using visual determinations ("eyeball"/caliper techniques), digitizing methods, and/or on-screen computerized methods. Visual determinations/ caliper techniques are considered less accurate than digitizing methods. Some digitizing methods employ a digitizing pad, magnifying lamp, and pointing device to identify the beginning and end of the QT/QTc interval for automatic recording in the ECG database. A more technologically advanced option is to display digitally recorded ECGs on a computer screen, where they can be measured using computer-driven, on-screen calipers. Scanned paper-recorded ECGs can also be subjected to on-screen measurements. For a given trial, the sponsor should describe the accuracy and precision of QT/QTc interval measurements using the selected system. All ECG readings should be performed by a few designated cardiologists operating from a Centralized (Core) ECG laboratory who are blinded to time, treatment and patient identity. The generation of multiple databases should be discouraged." (1)

Thus, the standard for 12-lead ECGs as recommended should employ a validated central ECG laboratory using digital acquisition, manual digitized analysis, and processing. This eliminates the site-to-site variability and provides for a more "definitive" Thorough ECG Trial. The FDA goes further and points out that it wants to actually review raw ECG data, especially from ECGs in the Thorough ECG Trial that is provided in a manner so that as part of their review they can actually see where the central ECG laboratory decided to mark the beginning of the QRS and the end of the T wave, etc. The actual details from the Concept paper (1) are: "For the purpose of validating assessments of ECG intervals and overall interpretations, it is necessary to review the placement of fiduciary marks on the ECG waveform. A standard format for the submission of annotated ECG waveforms is being developed in cooperation with the HL7 standards organization. When such a standard is available, annotated ECG waveform data may be submitted to supplement ECG interval and overall assessment datasets for any study, according to applicable guidance. However, it will be critical to have annotated ECG waveform data for those studies intended to definitively address the effects of a drug on ventricular repolarization." The standard format (*see* Chapter 16) is now available, and the FDA is now routinely requesting XML ECG files for review.

A New Technology to Record Standard 12-Lead Electrocardiographs

In addition to standard resting supine ECGs, new Holter technology allows for continuous ambulatory recordings of 12-lead digital ECGs for 24 h at a time. This Holter approach should prove useful for the assessment of ECG intervals, and especially cardiac repolarization at numerous discrete time points following drug administration or at baseline. The digital 12-lead Holter recorder also has additional applications for continuous beat-to-beat analysis, as well as for detecting cardiac arrhythmias. Validation that the 12-lead ECGs recorded by Holter technology rather than a standard ECG recorder is required to be certain that the new technology is comparable to the historic standard. Such a study has been conducted as has a technical validation in accordance with USC 21CFR11. This study compared the utility for QTc risk assessment of ECGs recorded by standard or digital 12-lead Holter devices, as well as the precision of QT and RR interval measurement by the manual digitized systems (digitizing board and digital onscreen calipers) on standard and Holter-derived ECGs *(10)* (*see also* Chapter 8).

This is the first study to compare the standard 12-lead ECGs to discrete ECGs derived from continuous digital 12-lead Holter recorder for their utility in the assessment of drug-induced changes in QT/QTc and RR intervals, measured on a very large number of serial ECGs (1600 simultaneously recorded pairs of ECGs). It is also the first study to compare the precision of QT/QTc and RR interval measurement by the two most relevant manual digitized methods (digipad and onscreen calipers).

The results of the study showed that the QT, QTcF, and RR data produced by digipad on standard ECGs were essentially equivalent to those from digital 12-lead Holter ECGs. There was a very small mean difference in the absolute QT and QTcF intervals (3.3 and −2.7 ms) and a negligible mean difference in the QT and QTcF change from baseline (0.5 and −0.3 ms) when digipad was applied to standard ECGs and Holter-derived paper ECG copies, respectively. Digipad RR data from standard ECGs were very similar to those from Holter-derived ECGs (mean differences, −3.5 ms for absolute RR and 7.3 ms for RR change from baseline), although with a considerably large standard deviation of difference. The mean difference of 7 ms between the RR changes from baseline produced by digipad on standard and Holter ECGs is so small relative to the total duration of RR interval that it would not affect the QT/RR relationship.

Overall, despite somewhat differences in lead positions (12-lead Holter ECG has electrodes only on the torso, whereas the standard ECG also uses the limb leads) and differences in the sampling frequency of ECG recordings, this study validated the utility of digital 12-lead Holter for the assessment of QT prolongation in clinical drug research. 12-lead ECG Holter will also make digital 12-lead ECG recordings available for retrospective analysis at critical time points after dosing that are difficult or impossible to capture by advance scheduling (maximum plasma concentration of the parent drug and active metabolites, clinical adverse events possibly related to QT prolongation). Numerous QT and RR intervals derived from continuous Holter ECGs will allow for easier employment of subject-specific QT correction formulae that are more accurate and preferred versus the Fridericia's in evaluating the true drug-induced QT effect at different heart rates.

One of the major advantages of using the 12-lead ECG Holter recorder in a Thorough ECG Trial is that the clinical site would not be involved in viewing the ECGs because they are recorded on a flash memory card. Thus, the cost of an investigator review and processing is eliminated. Some regularly recorded "safety" *ECGs* must be added for patient safety and should be done at screening, baseline, and certain days on-treatment. These *safety ECGs* should not be used in the formal analysis, but should be also manually analyzed by the central ECG laboratory because the data will be in the trial listings and available for regulatory safety review.

What Are the Electrocardiograph Deliverables From a Thorough Electrocardiograph Trial?

The central ECG laboratory must provide the sponsor with two sets of data:

1. The standard ECG intervals and morphological assessments of each ECG recorded in the trial. This dataset will be used to create the ECG tables of results so that the trial's endpoint can be defined and explained (*see* statistical plan below), and,
2. In addition, the central ECG laboratory must provide the sponsor with a set of XMLs that are in the form of the FDA Schema (*see* earlier), so that the FDA will have the ability to review the fiducial marks on the intervals made by the central laboratory. Freeware and more advanced software are available to view these XML ECGs and to manage the thousands of XML ECG files that will be recorded in a definitive ECG trial.

What Is the Role for Other Methods or End Points That Assess Cardiac Repolarization?

Many new methods are being proposed to look at cardiac repolarization (*see* Ch. 6). Unfortunately, before they can replace the standard 12-lead ECG they will have to show comparability data with standard 12-lead ECGs, because it is by this technique that drugs that have caused unacceptable cardiac responses (especially TdP) in the market have been identified. Prospective comparable trials need to require the addition of the new approach/method in conjunction with standard 12-lead ECGs, but the marketing experience will be needed to define whether a positive signal on the new method (with a negative 12-lead ECG dataset) is predictive. Likewise, a positive ECG signal but a negative new method evaluation will be a challenge for a regulatory authority to accept without a large scale trial to prove that the new method is more predictive or reliable.

Thus, I do not see the introduction of new methods for some time until "biological-epidemiological validation" is obtained.

THE STATISTICAL AND CLINICAL ANALYSES OF THE ELECTROCARDIOGRAPHIC RAW DATA FOR A THOROUGH ELECTROCARDIOGRAPHIC TRIAL

Calculation of Sample Size

As of 2002 *(1)*, the sample size of the Thorough ECG Trial is defined by the requirement of having enough power to detect a 5 ms (± 5 ms) QTc effect (change from baseline) with a power of 80% and an α of 0.05. A key determination of sample size is the variance of the QTc that can be assumed to be < 8 ms if > 36 ECGs are obtained at baseline and on-treatment. Sample size calculation will thus be in the range of 30–40 subjects per arm. Usually, the author recommends at least 40 subjects, half of which should be women because they appear to have increased sensitivity to drug-induced QTc effects. This allows for a gender analysis with a sample size of 20 women, a size likely to provide accurate endpoint data. Healthy volunteers are the assumed study population in this analysis since trying to employ the target population will add marked heterogeneity to the study in terms of disease magnitude, concomitant drugs, and comorbidities requiring a sample size of 100s in each treatment arm perhaps.

Descriptive Statistics Based on Change From Baseline Analysis vs a Standard Statistical (ANCOVA) Analysis

In defining ECG effects in the Thorough ECG Trial, consideration must be given to the type of statistical analysis that will be performed. Trying to analyze a specific time point at baseline to the same time point on drug analysis is dangerous if one only has one ECG at each of those time points because the power to eliminate spontaneous variability will be small, and thus a spurious result is likely. In fact, there is no reason to assume that any time point on one day has anything to do with the QTc duration of the same time point on another day as the result of the marked spontaneous variability in this ECG parameter. Thus, the author believes that the baseline should be defined as a means to define the best point estimate for each ECG interval duration. The QTc duration at baseline should be the mean duration of all the ECGs obtained on baseline, and all change from baseline should use that mean single duration value. One can explore the change from the baseline to Cmax or any other time point such as the maximum observed QTc duration, but if only one ECG is obtained at that on-treatment time point limited power to exclude a false negative or positive effect exists. Thus, more than one ECG should be obtained at each time point, and generally three ECGs around a time point (about 1 or 2 min apart) reduces the variance at that time (though some have used up to six ECGs at a time point—see the Vardenafil trial referred to earlier). The use of three instead of six ECGs per time point provides the most effect cost-benefit (*see* Fig. 1 in Chapter 14).

The author believes that the primary analysis is the central tendency or mean change from baseline (placebo-corrected) for each treatment arm in the trial. This produces the "treatment effect" for each arm. If the mean change shows no effect on cardiac repolarization, a drug is most unlikely to produce a valid positive outlier analysis. Of course, the mean change from baseline placebo corrected value "hides" outliers, and thus a categorical or outlier analysis is critical (*see* next paragraph). One form is the use of the maximum mean change in all treatments produces comparable data in my experience. This is done by looking at the largest positive change from baseline on-treatment at any time point (average the ECGs around that time point for better time point precision) in each subject and then calculate the mean "maximum" change for all subjects in each treatment arm. This approach may be considered the "time-averaged" analysis. There is ongoing discussion of using a maximum effect time-matched analysis as the primary endpoint for QTc effect in a Through ECG Trial. This process would select the time points on treatment and define the change from baseline for each of these time points by subtracting the ECG interval data obtained at the matched time point at baseline. Each resultant treatment time point change from baseline would be placebo corrected and a 95% confidence interval (CI) established. If any time point demonstraged a >8 ms change in QTc duration at the upper CI, the drug under investigation would be declared as having an effect on cardiac repolarization. This interesting approach has statistical merit but for clinical meaningfulness requires correlation with prior ECG QT data sets from drugs with known regulatory outcomes.

The outlier or categorical analysis is defined as determining what percentage of the patients on each treatment demonstrate a change from baseline in QTc (and all other ECG intervals) that is of a particular magnitude that identify them to be at potential risk because of the QTc effect. This is done by taking the largest positive change from the baseline value for each ECG interval at whatever time point on-treatment that this occurs (take the mean of the 3 ECGs used around that time point to establish that point's ECG interval value). Most clinicians use a QTc of 500 ms or more in duration as a clinical risk requiring re-evaluation of drug dose or risk benefit of the therapy *(11)*. Thus, the specific clinical criterion is a new > 500 ms QTc duration or the observation on drug or an abnormal T–U wave often thought to represent an early afterdepolarization that may be a harbinger of TdP. Statistically, a change in QTc of > 60 ms from baseline in an individual is considered as a specific outlier criterion. An often too sensitive (too many subjects on placebo will show this effect) criterion is a 30–60 ms change from baseline *(12)*. The use of other QTc outlier criteria such as normal to abnormal, percentage of subjects > 440 or 480 ms, etc., in my opinion, adds little except that the more times you "slice data" the more the likelihood of a false or spurious response. I believe for QTc the criteria to look at are:

- 30–60, > 60 ms change from baseline,
- new absolute 500 ms or more, and
- new abnormal U waves.

The more the number of ECGs obtained the more likely an outlier criterion will be met. However, placebo correction will generally reveal an imbalance as will as an analysis of QTc duration distributions between the treatment arms. Of course, all the ECG data are expressed in terms of means, standard deviations, ranges, and confidence intervals.

The use of an ANCOVA comparison that uses the ECG data just on-treatment (can virtually ignore the baseline ECG data) does provide for an assessment of whether the placebo, positive control, and the two doses of the new drug differ statistically when compared with one another in pairs. While this provides what I would call supportive data, in my opinion, the primary analysis of interest should be the analysis of each treatment arms' change from baseline as detailed earlier. The placebo needs to be close to 0 ms change from baseline if spontaneous variability has been controlled. The positive control drug should show a 5–10 ms effect, and then the new agent placebo adjusted is then viewed to see what if any QTc effect is present and if present what the dose response effect was.

What Is the Regulatory Implication of the Definitive Electrocardiograph Trial Result?

As detailed elsewhere (*see* Chapter 16) there is regulatory guidance on how much a magnitude of a QTc duration effect might be related to risk of TdP. This analysis has come from the experience of regulators over the past decade, mostly from approving QTc prolonging drugs and observing their effect in the market. The guidance from both Europe and the United States is based probably on the maximum mean change or QTc effect at Cmax. As noted in the FDA–Health Canada Concept paper *(1)* and elsewhere *(13),* general consensus that a magnitude of QTc duration effect of:

- 0 to 5 ms, imparts no risk of TdP.
- If the effect is over 20 ms, the risk is considered quite high for TdP.

Most would say that 5 to 10 ms effect for a drug is of minimal concern, but depends on the risk–benefit ratio of the particular drug. An effect between 10 to 20 ms is uncertain. Ziprasidone is an example of the drug with an approx 14 ms effect that was put in the market because of its risk–benefit ratio, and to date has not experienced a clear increase in TdP.

The decision for approval in reference to cardiac risk of the new drug's effect on the ECG (especially QTc duration-cardiac repolarization) depends on the total data available. The Thorough ECG Trial is the most important piece and trumps any preclincial cardiac safety data concerns. The Thorough ECG Trial must be viewed in the context of ECG data in the phase II–III target population where one looks carefully for the presence of unexpected outliers because the Thorough ECG Trial cannot be considered 100% definitive. The integrated summary of safety, taking all ECG data into analysis, provides the target population information that hopefully will be in harmony with the Thorough ECG Trial's results. The frequency of TdP is so uncommon (generally less than 1/100,000 to million background rate and in hospitalized patients about 4/100,000) *(14)* that it is not logical to argue that on the basis of a 5000 patient sample in a typical drug development program that there was no hint of a ventricular arrhythmia, and so the drug with a QTc effect is not clinically relevant.

When small QTc effects are noted either in the Thorough ECG Trial or in the target population, marketing approval can be expected but to be reasonably comfortable with the risk–benefit ratio, a simple large post-marketing study may need to be conducted (*see* Chapter 13).

POTENTIAL FUTURE MODIFICATIONS

It is now early in the history of the Thorough ECG Trial and changes with more experience are certain to emerge. When designs for this trial become more standardized as to sample size, population, numbers of ECGs, analysis methods, statistical approaches, and the like the need for a positive control arm may wane. Also, to date I have not personally seen any drug's effect in women reveal something not seen in men in the setting of this thorough trial, and thus the use of women in these trials (harder to recruit) may also not be necessary. The need for thousands (usually around 15,000 ECGs) of ECG samples in the Thorough ECG Trial begs the use of automated ECG analysis methods to define ECG interval durations to reduce costs. The possibility of using automatic computer analyzed ECG interval durations at present has not been recommended as a result of the difficulties of computer algorithms defining the end of low frequency waves, especially the T wave *(15)*. Perhaps improvements will allow this approach to gain acceptance in the future. Finally, the use of genetic assessments for selecting study populations is also enticing (*see* Chapter 5).

ACKNOWLEDGMENTS

The author expresses his appreciation for the careful review and comments provided by Norman Stockbridge, MD, and Rashmi Shah, BSc, MBBS, FRCP.

REFERENCES

1. Food and Drug Administration and Health Canada. The clinical evaluation of QT/QTc interval prolongation and proarrhythmic potential for non-antiarrhythmic drugs. Preliminary Concept paper, November 15, 2002.http//www.fda.gov/cder/workshop.htm#upcoming
2. Committee for Proprietary Medicinal Products (CPMP). Points to consider: the assessment of the potential for QT interval prolongation by non-cardiovascular medicinal products. The European Agency for the Evaluation of Medicinal Products, 17 December 1997.
3. Health Canada. Draft Guidance "Assessment of the QT prolongation potential of non-antiarrhythmic drugs." March 15, 2001 http//www.hc-sh.gc.ca/hpb-dgps/therapeut/htmleng/guidmain.html.
4. Morganroth J. Focus on issues in measuring and interpreting changes in the QTc interval duration. Eur Heart J Supplements 2001;3: K105–K111.
5. Morganroth J, Brown AM, Critz S, Crumb WJ, Kunze DL, Lacerda AE, Lopez H, Variability of the QTc interval: impact on defining drug effect and low-frequency cardiac event. Am J Cardiol 1993;72: 26B–32B.
6. Morganroth J, Brozovich FV, McDonald JT, Jacobs RA. Variability of the QT measurement in healthy men: with implications for selection of an abnormal QT value to predict drug toxicity and proarrhythmia. Am J Cardiol 1991;67:774–776.
7. Malik M, Färbom P, Batchvarov V, et al. Relation between QT and RR intervals is highly individual among healthy subjects: implications for heart rate correction of the QT interval. Heart 2002;87: 220–228.
8. Haverkamp W, Breithardt G, Camm AJ, et al. The potential for QT prolongation and proarrhythmia by non-antiarrhythmic drugs: clinical and regulatory implications. Report on a Policy Conference of the European Society of Cardiology. Cardiovascular Research 2000;47:219–33.
9. Shah RR. The significance of QT interval in drug development. Brit J Clin Pharmacol 2002;54:188–202.
10. Sarapa N, Morganroth J, Couderc J-P, Francom SF, Darpo B, Fleishaker JC, McEnroe JD, Chen WT, Zareba W, Moss AJ. Drug-induced QT prolongation in the electrocardiogram: ssessment by different recording and measurement methods. Ann Noninvasive Electrocardiol 2004;9:48–57.
11. Priori SG, Schwartz PJ Napoliatano C, et al Risk stratification in the long QT syndrome. N Engl J Med 2003;348:1866–1874.
12. Pratt CM, Ruberg S, Morganroth J, et al. Dose-response relation between terfenadine (Seldane) and the QTc interval on the scalar electrocardiogram: distinguishing a drug effect from spontaneous variability. Am Heart J 1996;131:472–480.
13. Shah RR. Drug-induced Prolongation of the QT interval: Regulatory Dilemmas and Implications for approval and Labelling of a new Chemical Entity. Fundam Clin Pharmacol 2002;16:147–146.
14. Darpö B. Spectrum of drugs prolonging the QT interval and the incidence of Torsades de Pointes. Eur Heart J 2001;3 (Suppl. K):K70–K80.
15. Funck-Brentano C, Jaillon P. Rate-corrected QT interval: techniques and limitations. Am J Cardiol 1993;72:17–22.

12

Use of ECGs in Support of Cardiac Safety in Phase II and III Clinical Trials

Martin P. Bedigian, MD

CONTENTS

INTRODUCTION

Drugs in clinical development that potentially have effects on cardiac safety based on nonclinical data or findings in phase I, may require systematic cardiac safety assessments throughout phases II and III. Of major concern are drugs which cause the lethal, but rare, ventricular arrhythmia, torsades de pointes (TdP). Indeed, drugs intended for the general population that cause a one in one million incidence of TdP can be a significant public health concern *(1,2)*. This risk cannot be adequately addressed in typical drug development programs by arrhythmia monitoring or adverse event reporting. However, drugs known to cause TdP are known to reproducibly perturb cardiac ventricular repolarization, an effect that is manifest on the standard 12-lead electrocardiogram (ECG) as prolongation of the QTc interval. Thus, QTc and the degree to which it is prolonged, is used as a surrogate marker for a drug's potential to cause TdP. This chapter will focus on the use of standard 12-lead ECGs in phases II and III clinical development to assess a drug's effect on cardiac intervals, durations, and morphologic patterns.

ELECTROCARDIOGRAPHIC ASSESSMENT OF CARDIAC SAFETY IN PHASES II AND III

In general, the "early" phases of drug development in humans are designed to provide information regarding pharmacokinetics, metabolism, pharacodynamics, and, importantly, tolerability and safety data. In "later" stage controlled clinical trials, in addition to delineating the range of the drug's effectiveness, the incidence of adverse events and the benefit to potential patient populations are evaluated. Recently, some have recommended that a development program should consider combining phase II and phase III trials that may reduce unnecessary delays to approval for some drugs.

From: *Cardiac Safety of Noncardiac Drugs:*
Practical Guidelines for Clinical Research and Drug Development
Edited by: J. Morganroth and I. Gussak © Humana Press Inc., Totowa, NJ

The main goal of the electrocardiographic assessment in phases II and III is to identify any clinically relevant effects of the investigational drug, and any dose effect on cardiac intervals and durations and on morphology. These assessments are of great importance to a development program in that effects can be determined in patients in whom the drug is intended and compared with standard therapies for the disease or indication being studied.

When and How Many Electrocardiograms Should Be Acquired?

In general, ECGs should be obtained at important clinical and safety milestones of a trial. The visits and times at which ECGs are required should be consistent across all trials within a program to facilitate the creation of an ECG dataset. Thus, ECGs can be obtained at the following times:

- screening
- baseline
- after first dose
- at steady-state
- after long-term exposure
- after discontinuation
- during an adverse event
- at the end of a treatment period
- at final visit

A "screening" *ECG* is obtained prior to patient enrollment to evaluate inclusion and exclusion criteria. If the drug is either known or suspected to cause QTc interval prolongation, the following exclusion criteria should be considered:

- history of or family history of long QT syndrome
- ECG findings consistent with disorders of cardiac sodium channel abnormalities (e.g., Brugada Syndrome)
- QTc > 450 ms (males) and > 470 ms (females)
- advanced defects of the cardiac conduction system (e.g., bifascicular block)
- hypokalemia or hypomagnesemia at screening or baseline
- history of syncope

Exclusion criteria, which can be used to exclude high-risk patients, include the following conditions:

- concomitant use of drugs that effect cardiac repolarization
- history of heart failure
- history of ischemic heart disease
- history of cardiomyopathy
- chronic arrhythmias, such as atrial fibrillation
- implanted defibrillators
- implanted pacemakers with predominantly or entirely paced rhythms

Attention should also be paid to exclude patients in whom technically acceptable ECG tracings may be difficult. Examples of such "noisy" ECG tracings are neurological conditions, such as spasticity and Parkinson's disease.

A "baseline" *ECG(s)* should be obtained prior to and as close to the time of the start of active treatment as possible. Cardiac intervals, such as the QTc are known to have high intra-patient variability *(3)*. QTc variability is affected by:

- heart rate
- autonomic influences
- position
- activity level
- post-prandial status
- diurnal and time effects
- time effects

To account for this variability, multiple ECGs are required to adequately determine the best point estimate of an individual's baseline status. For trials that are conducted in outpatients, multiple ECGs within a visit even over a short time period will decrease QTc variance, so that a change from baseline can be more accurately obtained. Usually, averaging the QTc values obtained from three to six ECGs taken over even a short time period of minutes to hours (often called "replicates" around a time point) can significantly increase the precision of defining drug effects on cardiac repolarization at any given time point. For trials that are conducted in a domiciled setting, ECGs can be obtained at the respective pharmacokinetic and pharmacodynamic time points of interest throughout the dosing interval as repeated measures. The mean of the repeated measures at baseline provides a "summary measure" that accounts for most of the known factors influencing the variability of QTc duration.

The ECG plan for obtaining on-treatment ECGs should be customized for each drug program, tailored to a drug's unique pharmacokinetic, pharmacodynamic and metabolic profile. For example, for drugs with suspected concentration-response effects on cardiac intervals and durations, it is of greater value to obtain ECGs at pharmacokinetic and pharmacodynamic peaks rather than at trough. If effects on cardiac intervals and durations at any particular time point is to be characterized, replicates (3 or more ECGs) should be obtained to define the values at the time point in question with greater precision. Finally, if the assumption that effects on cardiac intervals and durations is maximum and does not wane after steady state is achieved is valid, then all ECGs obtained post steady state can be treated as repeated measures and averaged together. In this method, values for cardiac intervals and durations are obtained from multiple ECGs yielding higher precision than that from a single ECG tracing at a single visit. The repeated measures approach for measures of central tendency and categorical analyses of data, yet does not preclude concomitant use of singe ECGs for outlier analysis.

How Should Electrocardiographic Measurements and Interpretations Be Conducted?

Investigator or local ECG measurements and interpretation are subject to high inter-reader variability. This can be particularly problematic in multicenter and multinational trials where regional differences in interpretation can also play a role. Studies, which have compared investigator interpretations with those of the appointed central core ECG laboratory, have shown high discordance rates *(4,5)*. In addition, investigators can potentially be biased by knowledge of patient medical history and other clinical data, to which core lab personnel remain blinded. Use of centralized reading of ECGs with a core laboratory provides a uniform methodology that can be applied across all clinical sites throughout the entire drug development program. Core laboratories also facilitate the "near real-time" viewing of ECG data by electronic methods such as secure web-based portals.

How Should Electrocardiograms Be Acquired at the Clinical Site, and What Is the Role of Local Interpretation of Electrocardiographic Data?

ECGs should be acquired on well maintained and validated equipment. Clinical site personnel should be trained by the ECG core laboratory in proper patient preparation and ECG lead placement to ensure good signal quality and comparability of serial ECGs. Investigators may review the ECG locally for immediate patient care often using automated interpretations, which though frequently inaccurate, can be used for screening purposes. However, the investigator or local interpretations need not be collected as part of the clinical database, and should not be included in the central laboratory-defined ECG dataset that provides objective and consistent interpretations for analysis. An exception to this is when an ECG interpretation is necessary for an adverse event report, though the ECG core laboratory interpretation subsequently may be used to enhance or clarify the initial ECG impression.

How Should Electrocardiographic Data Be Analyzed?

An ECG safety database can be developed by integrating ECG data collected across a development program when the ECGs are obtained with the same schedule in all trials, and when the ECG interval and duration measurements and interpretations are conducted by an ECG core laboratory. The ECG cardiac safety data become more easily interpreted when the trial design includes placebo or active controls to distinguish the "background" incidence of spontaneous ECG changes caused by the changes in the state of the disease or comorbid conditions.

Cardiac interval duration measurements such as heart rate, PR, QRS, and QT can be analyzed as continuous variables and also as categorical dichotomous variables (outlier analyses). Descriptive statistics for the change from baseline to on-treatment QTc duration compared with or corrected by the placebo response is usually the primary analysis. If placebo controlled trials are not conducted, it is important to view the change from baseline QTc for the investigational drug along side the comparator for interpretation. It is useful to note the 95% confidence limit to determine the "worst case" of interval changes observed. Outlier analyses of the number and percent of patients with QTc changes > 30 ms and > 60 ms provide for the ability to depict at risk individuals that may not be reflected in the mean change from baseline analysis. Additionally, the proportion of patients with new on-treatment QTc values > 480 ms or > 500 ms are additional categorical limits used in the outlier analysis.

The change from baseline for PR and QRS as a continuous variable is calculated in the same manner as the QTc (mean change from baseline). However, outliers are determined differently. For PR and QRS, the number and percent of patients with a 25% increase over baseline to a value > 200 ms for PR and >100 ms for QRS is often used.

The interpretive parts of the ECG can be thought of in the following domains: rhythm, conduction, myocardial infarction, ST abnormalities, morphology, and T and U wave abnormalities. Findings in each of the domains can be treated as categorical dichotomous variables. The number and percent of patients with new findings can be expressed in a table with a row for each finding and columns for each treatment group, in the same manner as adverse event tables are structured.

In summary, standard 12-lead ECGs can provide important cardiac safety data for drugs in development when the number and schedule of ECGs incorporated in the trials is well thought out, the ECGs are acquired in a high quality manner, the analysis and interpretation are carried out centrally by an ECG core laboratory, and the resultant data are integrated with the analyses of both continuous and categorical variables.

REFERENCES

1. Frothingham R. Rates of torsades de pointes associated with ciprofloxacin, ofloxacin, levofloxacin, gatifloxacin, and moxifloxacin. Pharmacotherapy 2001;21:1468–1472
2. Lannini PB. Cardiotoxicity of macrolides, ketolides and fluoroquinolines that prolong the QTc interval. Exp Opin Dr Saf 2002;1:121–128.
3. Morganroth J, Brozovich FV, McDonald JT, Jacobs RA. Variability of the QT measurement in healthy men, with implications for selection of an abnormal QT value to predict drug toxicity and proarrhythmia. Am J Cardiol 1991;67:774–776.
4. Bertolet BE, Boyette AF, Handberg-Thurmond EM, Wolf RA, Deitchman D, Blumenthal M, Pepine CJ. Digital assessment of the epicardial electrocardiogram: novel methodology for a core laboratory for clinical studies..Clin Cardiol 1999;22:311–315.
5. Holmvang L, Hasbak P, Clemmensen P, Wagner G, Grande P. Differences between local investigator and core-laboratory interpretation of the admission electrocardiogram in patients with unstable angina pectoris or non-Q myocardial infarction (a thrombin inhibition in myocardial ischemia [TRIM] substudy). Electrocardiol 1998;31:126–127.

13 Cardiac Arrhythmia Assessment in Phase IV Clinical Studies

Gerald A. Faich, MD
and Annette Stemhagen

CONTENTS

INTRODUCTION

The safety and efficacy of a pharmaceutical product is evaluated during product development; however, safety surveillance must continue after marketing. One principal tool for post-marketing safety surveillance is the analysis of spontaneous (nontrial based) adverse reaction reports. Formal studies, either experimental or observational in design, are other means to further assess an approved product's safety. Although the term "phase IV studies" is used to describe studies conducted after a drug is marketed, this term does not reflect a particular study design. Epidemiologic cohort studies conducted in administrative databases are examples of study designs used to examine the safety of new products. Other powerful study designs, such as large and simplified clinical trials (SCTs), may also provide safety and effectiveness data to supplement pre-approval information. The purpose of this chapter is to describe limitations of the drug approval process and to discuss post-marketing methods useful for assessing cardiac arrhythmias, particularly as related to QTc interval prolongation.

LIMITATIONS OF THE FORMAL DRUG DEVELOPMENT AND APPROVAL PROCESS

Pharmaceutical product development and the regulatory approval process cannot provide full assurance of safety and effectiveness for all patients who will ultimately receive

From: *Cardiac Safety of Noncardiac Drugs:*
Practical Guidelines for Clinical Research and Drug Development
Edited by: J. Morganroth and I. Gussak © Humana Press Inc., Totowa, NJ

a drug. This is a result of inherent limitations in the testing process for new products, particularly in regard to identification of rare risks and risks in susceptible subpopulations that cannot be readily tested prior to marketing and widespread use.

Modern drug development and regulatory approval is based upon a stepwise process of evaluation beginning with in vitro testing, followed by animal experiments and finally testing in humans. While invaluable for screening out toxic compounds, in vitro and animal testing cannot fully predict how humans will respond to candidate compounds. Predication models from chemistry and other models, particularly for safety, are not well developed or reliable. Small changes in the structure of compounds can result in dramatically differing effects in various preclinical models compared to their effects in humans. Differing effects in animals and humans may occur because of differences in drug action including differences in absorption, distribution, and receptor distribution and function.

Human testing, or phase I, of the clinical development process usually begins with use of the investigational compound in healthy volunteers to examine human absorption, distribution, metabolism, and excretion. Additionally, tolerability, pharmacokinetics, dose–response, and adverse effects are studied during the early stages of human testing. This is generally followed by so-called phase II trials which examine "proof of concept" or efficacy in patients with the disease of interest. At this stage, further studies of the optimal effective dose are also often done. Finally, larger (phase III) trials that are typically double-blinded are done. A hallmark of such studies is the random assignment of exposure to the test drug or a comparator. When all testing is done, the data intended to demonstrate safety and efficacy are submitted to regulatory authorities for review and discussion with the product sponsors. This process ultimately leads to approval or nonapproval of the drug for marketing (1).

Some of the most important limitations of drug development and approval are found in phase III testing. This testing is focused on scientifically evaluating the effects of a candidate drug under relatively optimal conditions so that the biologic effects of the drug can be understood. Phase III trials are typically classic experiments carefully examining predefined effects or endpoints following patient exposure to a drug or comparator (often a placebo). Generally, both the physician investigator and the patient are unaware (blinded) of whether the patient has been randomly assigned to receive the investigational drug or the comparator. Visit schedules, testing methods, and frequencies are carefully considered and described in study protocols. Investigators with access to appropriate patients and expertise in the required testing and in protocol adherence are recruited and trained.

To conduct a "cleaner" experiment, reduce confounding by extraneous variability and minimize risk to patients, eligibility criteria for entry of subjects into a phase III trial are clearly defined and rigorously enforced. Typically, inclusion criteria elaborate the duration, characteristics, and severity of the disease being treated, set age boundaries, and define other subject characteristics. Exclusion criteria usually eliminate pregnant women, patients with advanced disease or any disease that may interfere with completion of the study, patients with unstable disease state, and those who must continue use of specific concomitant medications.

Even when eligibility criteria are broad, investigators tend to enroll relatively healthy or stable patients. The effect of the explicit and implicit criteria used to enter patients into trials is to limit our knowledge of the effects of the test drug in elderly, young, pregnant, complex, and poly-medicated patients. Of course, these are the very patients often

Table 1
Preapproval Trial Limitations

1. Patient management generally is more intense than that found in practice
2. Rare effects are not detectable
3. Subsets such as the elderly, the young and pregnant women are not studied
4. Late effects are not thoroughly studied
5. The desired effect may not be measured because surrogate endpoint measures are used

exposed to the drug after approval. Put another way, the aim of pre-approval clinical trials is to achieve internal validity of results in an efficient manner. As described, this entails careful specification of the protocol, procedures, selection of subjects, and size of the trials. However, as trials are made more structured, restricted, and focused their results become less generalizable to the patients who will be prescribed the drug after approval. That is, clinical trials study a drug under ideal circumstances and address the question of "can it work?" Whereas the question raised post-marketing is "does it work?" Table 1 gives a summary of some pre-approval trial limitations.

Phase III trials are highly structured with detailed procedures for patient testing and follow-up. These procedures often do not parallel those procedures followed in actual clinical practice. Generally, clinical researchers who may have more time, specific training and insight into drug effects than usual practitioners conduct trials. Study and testing visits are often more frequent, and thus heighten detection of emerging medical events and reinforce patient compliance. Once a drug is used in actual practice, the differing procedures and setting may have different outcomes. For example, in premarket testing of alendronate for osteoporosis, and in recognition of its esophageal irritative effects, patients were repeatedly cautioned to take the pill with a full glass of water and not to recline afterwards. In practice, these precautions were not adequately followed even though they were described in the product's package insert *(2)*. Another example is that study protocols may require baseline and end of study electrocardiograms (ECGs), whereas these may not be done in practice once the drug is approved.

Determining the number of subjects needed for a phase III trial is an important aspect of study design *(3)*. Sample size is typically determined by estimating the size of the effect that will be observed, the anticipated difference in the rates of that effect that will be seen in the two (or more) comparison groups, and the statistical precision needed to decide if the difference reaches statistical significance. There are many complexities that determine these power calculations. Because trials are expensive and much of the expense is linked to the number of subjects enrolled in a trial, an effort is made to assure that enough, but not too many, subjects are included.

Most new drug applications (NDA) submissions for product approval include a maximum total of 1000 to 5000 exposed patients. Whereas these are reasonable numbers to study side effects occurring with an incidence of up to 1 or 2%, such studies lack the power to detect and understand the rate of less frequent effects, i.e., those occurring at rates below 1 or even 0.1%. A total sample of 3000 patients exposed to an investigational drug is needed to have 95% confidence that one adverse event will be seen if the event occurs at a rate of 0.1%. Even more daunting, much larger sample sizes are needed to study whether such a rare event is occurring at rates above those for a comparator or placebo. Put another way, the relatively small size of trials greatly limits their detection ability. For therapies intended for chronic use, only a much smaller subset—a few hundred patients—are typically studied for a year or two. This relatively brief duration of study in a relatively small number of patients precludes the ability to reach firm conclusions about uncommon, latent effects.

Lastly, trials and the regulatory submission dataset often use surrogate endpoints, because these are easier to measure. Examples include measurements of blood pressure when the ultimate goal of a new antihypertensive is reduction in stroke and myocardial infarction, and use of T4 lymphocyte counts in lieu of survival in acquired immune deficiency syndrome (AIDS).

TRIAL LIMITATIONS IN REGARD TO
QTc INTERVAL PROLONGATION

It is now well recognized that preclinical testing for potassium ion channel effects of candidate drugs is a means to assess the likelihood of QTc interval prolonging effects in humans. Moreover, phase I testing for QTc effects has evolved to the point where screening can provide some assurance of safety for many drugs, and can identify compounds with evident and substantial QTc prolonging effects. Nonetheless, when the QTc prolongation is between 5 and 20 ms (or even longer with drugs with unique benefits) usual phase III trials will likely not provide adequate safety assurance. In this situation, post-marketing cohort studies and large simplified trials may have a role to play.

OPTIONS PROVIDED BY POST-MARKETING
SURVEILLANCE AND COHORT STUDIES

A critical tool used for post-marketing safety surveillance is the collection and interpretation of spontaneous, nontrial reports of possible adverse drug reactions (4). These reports are made by practicing physicians and patients to manufacturers or to regulatory authorities directly. In recent years, the volume of such reporting has increased enormously in the United States, now reaching nearly 300,000 reports per year. In reviewing spontaneous reports to evaluate QcT-related safety issues, the key indicators are those reports that describe syncope, sudden death, or ventricular arrhythmias. The signature arrhythmia of highest interest is torsades de pointes (TdP).

Use and interpretation of spontaneous reports is often difficult. When reviewing individual case reports, details from the patient history may be lacking, and the actual arrhythmia and other events may be poorly described or documented. It is not always possible to obtain documentation from the medical record or ECG testing. Furthermore, the actual rate of occurrence of a drug-event combination cannot be quantified from spontaneous adverse event surveillance. It is well understood that reporting is incomplete and varies over time, with publicity, the patient population, and other factors (5). Generally, for these reasons the reporting rate (i.e., the number of arrhythmia reports divided by the estimated drug use) is compared within a therapeutic class to see if the drug of interest has a much higher reporting rate. When such a signal is found further study is needed, and regulatory action such as labeling change or restrictions on use may be taken.

An example of the use of spontaneous reports in evaluating possible QTc interval prolongation was given by the sparfloxacin experience (6). This quinolone antibiotic had a relatively high reporting rate, after marketing, of ventricular tachyarrhythmias compared to other quinolones and macrolide antibiotics, and therefore was withdrawn from the market soon after its approval.

What about epidemiologic cohort studies to evaluate cardiac safety? A cohort study consists of identifying patients prescribed the drug in actual practice ("naturally") and following them to determine outcomes of interest. Those outcomes, in the case of QTc concerns, are as noted earlier in the review of spontaneous reports: syncope, sudden death, and ventricular arrhythmias. Theoretically, cohort studies have the advantage of involving larger numbers of patients than can be readily studied pre-approval. Typically, for efficiency purposes, large linked, longitudinal databases, such as those established by managed care organizations or by Medicaid are used for such studies (7). Thus, patient baseline characteristics, exposures, and outcomes can all be determined "automatically" with validation through chart review. An excellent example of this type of study is given by an analysis of cardiac arrest and ventricular arrhythmias following several long-used antipsychotics done using the United Kingdom General Practice Research Database (GPRD) (8). However, for new drugs the databases are limited by the difficulties of collecting enough patients fast enough to provide timely data. The required sample size of many thousands of exposed patients is often not available for some time, until the drug is established on the formulary and until enough penetration or use happens. For example, a cohort study examining terfenadine-associated cardiac outcomes was feasible only after many years of extensive terfenadine use (9). For these reasons, cohort studies using linked databases are usually not of value in early phase IV when safety data are being sought soon after product launch.

USE AND CHARACTERISTICS OF SIMPLIFIED CLINICAL TRIALS

SCTs have a number of characteristics that distinguish them from phase III studies and demonstrate their utility (10). Many of these characteristics have been elaborated by Yusuf et al. (11) and colleagues in designing the International Study of Infraction Survival (ISIS) and other SCTs (12). The initial ISIS study examined over 16,000 myocardial infarction patients in 14 countries with random treatment allocation to atenolol or to usual care (i.e., no β-blocker). Other than demographic and risk factor data documented at enrollment, the main data collected were "hard endpoints" of 7-d and 30-d survival. In this way, the improvement of survival by β-blockade was shown.

It is important to note that there is no universal agreement on the nomenclature used for SCTs. They have been called mega trials, practical trials, public health trials, "low-tech" trials, and observational trials. The term "simplified clinical trials" is used here because it seems to most adequately cover the design being discussed. It must be emphasized that although "simpler" in terms of protocol and general procedures, SCTs are not simple to conduct and require careful planning and execution

In general terms, as was the case in the ISIS, SCTs are larger, more inclusive, more focused, and simpler than traditional phase III clinical trails out of necessity.

They are designed to detect rare events or relatively small effect size. Moreover, they are intended to include a heterogeneous patient population by having only minimal patient entry criteria. Thus, an SCT might include 5000 or more patients. The sheer numbers of patients is one of the reasons the study protocol and procedures must be simplified. Simplification means the use of a two- or three-page case report form instead of the 80-page form that attends most phase III studies. Data collection must be restricted to collecting relevant exposures, critical covariates, and the outcome of interest. This brevity is necessary as well because the majority of such trials are conducted in community practice settings rather than clinical research centers, and cannot be unduly burdensome to

Table 2
Aspects of Simplified Clinical Trials

1. Fewer patient exclusions (i.e., broad eligibility criteria)
2. Fewer variables collected
3. Definable "hard" endpoints
4. Ask only about major side effects (e.g., hospitalization, other forms of medical care, death)
5. Reduced onsite monitoring
6. Fewer and simpler protocol requirements and brief data collection instruments
7. Simple, noninvasive diagnostic techniques

the study site and participating physicians. The principle to be followed is to collect only information critical to the purpose of the trial and to avoid adding on "items of interest."

Several other features are common to SCTs. After (random) assignment of drug, much of the follow-up is "naturalistic" in that patients are followed in a manner consistent with usual practice. An exception is that every effort must be taken to ascertain each patient's status at the end of the study and to determine if the events of interest have or have not occurred. Table 2 summarizes some of the critical elements of SCTs.

SCTs share many attributes with prospective cohort studies. The major difference and the reason to classify such studies as trials is that exposure is assigned, whereas in cohort studies the treatments studied are "naturally" prescribed in usual practice and patients are enrolled only after the prescribing decision has been made. Thus, SCTs might be considered to be "quasi-observational." Initial data collection, large sample size, naturalistic follow-up, simple procedures, minimization of burden to the patient, and investigative site are all similar to methods typical of cohort studies (Table 3).

Because of their major differences from phase III trials, the application of standardized operating procedures and many other formulae used when conducting phase III trials are not appropriate for SCTs. However, even though simplified the specific aspects of study design and conduct are far from simple. Great care must be taken to decide on justifiable sample size and to consider the practical aspects of patient and physician recruitment. Use of a central human subjects review board (IRB) and formation of an endpoint adjudication group are usual features of SCTs. The number of subjects in SCTs and the potential need for interim analyses suggest that an independent safety monitoring board also be considered for these studies (13).

Comparators and Blinding in Simplified Clinical Trials

Some believe that only trials with randomized comparative exposures are true trials. In fact, for epidemiologists any "nonnatural" assignment of exposure with study of outcomes is a trial. Absent a comparator, SCTs may be deemed observational or surveillance studies. There is no universal agreement on nomenclature as previously noted.

What about blinding? If the study is of an endpoint not subject to observer bias, i.e., a "hard endpoint" such as death, then the need for blinding patients and physicians is lessened. In contrast to a phase III trial, conducting a SCT with blinded initial assignment of exposure and then "open-label" follow-up has at least two notable advantages. First, it is easier to prepare study supplies and distribution. Second, it facilitates enrollment of community practice sites and patients. Of course, knowing the exposure could result in diagnostic and other biases unlikely to happen in a blinded study. The likelihood of such biases and strategies to reduce their occurrence must be considered in planning a SCT.

Table 3
Means to Achieve Simplicity

1. Simplify entry criteria
2. Simplify patient management
3. Reduce/eliminate extra follow-up visits
4. Reduce the size and complexity of forms
5. Avoid ancillary studies and expensive investigations
6. Use simple treatment regimens

When Should Simplified Clinical Trials Be Considered ?

Peto and others *(11,12)* have listed the several features necessary to consider SCTs. These include the need to be treating a nonrare disease (otherwise enrollment of large numbers of patients will be impossible). Current therapy for the disease cannot be fully effective, which would make the conduct of the study unethical. The means to deliver and monitor the drug being used must be simple (e.g., oral therapy), because otherwise conduct of the study will be too complicated and study size will not be achieved. Simple and broad patient entry criteria must be definable.

Simplified Clinical Trial Examples

Perhaps one of the earliest SCTs was the trial of the Salk polio vaccine. Second-grade students were vaccinated and nonvaccinated children in the first and third grades served as comparator populations *(14)*. Another classic example of a SCT is the Physicians Health Study that enrolled 22,071 physicians, and randomized them to aspirin or placebo and to beta carotene or placebo (15). Follow-up was through mail surveys and national vital status records. Of course, this study showed the ability of low-dose aspirin to reduce the myocardial infarction rates.

Yet another study illustrating SCT principles was an assessment of the safety of pediatric ibuprofen conducted between 1991 and 1993. This was a randomized double-blind acetaminophen controlled trial with 84,192 children where the outcomes were hospitalizations for GI bleeding, acute renal failure, and anaphylaxis. These were initially assessed by mailed questionnaire or phone follow-up at 4 wk *(16)*.

There are many other examples of SCTs in a number of therapeutic areas. Castle *(17)* studied mortality associated with short- and long-acting bronchodilators in some 16,000 asthmatics. The series of infarction survival studies all used SCT principles as did many of the cholesterol lowering and mortality studies. Other examples include studies of therapies for congestive heart failure, AIDS, and benign prostatic hypertrophy.

Turning to studies of QTc interval prolongation, one "observational" trial of the quinolone antibiotic moxifloxacin is illustrative *(18)*. In 1999, the Food and Drug Administration (FDA) mandated this trial because of concern about a mean QTc prolongation of 6 ms for the drug. It was conducted as a single-arm (uncontrolled) study at about 3700 sites that enrolled and treated over 18,000 patients with bronchitis, sinusitis, or community acquired pneumonia. Follow-up of patient status was by return visit or telephone call. Detailed examination of all serious adverse events and hospitalizations, nonscheduled ECGs, syncope, arrhythmias, and cardiac events was done. There was limited monitoring of data collection at individual sites and central site coordination. ECGs were not required in the protocol. No life-threatening arrhythmias were found and only two sudden deaths were identified, one with many risk factors and one after one dose of drug. The rate of sudden death did not exceed the expected background rate for such events.

Distinguishing Simplified Clinical Trials From Seeding Trials

It is important to distinguish SCTs from so-called seeding studies. Seeding trials are "thinly veiled attempts to entice doctors to prescribe a new drug ... that serve little or no scientific purpose" (19). They are studies with features that distinguish them from SCTs including a design that does not support the stated research goal, disproportionately high payments to investigators, sponsorship by sales and marketing departments, and collection of data of little or no value. They are most often seen when a new drug enters a crowded therapeutic class. By contrast, SCTs clearly describe their purpose, justify the number of investigators and patients included, and provide investigator reimbursement proportionate to the work done by the investigators.

SUMMARY AND CONCLUSIONS

Because of inherent limitations in the drug approval process, it is likely that phase IV studies will be important in examining cardiac safety of pharmaceuticals. Arrhythmogenicity and other cardiac effects of new drugs may be relatively uncommon or occur in untested subgroups pre-approval. Spontaneous reporting after approval may raise signals of possible new safety concerns. To evaluate such signals or to anticipate potential safety questions, SCTs done after approval may be indicated. After a year or more of marketing, cohort studies such as those using administrative databases may be feasible.

REFERENCES

1. Mathieu M. New Drug Development: A Regulatory Overview , 4th ed. Waltham, MA: Parexel International Corp., 1997
2. Liberman UA, Hirsch LJ. Esophagitis and alendronate. N Engl J Med 1996;335:1069–1070.
3. Meinert CL. Clinical Trials. Design, Conduct and Analysis. NY: Oxford University Press, 1986.
4. Faich GA. Adverse drug reaction monitoring. New Engl J Med 1986;314:1589–1592.
5. Faich GA. US adverse drug reaction surveillance 1989–1994. Pharmacoepidem and Drug Safety 1996;5:393–398.
6. FDA/Pharma Task Force to Assess QT Risk, FDC Weekly (Pink Sheet). Nov 1, 1999, pp. 15–17.
7. Michels KB, Faich GA. Linked databases and epidemiology, J Clinical Research and Pharmacoepidemiology 1991;5:11–18.
8. Hennessy S, Bilker W, Knauss JS, Margolis DJ, Kimmel S, et al. Cardiac arrest and ventricular arrhythmia in patients taking antipsychotic drugs. Brit Med J 2002;325:1070.
9. Hanrahan JP, Choo PW, Carlson W, Greineder D, Faich GA, Platt R. Terfenadine-associated ventricular arrhythmias and QTc interval prolongation. A retrospective cohort comparison with other antihistamines among members of a health maintenance organization. Ann Epidemiol 1995;5:201–209.
10. Lesko SM, Mitchell AA. Use of randomized controlled trials for phramacoepidemiology studies. In Pharmacoepidemiology 3rd ed. Strom BL, ed. NY: John Wiley & Sons, 2000, pp. 539–552.
11. Yusuf S, Collins R, Peto R. Why do we need some large simple randomized trials? Stat in Med 1984; 3:409–420.
12. Peto R, Collins R, Gray R, Large-scale randomized evidence: large, simple trials and overviews of trials. J Clin Epidemiol 1995;48:23–40.
13. Ellenberg S, Fleming TR, DeMets DL. Data Monitoring Committees in Clinical Trials. NY: John Wiley & Sons, 2003.
14. Franceis T, Korns R, Voight R, et al. An evaluation of the 1954 poliomyelitis vaccine trails. Am J Public Health 1955;45:1–50.
15. Steering Committee of the Physicians Health Study Research Group. Final report on the aspirin component of the ongoing Physicians Health Study. New Engl J Med 1989;321:129–135.

16. Lesko SM, Mitchell AA. An assessment of the safety of pediatric ibuprofen. A practitioner-based randomized clinical trial. J Amer Med Assoc 1996;275:986.

17. Castle W, Fuller R, Hall J, Palmer R. Comparison of salmeterol with salbutamol. J Brit Med 1993;306: 1034–1037

18. Faich GA, Morganroth J, Whitehouse AB, Brar JS, Arcuri P, Kowalshy SF, Haverstock DC, Celesk, RA, Church DA. Clinical experience with moxifloxacin in patients with respiratory tract infections. Ann Pharmacother 2004;38:140.

19. Kessler D, Rose L, Temple R. et al. Seeding trials—Therapeutic class wars—drug promotion. New Engl J Med 1994;331:1350–1353.

14 Statistical Analysis Plans for ECG Data

Controlling the Intrinsic and Extrinsic Variability in QT Data

Alan S. Hollister, MD, PhD
and Timothy H Montague

CONTENTS

INTRODUCTION

The safety and regulatory needs to detect small drug-induced changes in the QT interval have created many challenges for the design and analysis of "thorough" QT studies. The measurement techniques available, the correlation between the RR interval and the QT interval, and the high variability in the QT interval have made the detection of changes in the QT interval difficult, and the verification of a lack of an effect on the QT interval even more difficult. The purpose of this chapter is to provide statistical and empirical rationales for key elements of study design, and statistical analysis that will control for sources of QT variability and will enhance study sensitivity. We will identify study design and statistical techniques to reduce QT variability, discuss the assumptions inherent in many of the choices available in study design, and recommend study designs based on these principles.

The QT interval, and its heart rate corrected value (QTc) varies widely throughout the day in normal individuals with reports ranging from 76 ms to 117 ms *(1,2)*. Numerous groups have reported the influence of meals, sleep, age, autonomic tone or balance,

From: *Cardiac Safety of Noncardiac Drugs:*
Practical Guidelines for Clinical Research and Drug Development
Edited by: J. Morganroth and I. Gussak © Humana Press Inc., Totowa, NJ

gender, body position, electrolyte abnormalities, exercise, and insulin levels, as well as the effects of drugs, disease, and genetic abnormalities on the QT interval *(2–11)*. Despite study designs that control for many of these factors, several factors may change during the course of a study, and a time or sequence effect may be present in both the QT variability as well as the absolute value of the QT. It is also important to understand that it is not known whether the diurnal variation in the QT is a pattern or rhythm that is reproducible day to day within individuals. In general, minute-to-minute variations in the QT interval are less than day-to-day variations, and much less than week-to-week variations *(12)*.

The sensitivity of a study is dependent on the ratio of the change in the QT to the variability of that change. The magnitude of the change in QT is dependent on the drug, dose, and occasionally the study population, but is often limited by drug tolerability and/or safety. Thus, study designs that minimize the variability of the QT and reliably measure the QT at the time of maximal drug-induced changes will most efficiently detect the change, and will require the smallest sample size.

STATISTICAL LIMITATION OF THE QT VARIABILITY

The simplest and easiest technique for reducing the minute-to-minute variability in the QT is to standardize which complexes are measured within an electrocardiogram (ECG), to measure two or more complexes, and to average values from two or more ECGs. Typically, the QT interval is measured on three consecutive complexes from the same ECG lead during a period of stable heart rate and rhythm, and the QT and its corrected value averaged from the three complexes. Duplicate or triplicate ECGs are obtained at 1-to-5 min intervals and the values of these are all averaged to estimate the QT and QTc values. In this fashion, the minute-to-minute variability in the QT is reduced by the square root of the number of complexes and the number of ECGs measured. The effect of this technique on reducing the variability (standard deviation) of the change in QT, as well as on the sample size, is shown in Fig. 1.

The bars represent the standard deviation for the change in QTc from a model data set where the true difference between baseline and on-drug QT values is 10 ms and the within-subject standard deviations at both baseline and on-drug are 15 ms. Note how the standard deviation decreases in an exponential fashion as the number of replicate ECGs increase. The numbers above the bars indicate the number of subjects required for an 80% probability of finding a $p < 0.05$ difference between baseline and on-drug QTc by the *t*-test. Multiple iterations of this model found a statistically significant reduction in the standard deviation between one and two ECGs per time point, and a $p = 0.07$ reduction between two and three replicate ECGs per time point. Thus, the QT and QTc averaged from two or more ECGs per time point is a simple and effective method for increasing study sensitivity and reducing sample size.

CHOICE OF BASELINE

The baseline against which the effect of drug is to be compared needs to be chosen carefully. Factors to consider in this choice are listed previously and include the time of day, meals, period of awakening, familiarity of the experimental surroundings, and the time interval between the baseline and on-drug measurements. The assumption present in the choice of baseline is that it should neither increase nor decrease the magnitude of

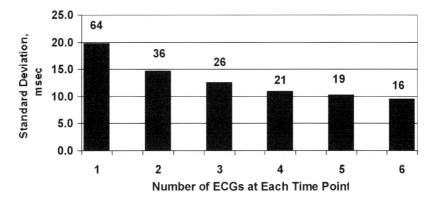

Fig. 1. Effect of the number of replicate ECGs per time point on the standard deviation of the change in QTc.

the QT change, and it should minimize the variance of the estimate of the QT change. There is some debate about what is the "best" baseline: a predose value of the QT or an on-placebo, time-matched QT value. The predose baseline may be collected immediately before dosing, or may be an average of baselines over several periods (as proposed in the original Canadian/FDA draft of the ICH document). The on-placebo baseline may be the QT obtained at the same time of day as the on-drug measurement (i.e., time-matched), or an average of QTs over the course of multiple measurements on a placebo day. Each of these options makes one or more assumptions about QT variability:

1. Predose QT as baseline: assumes time proximity to the drug-induced change minimizes the variability, no diurnal pattern of QT changes, no study protocol-induced QT changes.
2. Multiple predose baselines over several days or periods: assumes no difference in the absolute QT value or its variance between days (or weeks) compared to within day, no sequence effect, no difference in QT or its variability caused by diurnal changes.
3. Same time of day on placebo day: assumes a stable, reliable pattern in QT with time of day and study conditions, no sequence effect, stable day-to-day variability, stable QT–RR relationship between the placebo day and the active drug day, and no effect of time interval on magnitude of QT change.
4. Multiple ECGs averaged over a period of time on a baseline/placebo day: assumes stable and consistent QT variability from day to day, with limited within day variability.

In the experience of the authors, the within subject moment-to-moment QT variability (average SD = 6–9 ms) is slightly less than within day variability (SD = 9–10) which is less than day-to-day variability (SD = 9–13) and less than between week variability (SD = 10–15). A sequence effect has been noted in some studies, and the time-matched placebo as baseline has been criticized for a lack of sensitivity and reliability *(13)*. In addition, the apparent magnitude of the QT change increases with the interval between the baseline and on-drug measurements. Figure 2 illustrates the effect of time between baseline and on-drug measurement of the Fridericia's corrected QT (QTcF) change caused by a single 400 mg oral dose of moxifloxacin (data taken from three studies reported in the 4/27/01 Summary Basis for Approval for moxifloxacin *[14]*).

Figure 2 illustrates the change in QTcF at the time of drug Cmax when the time between baseline and on-drug measurements was 0 (predose on the same day as drug dosing), 1 d, 1 to 3 wk, and 1 to 5 wk. The diamond symbols are data from single ECG

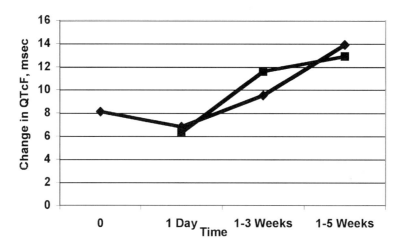

Fig. 2. Effect of time between baseline and on-drug measurement of the change in QTcF at Cmax after oral doses of 400 mg moxifloxacin.

determinations of baseline, and the squares are data from multiple ECG determinations of baseline. These results suggest that the greater the interval between the baseline and on-drug measurements of QTc, the greater the apparent effect of the drug. This phenomenon was observed in three studies designed *a priori* to test for this effect, and warrant consideration in the design of crossover studies or in parallel design studies requiring longer periods between predose baseline and drug steadystate concentration levels.

A similar effect was observed in the variability of the change in QTc in these moxifloxacin studies. Figure 3 illustrates the standard deviation for the change in QTcF at Cmax for moxifloxacin plotted against the time between the baseline and on-drug measurements. The diamond symbols are data from single determinations of the baseline QT, and the squares display data from multiple ECG determinations of baseline. Although the differences between single and multiple ECG measurements is clear, there is also a trend for greater variability in the group standard deviation when the time between baseline and on-drug measurements increase. This increase in variability as the time between baseline and on-drug measurements increases will impact the sample size (number of subjects) necessary to detect a drug effect in longer term studies.

In summary, whether the drug effect is expressed as a change from baseline or a change from placebo, there are multiple assumptions inherent in the choice. For data transparency, display of data as a change from the predose baseline for both drug and placebo will enhance the understanding of the drug effect as well as effects related to experimental conditions. As indicated by the experience with moxifloxacin, the closer in time the baseline is to the on-drug measurements of QT, the lower the magnitude of QT change, and the lower the variance of the change. There appears to be little difference between same day and preceding day baselines, but longer intervals have the potential to falsely elevate the magnitude of QT effect, increase the variability of the estimate of this effect, and will require larger sample sizes. This will be of particular concern in the design of "thorough" QT studies with drugs or metabolites that have long half-lives, or that require titration to reach the tested dose. Parallel designs that incorporate assessment of the interval and sequence effect may be the best approach for evaluation of these drugs.

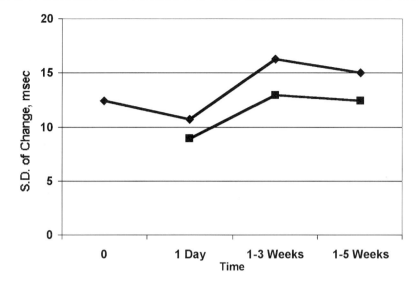

Fig. 3. Effect of time between baseline and on-drug measurement of QTcF on the standard deviation of the change in QTcF.

QT CORRECTION METHODS

The RR and QT intervals are highly correlated, with the QT interval increasing with increasing RR interval. As such, an observed increase in the absolute QT interval could be the results of changes in the RR interval rather than a drug effect. Several methods have been proposed to "correct" the QT interval with respect to the RR interval, such that the corrected QT interval (QTc) is independent of the RR interval *(15)*.

Figure 4 illustrates the relationship between the RR interval (*x*-axis) and the QT interval (*y*-axis), showing a clear trend for the QT interval to increase with increasing values of the RR interval. An appropriate correction method should show no trend in the data when the corrected QT (QTc) is plotted vs the RR interval.

All methods are based on defining the RR–QT relationship, and then standardizing the QT interval around an RR value of 1 s (equivalent to a heart rate of 60 bpm). In this chapter, "population" and "individual" correction methods will be reviewed, as well as a method that requires no correction. Finally, a brief overview of the use of Holter ECGs and their analyses will be provided.

Population corrections are the most common and historically used methods. The oldest of these is Bazett's, $QTcB = QT/(RR^{1/2})$, where RR is in seconds and QT in milliseconds. Another common correction, is Fridericia's, $QTcF = QT/(RR^{1/3})$. These methods assume a log-linear QT–RR relationship. The problem with these "fixed" corrections is that if the actual QT–RR relationship differs from the fixed relationship, then the estimate of treatment effects will be biased. In the case of Bazett's correction, it is widely recognized that Bazett's over-corrects for the RR interval at higher heart rates, resulting in an increase in false positive effects. Fridericia's typically performs a bit better, but also is susceptible to both over- and under-correcting, leading to both false positive and negative conclusions, respectively.

Figure 5 illustrates that there is an inverse relationship between the RR interval (*x*-axis) and the Bazett's corrected QT (QTcB) interval (*y*-axis). The QTcB interval decreases

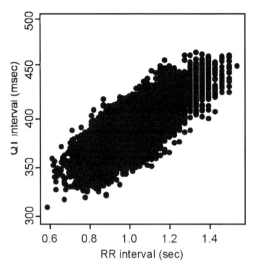

Fig. 4. QT–RR relationship.

Table 1
Linear and Log-Linear Models of QT–RR Relationship
and Corresponding Formulae for Corrected QT (QTc)

	Model QT	*Calculation of QTc*
Linear	$QT = \alpha + \beta RR$	$QTc = QT + \beta(1{-}RR)$
Log–linear	$\log(QT) = \alpha + \beta\log(RR)$	$QTc = QT/(RR^{\beta})$

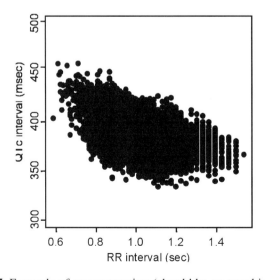

Fig. 5. Example of overcorrecting (should be no trend in QTc).

with increasing values of the RR interval, indicating that Bazett's correction over-corrected for the RR interval.

An alternative to the fixed population methods is to define the QT-RR relationship based on the observed study data. It is recommended that one use off-treatment data (baseline or baseline + on-placebo data). The first step is to model QT as a function of RR (linear or log–linear) and estimate the slope parameter, β. Then QTc is calculated using this estimate of the slope parameter.

In Table 1, the second column shows the model for the QT-RR relationship. The third column shows the formulae for calculating the corrected QT interval (QTc) based on the estimated parameters from the model for the QT-RR relationship. Note, for Bazett's and Fridericia's corrections, the slope parameter, β, equals 0.5 and 0.33, respectively, for a log-linear model.

The limitations of the population corrections are that they require the following assumptions:

1. stable and constant QT–RR relationship across subjects
2. stable and constant QT–RR relationship across time, days, and/or sessions
3. stable and constant QT–RR relationship across treatments

There are data to suggest that the QT–RR relationship varies from subject to subject and varies over time (when awakening, within a day, across days, weeks, months) *(2,4,6,7,16,17)*. Additionally, the QT–RR relationship may be altered by external factors such as autonomic balance, drugs, and other external factors, as reviewed earlier.

Individual correction methods relax the assumption about stable and constant relationships across subjects, by determining a unique relationship for each individual subject. The only assumption across subjects is that the form of the relationship (linear or log-linear) is the same. The correction is similar to the population approach, but a unique slope parameter, β, is calculated for each subject. Thus, only assumptions 2 and 3 from above are made. As with a population correction, it is recommended that individual corrections be based on off-treatment data.

The limitations of the individual correction are the need for a sufficient number of observations and a sufficient range of RR intervals. If either or both are insufficient, the QT–RR relationship may be poorly defined, adding both bias and variability to treatment effects. Figure 6 provides two such scenarios. Figure 6 illustrates two examples of insufficient data for determining an individual correction. Off-treatment RR interval (*x*-axis) vs QT intervals are plotted with the dashed line representing a "best" fit log–linear model. In the figure on the left, the data are clustered around a small range of RR values. In this case, one could imagine that any line would have provided a reasonably good fit to the data. In addition, one would not have much confidence in the modeled QT–RR relationship for an RR interval greater than 1.2 s. The figure on the right illustrates that a single observation (at RR 1.1 s) can impact the slope of the curve for sparse data. If that point was not there, the slope of the curve might be quite different, leading to a different set of corrected QT values.

The authors recommend that 20 to 50 off-treatment observations per subject are needed for use of an individual correction, with more being better. For a crossover design this should not be an issue, but it may be a limitation for parallel group designs. QTs distributed over a sufficient range of RR intervals, approx 0.7 to 1.1 s (heart rate of 55 to 86), are necessary for an adequate estimate for each individual's correction. However, a well-controlled trial by design is going to limit the range of RR intervals for a subject, by

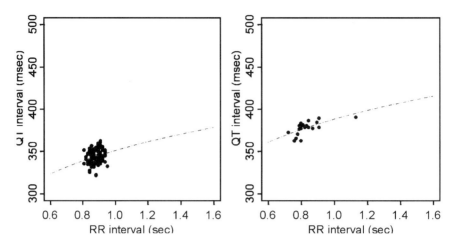

Fig. 6. Insufficient data for individual corrections.

controlling the external factors that may affect the RR interval. As such, care should be taken when using an individual approach.

As all correction methods are flawed in some manner, two statisticians have proposed using a repeated measures analysis that does not require a correction of the QT interval *(18)*. This is desirable as it avoids the potential for adding bias and variability to treatment effects caused by the correction method, and it can account for potential treatment effects on both the RR interval and the QT–RR relationship. The proposed method also allows for assumptions that the QT–RR relationship may vary over time and treatment, and takes into account the correlation between observations within a subject. As with population and individual correction methods, the QT interval is modeled as either a linear or log-linear function of the RR interval, with a unique set of parameters being determined for each sampling time (i.e., pre- and post-dose) and each treatment (i.e., placebo and each active dose). Treatment differences are then calculated for the QT interval based on the estimates of the model parameters for a given RR interval. For further description of this approach the reader is referred to the method description *(18)*. Graphically, this analysis is illustrated in Fig. 7. The placebo is represented by the circles and the experimental drug by the triangles. Open symbols are predose or baseline values and filled symbols are post-dose values. The treatment effect is the difference between experimental drug post-dose and predose values and placebo post-dose and predose values ([▲ - △] – [● - ○]).

As the QT–RR relationship is no longer restricted to be the same for each treatment and time point, treatment effects must be evaluated at a range of values for the RR interval. Specifically, if the QT–RR relationships are not parallel across treatments and time, then the treatment effect will vary with the value of the RR interval. In the left part of Fig. 7, the treatment effect increases with increasing RR interval. This may confound the study results, leading to a false negative conclusion. Because many QT-prolonging drugs change the QT–RR relationship and exhibit greater QT prolongation at slow heart rates ("reverse rate dependency"), the assumptions of this method may underestimate drug effects. When the method assumes parallel lines (i.e., assume stable and constant QT–RR relationship across time and treatment) illustrated in the right part of Fig. 7, the treatment effects are calculated by a linear combination of intercepts for the various

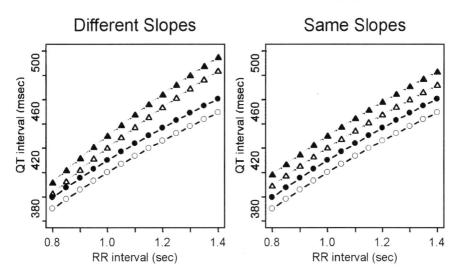

Fig. 7. QT analysis without heart rate correction: model options.

treatments and time points. By imposing parallel lines, this method provides results similar to data based on a population correction.

The draft ICH guidance document *(19)* recognizes that none of the discussed methods can be identified as "best" for all situations. As such, the guidance recommends and allows for multiple correction methods to be used, with Bazett's and Fridericia's being the standard methods. The authors recommend data-driven corrections (population or individual) or repeated measures analysis on uncorrected QT values.

One recently validated method to avoid the use of correction factors is the so-called "Holter bin" method *(20)*. This method uses continuous ECG recordings via a Holter monitor over a period of maximum pharmacodynamic effect of the drug. All of the PQRST complexes from 10 ms RR intervals ("bins") are averaged electronically and the resulting high fidelity trace is measured for the QT interval. This allows for the comparison of placebo and on-drug QT intervals at every heart rate recorded, generating the QT–RR relationship for both drug and placebo during the period of maximum drug effect. The drug and placebo QT can be compared at the same heart rate (e.g., an RR of 1000 ms = a HR of 60 bpm), across all heart rates recorded, from the RR bin where the greatest number of complexes were recorded for placebo and drug, and/or a regression of the QT–RR relationship. Because of the large number of complexes averaged within each RR bin, the within subject variability of the QT interval and its change is one-half to one-third that of replicate ECGs. This results in a large increase in the sensitivity for identifying a QT effect of a drug. The limitation of the "Holter bin" method is that recording must be performed over a period of time (2–4 h) covering the peak effect of the drug. This may dilute the maximum effect of a short half-life drug that exhibits a short-lived peak. The marked advantage of the Holter bin method is that it allows within-subject analysis via the repeated measures method using many more data points than can be obtained with ECGs. It also avoids the increases in variability caused by correction methods.

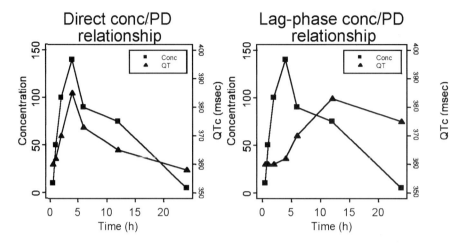

Fig. 8. Direct and lag-phase concentration QT relationships.

CENTRAL TENDENCY ANALYSIS

The draft ICH guidance recommends that the "thorough" QT trial to evaluate repolarization be designed to either detect a minimal mean effect or to "rule out" a mean effect. In either case, the mean effect can be defined by a summary measure of the time course of ECGs measured after each treatment. Possible summary measures or central tendency parameters include:

1. change at observed drug Cmax/Tmax (maximum plasma concentration and time to maximum concentration)
2. change at anticipated Tmax
3. maximum change regardless of drug concentration or time
4. average change over a specific period
5. area under the curve (or more properly, the area under the effect curve [AUEC]) of QT for a specific period.

As the QT, RR, and corrected QT (QTc) are highly correlated, all should be summarized in the same manner and analyzed at the same time points or periods chosen. The choice of the parameter depends on the experimental drug's pharmacokinetic (PK) characteristics (time and duration of Cmax, variability of Tmax, half-life) and its concentration/QTc relationship (direct or lag-phase). If the experimental drug has active metabolite(s), the PK and PK/QTc relationship should also be considered. For example, Fig. 8 illustrates a direct concentration/QT relationship (left) and lag-phase (or indirect) relationship (right). On the left, both the time profiles of the concentration data and the QT interval are similar, with peaks occurring approximately at the same time. While on the right, the time profiles are different, with the peak of the QT profile occurring several hours after the peak of the concentration profile. It is easy to see that using the change at Tmax for a compound with a lag-phase concentration–QT relationship could result in a false negative conclusion.

The change from baseline at observed Tmax or anticipated Tmax (option 1 or 2) is an appropriate parameter when the drug has the following characteristics: The concentration-QTc relationship is a direct one (i.e., no lag-phase as in the left figure); Tmax is well defined with low variability; the half-lives of the drug and its pharmacodynamic effect are fairly

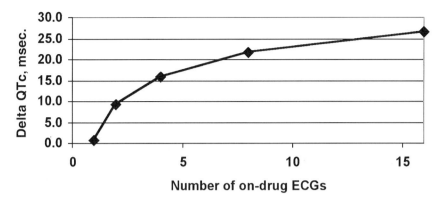

Fig. 9. False positivity magnitude with the maximum change in QTc.

short (< 24 h); and the drug either has no active metabolite or the active metabolite(s) have both a similar PK profile as the parent and direct concentration–QTc relationship.

The change from baseline at the anticipated Tmax is more easily implemented during a study than the change from baseline at the actual Tmax, especially for parallel group designs. For the change from baseline at observed Tmax, it is recommended that the placebo comparator be time-matched to reduce bias caused by diurnal variation. For a crossover trial, this would entail for each subject that the placebo comparator be the change from baseline to the same Tmax of the active treatment. Although parallel group designs cannot be analyzed in this manner, a Hodges-Lehmann-Moses non-parametric approach can be used to estimate a time-matched comparison between active and placebo treatments *(21)*. Again, the change at Tmax parameter is only valid when there is a good correspondence between the PK and the pharmacodynamic effect of the measured drug (the left part of Fig. 8).

Another concern with using the change at observed or anticipated Tmax is that the Cmax is typically the most variable PK parameter. As such, this variability will contribute to the variability of the QT parameters. This is especially important when designing parallel group designs. To help minimize variability, the study should be designed to ensure that experimental conditions are optimal at the time of maximum concentration. For example, one would not want to feed subjects within 2 h of the anticipated Tmax.

If the Tmax is highly variable, if there is a lag-phase in the concentration–QT relationship, and/or if active metabolites have a different PK profile than the parent, then the maximum change from baseline may be the appropriate measure of drug-induced QT change. For the QTc interval, the maximum change is just the maximum post-dose QTc value minus the baseline value, regardless of time and pharmacokinetics. For the QT and RR intervals, the authors recommend that the change from baseline be time-matched to the time at which the maximum QTc value occurred, so that one can assess and relate effects on QTc to those of the QT and RR interval appropriately. This parameter is dependent on both the sampling scheme for the ECG (number and timing) measurements and the experimental conditions (evaluation time, meals, sleep, etc.). Too few sampling time points may result in missing the maximal drug effect, whereas too many samples can increase the probability of spurious effect (false-positive). This is illustrated in Fig. 9, which demonstrates that the magnitude of the "maximum change in QTc" parameter is dependent on the number of ECGs obtained after drug administration, as a result of simple statistical variabil-

Table 2
Difference in Change From Baseline @ Tmax vs Maximum Change From Baseline

Drug	Δ QTc @ Cmax (mean ± SE)	Tmax (h)	Max Δ QTc (mean ± SE)	Time of max QTc (h)
X 1x	9 ± 15	2	24 ± 15	5.2
X 2x	20 ± 18	2.4	32 ± 17	4.3
Y 1x	5 ± 14	1.5	22 ± 14	5.5
Y 2x	7 ± 15	1.5	21 ± 12	5.3
Z	3 ± 14	1.3	21 ± 13	5.9
Placebo	−5 ± 15	—	16 ± 14	6.1

ity. The magnitude of this change may be reduced if replicate ECGs are obtained at each time point, but the risk of a falsely positive result is still present. The use of the maximum change in QTc parameter will consistently overestimate the magnitude of drug-induced QTc changes, and is only of value when changes can be compared to placebo data, or when hysteresis curve analysis indicates a disjunction between the pharmacodynamic effect (PD) and the PK of the measured drug. Additionally, the parameter is susceptible to diurnal variation with the sampling times chosen, another cause of false-positive results. As with the change at observed Tmax, it is recommended that the placebo comparator be time-matched to reduce bias caused by diurnal variation.

A potential pitfall of the maximum change from baseline is that, as a result of the high variability of the QT interval, often the maximum change from baseline does not occur at the same time as Tmax, even for drugs with a well defined Tmax of low variability, direct PK/PD relationship and no active metabolites. This is illustrated in the Table 2 of actual data taken from the moxifloxacin Summary Basis of Approval for three different drugs and placebo.

Table 2 demonstrates the large difference between the change in QTc at the time of Cmax compared to the maximum change in QTc at any time after drug administration. All three of these known QT-prolonging drugs (and even placebo) had their effects confounded by the parameter "maximum change in QTc." The time of Tmax and true drug QT effect occurred at about 2 h for each drug, whereas the time of the maximum change in QTc varied over the entire 12 h of data collection after drug administration. The consistent 12 to 20 ms difference between these two estimates of drug effect demonstrates the problems of false positivity with the maximum change in QTc parameter, and is completely predictable as in Fig. 9.

If the drug has a long pharmacokinetic or pharmacodynamic (QTc) half-life, then the average QTc change or the QTc area under the effect curve (AUEC) over a specific time period may be considered as the response parameters. Similar to the maximum change, the sampling scheme and experimental conditions may bias these parameters. Whereas these parameters are useful for evaluating whether a drug has a sustained effect over time, they have not been independently validated and as such are not considered sufficient for drug approval when used alone. Specifically, these parameters are not appropriate for drugs that have a direct concentration–QT relationship with a short half-life, as they may provide a false-negative result.

The statistical model for all of these central tendency parameters is similar. For a crossover design, the authors recommend a mixed effect model fitting a random term for subjects and fixed terms for sequence, period, and treatments. Additionally, baseline

Table 3
Clinical Interpretation of Mean Changes in QTc

Change from baseline	Relative risk of TdP
< 5 ms	So far no TdP
5–10 ms	No clear risk
10–20 ms	Uncertainty
> 20 ms	"Substantially" increased likelihood of being pro-arrhythmic

TdP, torsade des pointes.

Table 4
Null and Alternative Hypotheses for Two Statistical Approaches to Definitive QT Study

	To detect an effect	To rule out an effect
Null hypothesis	Ho: $\theta = 0$	Ho: $\theta \geq \delta$
Alternative hypothesis	Ha: $\theta \neq 0$	Ha: $\theta < \delta$

θ represents the difference between the experimental drug and placebo.
δ represents a clinical relevant difference, e.g., the change from baseline in Table 3.

(predose) values should be fit as a covariate to further reduce variability. For a parallel group design, an analysis of covariance (ANCOVA) is recommended, fitting a single fixed term for treatment and baseline as a covariate. As appropriate to the study design, fixed terms for other factors such as gender and age can also be included in either model.

INTERPRETATION OF THE OBSERVED CENTRAL TENDENCIES IN QTc

There are two aspects to interpreting the observed central tendencies in QTc of an experimental drug; statistical and clinical. The statistical interpretation is based on the statistical hypothesis being tested. For a "thorough" QT study, this will either be to detect a specific effect or to rule out a specific effect. The specific effects should be clinically meaningful changes in QTc.

The ranges and associated risks in Table 3 are from the draft ICH guidance and are based on clinical experience. It should be noted that there are other factors that may mitigate or enhance the risk of TdP. In addition, these ranges do not take into account the variability of the measurement, method of measurement, or correction factor. Finally, these are based on historical data using Bazett's corrected QT.

As mentioned earlier, the "thorough" QT study can be designed to test one of two hypotheses: to detect a specific difference or to rule out a specific difference. The mathematical expressions of these hypotheses are shown in Table 4.

The former is the more traditional statistical hypothesis (similar to that used to demonstrate a drug is superior to placebo in a pivotal trial). The latter is similar to that used for a bioequivalence trial or a noninferiority trial. The draft ICH document recommends that the study be designed to detect a 5 ms difference or to rule out a 5 or 7.5 ms difference. For both hypotheses, the study should be adequately powered. In general, to rule out an effect is a more stringent test and will require a larger sample size than that needed to detect a difference.

For either of these hypotheses, the comparison of interest should be between the change in QTc by the experimental drug vs the change in QTc on placebo. The draft ICH guidance does not indicate for which dose, therapeutic or supratherapeutic, of the experimental drug the hypotheses should be tested. If the hypotheses are to be tested for more than one dose, then the type I error rate, α, needs to be controlled for multiple comparisons.

For all comparisons of interest, $100(1-\alpha)\%$ confidence intervals, rather than p values should be employed to interpret the results, where α is the type I error rate. For the hypothesis to detect a difference, the confidence interval should not include 0. For the hypothesis to rule out an effect, the upper bound of the confidence interval should be less than the clinically relevant difference, δ. For comparisons for which no hypotheses are being tested, confidence intervals provide a range of plausible values. In addition, it is recommended that point estimates and $100(1-\alpha)\%$ confidence intervals be provided for mean effect of each treatment including placebo.

As changes in the QTc interval may be confounded with changes in the heart rate (RR interval), effects of the drug on both the QT and RR (or HR) intervals should be examined. Whereas there is no current guidance to interpret changes in the QT and RR intervals, an increase in the RR interval should correspond to an increase in the QT interval, although the magnitude of the increases should not necessarily be the same. Another signal that drug effects may be confounded is when there are differences in the results depending on the method of correcting QT for the RR interval. Bazett's method tends to overcorrect the QT interval when there are increases in heart rate. Thus, for a drug that increases the heart rate, Bazett's method may yield a larger estimate of drug effect on QTc than either a Fridericia's or population-based QT correction would.

There are two other analyses that might be done to help further assess the effect of experimental drugs. The first is to examine the dose- or concentration–response relationship, and the second is to look at individual subject changes from baseline. These are discussed in the next two sections.

DOSE–RESPONSE AND CONCENTRATION–RESPONSE MODELING

Understanding the dose–response and/or concentration–response of an experimental drug is essential to assessing the risk of QT prolongation. A shallow dose- or concentration–response may indicate a low risk of prolongation. To adequately model a dose–response of an experimental drug, a minimum of three doses should be studied, which has not been employed in "thorough" QT studies submitted to the regulatory agencies *(22)*. However, a concentration–response can be done with two doses, such as the therapeutic and supratherapeutic doses. If pharmacokinetic samples are taken over a range of times following dose, this should provide a range of concentrations from very low to supratherapeutic levels.

It is recommended that the following plots be generated to better understand the concentration–response:

- individual hysteresis plots of concentration vs QTc
- population scatter plots of drug concentration vs QTc
- mean time course plots of both concentration and QTc

Hysteresis plots account for time, and thus are useful in helping to assess whether there is lag-phase or prolonged effect on QTc. Figure 10 provides an example of what a hysteresis plot might look like for a drug with a direct concentration–response relation-

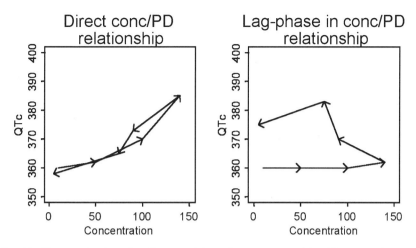

Fig. 10. Hysteresis plots for direct and lag-phase concentration/QTc relationships.

ship (left) and for a drug with a lag phase (right). These plots can also provide insight into the shape of the concentration–response relationship, will validate the adequacy of the frequency and timing of ECG collection, and may reveal additional factors (e.g., active metabolites, distribution phase, etc.) that will influence the interpretation of the results.

Figure 10 shows hysteresis plots for direct (left) and lag-phase (right) concentration–QTc relationships. Paired concentration (x-axis) and QTc interval (y-axis) values are plotted, with > indicating the time sequence of the paired observations. The figure on the left shows that concentration and QTc move together over time, whereas the right figure shows that there is delay.

Plots of the mean time courses of both concentration and QTc provide a visual assessment of the presence of a lag phase in the concentration–response relationship as illustrated in Fig. 8. These are then enhanced by the hysteresis plots of the concentration–PD effect relationship illustrated earlier.

Scatter plots of concentration vs QTc provide a visual assessment of a direct concentration–response. It is recommended that scatter plots include data from all doses of the experimental drug.

Figure 11 illustrates the concentration–response relationship for an experimental drug (open circles). A linear relationship was assumed that is represented by the solid line.

If the relationship between the drug concentration and the QTc change appears to be well defined and without a lag phase, a simple linear or nonlinear regression can be used to model the concentration–response relationship. The model should account for the study design (crossover or parallel group), for correlation between observation and within and between-subject variability. Whether three doses are tested or a concentration–response model is used, this approach rapidly increases the power of the study and minimizes the sample size.

The balance between the number of subjects and the frequency of data collection can be estimated using techniques described by Ahn and Jung *(23)*. In the presence of a lag phase, modeling of the concentration–response relationship can be performed using software designed for this purpose (e.g., Non-Mem, Win Non-Lin) and the model results tested for significance of the relationship. The model then can be

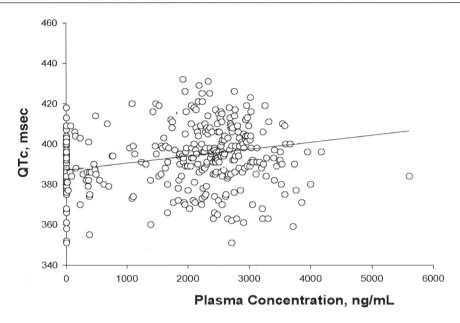

Fig. 11. Scatter plot of concentration and QTc intervals.

used to provide predictions for various concentrations or to predict at what concentration a threshold or target effect occurs. As a general rule, predictions should only be made for concentrations that fall within the range of observed concentrations, and care should be taken in interpreting results for concentrations outside this range. As a result of the large number of observations employed for concentration–response modeling, this approach may avoid some of the inherent problems with the central tendency analyses for drugs with variable Tmaxs. However, this analysis is not sufficient for drug approval and should be considered a supplemental analysis to the central tendency analyses.

CATEGORICAL AND OUTLIER ANALYSIS

One further way of assessing a drug's effect on the QT interval is to look at the individual values, as well as individual changes from baseline of QT and QTc. Both the draft ICH guidance document and a CPMP Points to Consider document *(24)* provide categories (Tables 5 and 6).

These categories are based on published clinical data and/or clinical experience, and most recently have been influenced by the terfenadine data. As with other critical ranges for QTc, these are primarily based on data using Bazett's correction and single ECG QT measurements. These may not be applicable to alternative correction factors, and specifically should not be employed for QT data averaged from two or more ECGs. Additionally, they may not account for the variability of the measurement, differences between males and females or the method of ECG measurement.

A simple way to display the data is to generate tables with a row for each category and column for each treatment arm (placebo and experimental drug). Each cell of the table should include both the number and frequency/percentage. Additionally, a total row and column is recommended (*see* Table 7).

Table 5
Categories of Risk for Absolute Values of Individual QT/QTc Intervals

Absolute QTc values	Relative risk of TdP
≤ 450 ms	So far no TdP
> 450 and ≤480 ms	No clear risk
> 480 and ≤ 500 ms	Uncertainty
> 500 ms	"Substantially" increased likelihood of being pro-arrhythmic

TdP, torsade des pointes.

Table 6
Categories of Risk for Changes From Baseline of Individual QT/QTc Intervals

Change from baseline	Relative risk of TdP
≤ 30 ms	No clear risk
> 30 and ≤ 60 ms	Uncertainty
> 60 ms	"Substantially" increased likelihood of being pro-arrhythmic

TdP, torsade des pointes.

Table 7
Sample Table of Categorical Summary of Individual Changes From Baseline

Change from Baseline	Placebo	Drug X, dose 1	Drug X, dose 2	Active control	Total
≤ 30 ms	25 (50%)	23 (46%)	20 (40%)	20 (40%)	88 (44%)
> 30 and ≤ 60 ms	20 (40%)	19 (38%)	20 (40%)	23 (46%)	82 (41%)
> 60 ms	5 (10%)	8 (16%)	10 (20%)	7 (14%)	30 (15%)
Total	50	50	50	50	200

As with some of the central tendency parameters, these tables may be dependent on the sampling scheme for ECGs and experimental conditions. Again, drugs that require a longer evaluation time in which meals, sleep, etc. will occur, may result in more observations in the higher categories. However, if the drug has no effect, numbers and frequencies should be similar to placebo.

SUMMARY AND RECOMMENDATIONS

A large number of factors influence the QT interval and its variability within and between subjects. Appropriate experimental design and conditions can limit those that are intrinsic to the individual (e.g., meals, sleep, physical activity, minute-to-minute QT variations, etc.). Those extrinsic factors, such as ECG data collection and measurement, correction factors, use of data from Cmax or anticipated Tmax, choice of baseline, and the time between baseline and on-drug measurements, must all be carefully controlled in order to enhance the power and efficiency of QT study design. Because the dose range employed in QT studies is often limited by subject tolerability, virtually all of the design decisions in "thorough" QT studies must be directed toward reducing the QT variability and toward the use of the most powerful statistical analyses available. The choice of many of the study design options is often a trade-off, and the assumptions inherent in these choices must be understood and incorporated into the data analysis and interpretation.

We offer the following recommendations for the design and statistical analyses of "thorough" QT studies:

1. The experimental design and setting should minimize known sources of QT variability. The period of peak pharmacodynamic effect should avoid the post-prandial period, exercise, and sleep. Because of altered QT–RR relationships during sleep, QT data should not be compared between awake and asleep periods, nor for approx 1 h after awakening. Balancing male and female subjects and studying subjects evenly distributed throughout the age range of the intended patient population will allow these factors to be added as covariates in the statistical analysis. At least two and preferably three doses of the drug should be tested to gain the marked increase in statistical power of a dose–response or a concentration–response analysis. Crossover designs offer enhanced power by controlling for intersubject variability, but may not be practical for long half-life drugs and active metabolites, or for drugs requiring dose titration.

2. Computer-assisted manual over-read of QT intervals from at least two replicate ECGs at each time point is the most effective way to reduce QT variability. The same ECG lead should be used within subjects for estimation of QT changes.

3. The preferred baseline is a predose time point on the same day as, or as close as practicable to the on-drug ECG recordings. Data for both placebo and drug should be reported prior to any "placebo-adjusted" calculations. For long half-life drugs requiring parallel study designs, careful control for sequence effects in both the drug and placebo groups should be incorporated in the data collection.

4. The Bazett's and Fridericia's corrected QT intervals are requested by regulatory agencies, however, the QT–RR relationship of the study population should be inspected. Where necessary, a population or individualized correction factor should also be employed to avoid the increases in variability caused by standardized equations. A "Holter bin" analysis that constructs the QT–RR relationship for each subject on drug and on placebo is a highly sensitive and informative method that was accepted the FDA as supporting evidence for the alfuzosin NDA in 2003. Alternative statistical methods that avoid correction of the QT interval have been proposed but, as of the time of this manuscript, have not been the basis for regulatory approval.

5. The ICH draft document proposes that the ECG obtained at drug Cmax or anticipated Tmax is the first central tendency parameter to use. This is of value when the plasma pharmacokinetics of the drug and/or measured metabolite corresponds to the pharmacodynamic effect of the drug. The alternative parameter, the maximum change in QT, has a high false positive rate and is randomly distributed over the time of observation even in the presence of a moderate, true drug effect. The high false positive rate can be reduced by obtaining replicate ECGs at each time point, and by performing an hysteresis analysis. When hysteresis analysis indicates a correlation between drug or metabolite and the maximum change in QT, the data at this time point may be considered as valid.

6. Dose–response and concentration–response modeling analysis offers powerful statistical tools to increase the sensitivity of the "thorough" QT studies and to enhance the ability to assess risk. When careful attention is paid to the timing of the concentration–response relationships, this method is the most effective way to reduce sample size and increase statistical power.

7. The categorical analyses should be limited to comparative frequency tables between drug and placebo for individual (i.e., nonaveraged) ECG QT data.

REFERENCES

1. Morganroth J, Brozovich FV, McDonald JT, Jacobs RA. Variability of the QT measurement in healthy men, with implications for selection of an abnormal QT value to predict drug toxicity and proarrhythmia. Am J Cardiol 1991;67:774–776.
2. Molnar J, Zhang F, Weiss J, Ehlert FA, Rosenthal JE. Diurnal pattern of QTc interval: How long is prolonged? J Am Coll Cardiol 1996;27:76–83.
3. Widerlov E, Jostell KG, Claesson L, Odlind B, Keisu M, Freyschuss U. Influence of food intake on electrocardiograms of healthy male volunteers. Eur J Clin Pharmacol 1999;55:619–624.
4. Browne KF, Prystowsky E, Heger JJ, Chilson DA, Zipes DP. Prolongation of the Q-T interval in man during sleep. Am J Cardiol 1983;52:55–59.
5. Vrancianu R, Filcescu V, Ionescu V, Groza P, Persson J, Kadefors R, Petersen I. The influence of day and night work on the circadian variations of cardiovascular performance. Eur J Appl Physiol 1982; 48:11–23.
6. Lande G, Funck-Brentano C, Ghadanfar M, Escande D. Steady-state versus non-steady-state QT–RR relationships in 24-hour Holter recordings. PACE 2000;23:293–302.
7. Extramiana F, Maison-Blanche P, Badilini F, Pinoteau J, Deseo T, Coumel P. Circadian modulation of QT rate dependence in healthy volunteers. Gender and age differences. J Electrocardiol 1999;32:33–43.
8. Rautaharju PM, Zhou SH, Wong S, Calhoun HP, Berenson BS, Prineas R, Davignon A. Sex differences in the evolution of the electrocardiographic QT interval with age. Can J Cardiol 1992;8:690–695.
9. Ahnve S, Vallin H. Influence of heart rate and inhibition of autonomic tone on the QT interval. Circulation 1982;65:435–439.
10. Roden DM. Drug-induced prolongation of the QT interval. New Engl J Med 2004;350:1013–1022.
11. Camm AJ, Janse MJ, Roden DM, Rosen MR, Cinca J, Cobbe SM. Congenital and acquired long QT syndrome. Eur Heart J 2000;21:1232–1237.
12. Sun H, Chen P, Kenna L, Lee P. The chaotic QT interval variabilities on risk assessment trial designs. Clin Pharm Ther 2004;75:P55.
13. Lee SH, Sun H, Chen P, Doddapaneni S, Hunt J, Malinowski H. Sensitivity/reliability of the time-matched baseline subtraction method in assessment of QTc interval prolongation. Clin Pharm Ther 2004;75:P56.
14. Summary Basis of Approval, moxifloxacin hydrochloride, April 21, 2001. FDA document.
15. Hnatkova K, Malik M. "Optimum" formulae for heart rate correction of the QT interval. PACE 1999;1683–1687.
16. Malik M, Farbom P, Batchvarov V, Hnatkova K, Camm AJ. Relation between QT and RR intervals is highly individual among healthy subjects: Implications for heart rate correction of the QT interval. Heart 2002;87:220–228.
17. Batchvarov VN, Ghuran A, Smetana P, Hnatkova K, Harries M, Dilaveris P, Camm AJ, Malik M. QT–RR relationship in healthy subjects exhibits substantial intersubject variability and high intrasubject stability. Am J Physiol 2002;282:H2356–H2363.
18. Dmitrienko A, Smith B. Repeated-measures models in the analysis of QT interval. Pharmaceut Statist 2003;2:175–190.
19. The Clinical Evaluation of QT/QTc Interval Prolongation and Proarrhythmic Potential for Non-Antiarrhythmic Drugs: Preliminary Concept Paper, November 15, 2003. http://cdernet.cder.fda.gov/QTWG/ QT%20Workshop/qt4jam.pdf.
20. Badilini F, Maison-Blanche P, Childers R, Coumel P. QT interval analysis on ambulatory electrocardiographic recordings: A selective beat averaging approach. Med Biol Eng Comput 1999;37:71–79.
21. Hollander M, Wolfe DA. Non-parametric Statistical Methods, Wiley Series, 1999, pp. 125–133.
22. Kenna LA, Parekh A, Jarugula V, Chatterjee DJ, Sun H, Kim MJ, Ortiz S, Hunt JP, Malinowski H. Experience evaluating QT prolongation data. Clin Pharm Ther 2004;75:P7.
23. Ahn C, Jung S-H. Efficiency of general estimating equations estimators of slopes in repeated measurements: Adding subjects or adding measurements? Drug Info J 2003;37:309–316.
24. Points to Consider: The Assessment of the Potential for QT Interval Prolongation by Non-Cardiovascular Medicinal Products. Committee for Proprietary Medicinal Products, EMEA, December 17, 1997.

15 Interpretation of Clinical ECG Data

Understanding the Risk From Non-Antiarrhythmic Drugs

Rashmi R. Shah, MD

CONTENTS

INTRODUCTION

Prolongation of the QTc interval on the surface electrocardiogram (ECG) reflects a delay in ventricular repolarization, and, when drug-induced, it is almost always a result of inhibition of the rapid component of the delayed rectifier potassium current (I_{Kr}). The other current that is infrequently inhibited is its slow component (I_{Ks}). Drug-induced prolongation of the QTc interval, when excessive in the right setting, can be pro-arrhythmic and degenerate into torsade de pointes (TdP), a potentially fatal and unique form of polymorphic ventricular tachycardia. One review in 1993 concluded, "At present, our knowledge base about the relation of the QT interval and torsades de pointes is grossly incomplete" *(1)*. Unfortunately, despite extensive research for more than a decade since, this still remains the case today. It is therefore not surprising that more than any other drug-induced adverse reaction, it has been responsible in recent times for the withdrawal of many drugs from the market.

From: *Cardiac Safety of Noncardiac Drugs:*
Practical Guidelines for Clinical Research and Drug Development
Edited by: J. Morganroth and I. Gussak © Humana Press Inc., Totowa, NJ

Significance of Drug-Induced QTc Interval Prolongation for Drug Development

Prolongation of the QTc interval is inevitable with class III antiarrhythmic drugs which, by design, are intended to produce their desired therapeutic benefit by delaying ventricular repolarization, and thereby increasing myocardial refractory period. As might be expected, these class III antiarrhythmic drugs are frequently associated TdP. Unfortunately, the potential to prolong the QTc interval and induce TdP is not confined to class III antiarrhythmic drugs. A number of class I antiarrhythmic drugs and antianginal agents as well as many noncardiovascular drugs carry what has been termed the "QT-liability." There are now well over 10 antianginal and 90 noncardiovascular drugs recognized to have this liability (2), and the number of such drugs continues to increase almost daily. Over the last decade, regulatory authorities have rejected many new drugs or placed restrictions on the use of many old and new drugs because of concerns arising from their potential to prolong the QTc interval. Regulatory focus on drug-induced QTc interval prolongation has changed from one of a potentially desirable antiarrhythmic mechanism to that of a potentially fatal torsadogenic/pro-arrhythmic proclivity. QT interval prolongation has been regarded as a liability since it is the one measure that has been used most frequently as a marker of delayed ventricular repolarization. As will become apparent later in this chapter, assessment of clinical risk following drug-induced delay in ventricular repolarization by an NCE should be an integrated evaluation of all parameters indicative of changes in repolarization and not just the QT interval.

The frequency of TdP with noncardiac drugs is largely unknown but it is typically well below 0.1% of the patients receiving such a drug. Trials conducted during the clinical development of a new chemical entity (NCE) usually include 1500 to 3000 plus highly selected patients showing little pharmacokinetic or pharmacodynamic variability. Whereas vigorous monitoring of these patients may provide information on the potential of the NCE to prolong the QTc interval, these trials are unlikely to identify its potential to induce TdP. A database of 1500 patients will barely detect an event that occurs at the rate of 1 in 1000 and almost certainly miss the one that occurs with a frequency of 1 in 5000 or less (α error of 0.05 and β error of 0.05). Long-term safety studies also do not usually include adequate ECG monitoring at peak plasma concentrations of the drug or its metabolites. Therefore, it is highly desirable that NCEs that have systemic bioavailability should be tested during their development for their effect on ventricular repolarization with a more robust, efficient, and rational approach.

Regulatory Guidance on Investigating Drug-Induced Prolongation of the QTc Interval

In December 1997, the European Union's Committee for Proprietary Medicinal Products (CPMP) was the first regulatory authority to issue a formal guidance note on a strategy by which all NCEs should be investigated for their effect on QTc interval (3). This guidance includes recommendations on a set of nonclinical as well as clinical investigations. All strategies devised subsequently are an elaboration of, or minor variations on, the broad pattern set by the CPMP.

On November 15, 2002, the U.S. Food and Drug Administration (FDA) and Health Canada (HC) issued a joint document on clinical strategies for evaluating the effects of NCEs on QT/QTc interval prolongation (a preliminary concept paper for discussion) (4). The detailed strategy described in this document was discussed in great depth at an international Workshop hosted by NASPE/FDA/HC/DIA in January 2003. Following a number of amendments, it was entered into the International Conference on Harmonization (ICH) process in February 2003 for adoption as a topic that merited harmonization (ICH topic E14). This ICH initiative is currently in progress and a draft document, agreed in June 2004, is out for consultation with a view to harmonizing internationally the regulatory recommendations and strategies for evaluating an NCE for its ECG effects with a focus on the QTc interval. The draft strategy proposed anticipates clinical evaluation of almost all NCEs for their effect on QTc interval. For each NCE, this will involve a single trial (typically in healthy volunteers) designed and dedicated for this purpose, and referred to as the "thorough QT/QTc study." The result of this "thorough QT/QTc study" will usually influence the ECG evaluation during the subsequent drug development. Since the ICH E14 guidance note is still evolving, the reader should consult the most current version for details of the design of the study and what constitutes a positive or negative study.

Regulatory expectations of a better pre-approval characterization of NCEs for this potential risk have inevitably had a very profound influence on the drug development process. Whether or not such evaluation should routinely include a single dedicated clinical trial (typically in healthy volunteers) depends on the integrated risk assessment from nonclinical studies, and whether other drugs in the same pharmacological or chemical class have been associated with QTc interval prolongation with or without TdP. However, as will be discussed later this point of view does not enjoy a universal support, and therefore there are regional differences in regulatory expectations.

Issues surrounding the techniques of recording, measuring, and correcting the measured QT interval for heart rate and of investigating other parameters of ventricular repolarization in man have been dealt with elsewhere in this book. Important for the purpose of this chapter is a reminder that changes in QT inteval lag behind the changes in heart rate by a period of 2–3 min giving rise to hysteresis. It is important to take account of this QT/RR hysteresis when correcting the measured QT interval for changes in heart rate. This chapter will focus on interpretation of clinical ECG data, gathered reliably and accurately from all clinical studies including a single trial dedicated to evaluating the effect of an NCE on the QTc interval, in understanding and assessing the risk of TdP from non-antiarrhythmic drugs. There will be a particular emphasis on the strengths and limitations of various QTc-derived indices, and on the need to consider other properties of the drug that may significantly modify the pro-arrhythmic risk from a prolonged QTc interval.

SOURCE OF CLINICAL ELECTROCARDIOGRAM DATA
Correlations Between Nonclinical and Clinical Data

Native I_{Kr} is a co-assembly of human ether-a-go-go related (hERG) α-subunits encoded by the *KCNH2* gene and MiRP1 β-subunits encoded by the *KCNE2* gene. These subunits co-assemble to form a functional heteromultimeric channel complex. All the drugs that reduce I_{Kr} current have been shown to exert their effect by binding to the hERG α-subunits *(5–8)*. Another draft ICH guidance regarding nonclinical strategies (ICH topic S7B) for evaluating the effects of NCEs on ventricular repolarization envisages the use of in vitro I_{Kr} assay and in vivo QT assay (in dog) as the core components of nonclinical integrated risk assessment. When positive at low concentrations, the most direct benefit of these studies is the guidance they provide for ECG monitoring in early human studies.

There have been a number of comprehensive analyses correlating clinical and extensive, retrospectively and prospectively gathered, nonclinical data. Although one can debate *ad infinitum* what constitutes a "negative nonclinical" data package and a "positive clinical study," these analyses have shown so far that: (1) drugs prolonging the QT interval to a clinically relevant duration in humans have always been positive in nonclinical studies, and (2) there are no examples to date of drugs negative in nonclinical studies that have proved to be arrhythmogenic in humans. Both ICH E14 and S7B guidance notes recognize that the subject of drug-induced changes in cardiac repolarization is one of active research and as further data (nonclinical and clinical) accumulates in the furture, their contents may be reevaluated and revised. Nevertheless, all regulatory authorities believe that adequately conducted nonclinical studies provide important evidence of safety that requires to be corroborated by data from clinical trials.

Clinical Data

However, because there is no universal agreement at present on the extent to, or the findings by, which nonclinical testing can exclude a clinical risk, regulatory authorities in some regions of the world will require clinical evaluation of an NCE in a single trial (typically in healthy volunteers) dedicated to evaluating its effects on ECG with a focus on the QTc interval for almost all NCEs. For the European and the Japanese regulatory authorities, this single dedicated clinical trial is required only if the nonclinical studies are positive or equivocal and if other drugs in the same pharmacological or chemical class have been associated with QTc interval prolongation with or without TdP. In the absence of a single dedicated clinical trial, provided the quality of ECG monitoring is acceptable and of high standard, these authorities would be content with evidence gathered from well-conducted clinical pharmacology studies in healthy volunteers and from an integrated summary of all ECG data across all trials, as long as the information on the effect of the NCE on QTc interval includes data on its dose–concentration–response relationship. Other factors that could influence the need for or the design of such a study include durations of the pharmacodynamic action of a drug and treatment with it, the metabolic profile of the drug and previous experience with other members of the same chemical or pharmacological class.

Dedicated QTc Clinical Trial in Perspective

Doubtless, a single dedicated clinical trial has much to recommend to it. Apart from the use of a placebo and a positive control to facilitate evaluation of a drug effect, a single dedicated clinical trial allows study designs, sample sizes, and drug administration protocols to be optimized to suit the pharmacokinetics of the NCE. Techniques for recording ECGs and measuring the QT interval can be robust and standardized whereas correction of the measured QT interval for changes in heart rate can be made more reliable by employing additional correction formula, derived during placebo administration, for each individual or for the study population as a whole. A single dedicated clinical trial is also ideal for gathering prospectively all the data needed in a format that allows comparison across different drugs.

However, these benefits of a single dedicated clinical trial must be seen in the context of its impact on the safety evaluation of the NCE, availability of future new drugs (2,9) and the cost of developing new drugs (10). Recently, these studies are being undertaken more frequently and it will be interesting to see if any drug with a high nonclinical safety margin (e.g., a ratio of ≥ 30 between IC_{50} for hERG or I_{Kr} and maximum free therapeutic plasma concentrations) is found to induce a clinically relevant effect on QTc interval in healthy volunteers; in other words, defining the contribution of the single dedicated clinical trial when nonclinical data are neither positive nor equivocal. As will be discussed later, moxifloxacin that is now routinely used as a safe positive control has a safety margin of about 22 *(11)*. Other important issues are whether such a study provides information that cannot be gathered otherwise, and whether results from healthy volunteers can be readily extrapolated to patients with diminished repolarization reserve (e.g., individuals with hypokalaemia, heart failure, enhanced pharmacodynamic susceptibility associated with some comorbidities or carrying silent mutations of potassium channels). When using the drug concerned in such patients, a "negative" dedicated clinical trial in healthy volunteers may well impart a false sense of clinical security. A typical phase I study for a single compound with nonclinical QT signal is estimated to cost US $1 million and if the drug proceeds to phase II, the cost is estimated to increase six-fold *(9)*. These costs are of no relevance when there are real safety concerns from nonclinical studies. However, when there are no nonclinical signals of what is a mechanism-based toxicity, these costs are not insignificant when one considers that the commonly stated average cost of US $802 million for researching and developing an NCE has been seriously challenged as a gross over-estimate *(10)*.

QT INTERVAL PROLONGATION VS TORSADE DE POINTES

QTc interval prolongation per se is neither harmful nor does it adversely affect myocardial pump function. The relationship between QTc interval prolongation on the ECG and the clinical risk of TdP is complex. Unless this relationship is better appreciated, there is a risk that many valuable drugs may be denied an approval.

Mechanisms of Torsade de Pointes

Typically, drug-induced TdP is characterized by a syndrome of prolonged QT interval and the long coupling interval of the initial premature beat *(8)*. Delayed or prolonged ventricular repolarization in this setting gives rise to the development of early afterdepolarizations (EADs) at the levels of ventricular midmyocardial M-cells and the Purkinje fibres. The emergence of these EADs is favored by calcium loading during the late Phase II of the prolonged action potential (9). The amplitude of EADs is cycle length dependent and there is a strong correlation between the preceding RR interval and the amplitude of EADs that follow. When the amplitude of the EADs reaches a critical threshold, the resulting ectopic beat triggers a repetitive burst of electrical activity that forms the basis of TdP. The other hypothesis relies on the known uneven distribution of I_{Kr} across the ventricular wall and proposes an increase in transmural dispersion of action potential duration (APD) throughout the ventricle, and this is claimed to facilitate induction of TdP and other ventricular tachyarrhythmias by creating the conditions for re-entry *(12)*. However, these two hypotheses are not mutually exclusive and, indeed, appear to be even complementary.

QTc Interval as a Surrogate of Torsade de Pointes

QTc interval prolongation has come to be recognized as a surrogate marker of the risk of TdP, albeit an imperfect one; however, it is at present the best and the simplest clinical measure that is available. When interpreting data from a study designed to evaluate the effect of a drug on QTc interval, it is important to appreciate that QTc interval prolongation per se does not constitute a direct risk, e.g., hypocalcaemia frequently produces QTc interval prolongation, but is not typically associated with TdP. Similarly, myxoedema and treatment with amiodarone are often associated with prolongation of the QTc interval, but only rarely are they associated with TdP.

The apparently all-exclusive and hitherto persuasive association between QT interval prolongation and TdP is partly the consequence of the very definition of this unique polymorphic ventricular tachyarrhythmia *(13)*. Ventricular tachyarrhythmias, even when meeting the morphological criteria of TdP, are not labeled by many clinicians as TdP unless preceded by QTc interval prolongation *(14–16)*. In reality, not all agents that have been linked with ventricular tachyarrhythmias morphologically similar to TdP or short-coupled variants of TdP cause significant lengthening of the QTc interval *(17–24)*. It is of course possible with regard to these drugs that, although the QTc interval may be normal a few seconds before, it may be prolonged immediately before the induction of true TdP. During 43 episodes of TdP in seven patients with drug-induced QT interval prolongation, the QTc intervals measured immediately before the episodes of TdP were significantly longer than those 6–24 h before the episodes (690 ms vs 560 ms) *(25)*. It is also important to note that TdP does not develop invariably in all individuals with equivalent prolongation of the QTc interval, and that not all drugs that prolong the QTc interval to an equivalent duration carry the same risk of inducing TdP. Nevertheless, concerns on the effect of a drug on QTc interval duration arise from its frequently observed association with TdP. Numerous clinical and experimental data have established that QTc interval prolongation is a major precursor of drug-induced TdP.

With regard to assessing the risk of TdP following prolongation of the QTc interval, and its use as a surrogate of TdP, it is helpful to recognize a number of properties and limitations of QTc interval. One property of the QTc interval that complicates the risk assessment is its inter-individual, and to a much lesser extent its intra-individual, variability *(26)*. Intra-individual variability is an important confounder in risk assessment and its magnitude is dependent on a number of technical details related to recording, measuring, and correcting the QT interval. Morganroth et al. *(27)* reported a large degree of intra-individual variability with a mean difference between the longest and the shortest QTc interval being 76 ± 19 ms. Although this variability was determined using Holter monitoring, it does illustrate the point. Using standard 12-lead ECGs, Ganput et al. *(28)* also demonstrated similar variability. When a change in the duration of QTc interval is observed following drug administration, a decision is required as to whether it is drug-induced or just a spontaneous normal variation. An inappropriate conclusion may result in either restriction in the use (or even rejection) of a potentially beneficial drug or approval of an otherwise hazardous drug without the restrictions required to promote its safe use.

The other property is the magnitude of the duration of QTc interval at which the risk of TdP begins. The risk varies not only between drugs but also between individuals and even within an individual, depending on the presence of any one of many inter-current risk-modifying factors *(see* below). Therefore, TdP is essentially a moving target. Although the risk of TdP most frequently begins when the QTc interval is about 500 ms and rises exponentially thereafter, isolated cases of TdP have been reported with QTc intervals in the range of 450 to 500 ms *(29)*. As will be discussed later, autonomic properties and other ion channel blocking activities of a drug also significantly modulate the torsadogenic risk associated with a given degree of QTc interval prolongation produced by that drug. Therefore, although evaluating the effect of an NCE on the QTc interval is important, conclusions on the potential clinical risk of TdP associated with its use, based solely on its ability to prolong the QTc interval, might turn out to be highly flawed.

It is plainly evident that the balance between a therapeutic antiarrhythmic and potentially fatal pro-arrhythmic prolongations of the QTc interval is a very delicate one, depending not only on the drug concerned and its plasma concentration but also on a number of host factors that modify the risk. These factors include female gender, electrolyte imbalance (especially hypokalemia), myocardial ischaemia, congestive heart failure (CHF), bradycardia with or without heart block, and pre-existing prolongation of QTc interval to list just a few.

Assessment of risk should also take into account other drug-related factors such as formulation. Sotalol is a β-adrenoreceptor blocking drug with a chiral center. Its class III activity resides in both isomers whereas the β-adrenoreceptor blocking activity resides only in the (–)-(R)-isomer. Not surprisingly, while the racemic drug is predominantly antiarrhythmic, the (+)-(S)-isomer ("d-sotalol") is predominantly pro-arrhythmic. Additionally, a fixed combination product of sotalol with a thiazide diuretic (Sotazide) that was indicated for hypertension proved to be highly pro-arrhythmic (because of the contribution of hypokalaemia induced by the thiazide component). Needless to say, this product has long been removed from the market. Relative to their oral formulations, intravenous formulations of haloperidol or erythromycin are significantly more torsadogenic as attested to by reports.

Significance of a Short QTc Interval

One issue that is certain to emerge in the future is whether a short QTc interval is pro-arrhythmic. Early evidence suggests that just as prolongation of QT interval can be pro-arrhythmic, shortening of QT interval can also be pro-arrhythmic. Idiopathic short QT interval as a new clinical syndrome was first described by Gussak et al. *(30)* in three members of one family. One family member, a 17-yr-old female, required cardioversion for several episodes of paroxysmal atrial fibrillation. Similar ECG changes were also seen in an unrelated 37-yr-old patient who experienced sudden cardiac death *(30)*. There are now a number of reports associating short QT interval with proarrhythmias. Gaita et al. *(31)* described several members of two different families with short QT interval (QTc interval ≤ 300 ms) who were referred for syncope, palpitation, and resuscitated cardiac arrest in the presence of a positive family history of sudden cardiac death without any structural heart disease. Five of these patients have been successfully treated with implantable cardioverter defibrillators *(32)*. Makarow et al. *(33)* reported 11 children aged 3–16 yr from families with cases of sudden deaths at young age, and without any structural cardiac disease. Nine of these children had short QTc interval. Thus, congenital short QT syndrome may constitute a new clinical entity with an increased risk for arrhythmias and sudden cardiac death.

Bezzina et al. *(34)* conducted a large population study in German Caucasians, investigating an association between the common amino acid polymorphism K897T (A2690C) within hERG and QTc interval. They found a significant association between this polymorphism and QTc interval duration. Subjects with CC genotype had significantly shorter QTc interval (388.5 ± 2.9 ms) compared to AA homozygotes (398.5 ± 0.9 ms) and AC heterozygotes (397.2 ± 1.2 ms). After stratification by gender, the association of the genotype was significant in females only. Enthusiasts of pharmacogenetically driven therapy may note that in an earlier study in Finnish women, this polymorphism was found to prolong the QTc interval and increase transmural dispersion in repolarization in females of AC or CC genotype *(35)*. The QTc interval and transmural dispersions in AC/CC and AA genotypes were 477 and 441 ms and 143 ms and 116 ms, respectively. In males, there was no genotype-specific effect. The contradictory findings from these two studies emphasize the importance of confirming associations in different populations. This major disparity between the two studies could reflect differences in sample size or other population-specific differences in the occurrence of additional (functional) polymorphisms. Brugada et al. *(36)* described three families with hereditary short-QT syndrome and a high incidence of ventricular arrhythmias and sudden cardiac death. In two of them, they identified two different missense mutations resulting in the same amino acid change (N588K) in the cardiac hERG channel (KCNH2). The mutations dramatically increased I_{Kr}, leading to heterogeneous abbreviation of APD and refractoriness, and reduce the affinity of the channels to I_{Kr} blockers. Bellocq et al. *(36a)* have recently identified a mutation (V307L) in *KCNQ1* gene that is associated with gain of function in I_{Ks}, resulting in short QT interval and ventricular fibrillation.

DeSilvey and Moss *(37)* reported shortening of QT interval following treatment with primidone in three patients with congenital QT interval prolongation. Whether or not, following a normal QT interval at baseline, a pro-arrhythmic shortening of the QT interval can be induced by a drug remains to be seen. Nevertheless, these clinical observations have important implications for the use of only the prolongation of QTc interval as a surrogate of TdP and other associated pro arrhythmias.

CORRECTED VS UNCORRECTED QT INTERVAL

The longer the preceding RR interval, the longer is the measured QT interval. Because the measured QT interval varies inversely with heart rate, the QT interval duration requires a correction to obtain a rate-corrected QT interval—the QTc interval—in order to compensate for any changes in heart rate whether physiological or induced by an intervention. Among the 30 or more correction formulas that are available, the two most widely used are the Bazett formula and the Fridericia formula. Bazett formula corrects the measured QT interval by the square root of the preceding RR interval ($QTc = QT/RR^{0.50}$) while the Fridericia formula uses the cube root of the preceding RR interval ($QTc = QT/RR^{0.33}$). Issues surrounding the choice of the most appropriate rate-correction formula are complex. For a more detailed discussion the reader is referred to other chapters in this book.

Most drugs that cause TdP clearly increase both the measured (uncorrected) QT and the QTc intervals. However, it is often questioned whether the development of TdP is more closely related to an increase in uncorrected QT interval or the rate-corrected interval—the QTc interval. Available data suggest that QTc interval is a better predictor of risk than is the uncorrected QT interval.

In patients with bradycardia who have heart rates below 40 beats per minute, the measured QT interval often exceeds the duration thought to be pro-arrhythmic and, yet, there is no evidence that TdP is unduly frequent in these patients. When the measured QT interval is corrected for heart rate in these patients, the corrected interval is lower and generally well below the pro-arrhythmic threshold. It is noted, however, that the term "torsade de pointes" was first coined to describe this unique tachycardia in an elderly female patient with heart block *(13)*. From their meta-analysis of 332 patients with drug-induced TdP, Makkar et al. *(29)* reported that 80.2% of 212 patients had an uncorrected QT interval >500 ms whereas as many as 89.5% of the 258 patients had QTc interval > 500 ms while receiving the offending drug. These and other available data argue in favor of corrected QT interval—the QTc interval —being a better marker of the clinical risk.

The evaluation of an NCE for its effect on QTc interval is made more robust by investigating its dose–concentration–response relationship, together with evaluation of the effects of a placebo and a positive control. The reader is referred to other reviews for further discussion on characterizing this relationship. Briefly, however, the information required includes dose–concentration linearity, the threshold concentration at which QTc interval begins to increase, the slope of the concentration–response relationship, changes at the usual therapeutic concentrations and the anticipated maximal QTc interval prolongation. QTc interval data from clinical trials can be analyzed for risk of TdP by a variety of QTc-derived indices. The most frequently used are: (1) the number of subjects with categorical responses in QTc interval ("outliers" responding with $\geq$ 60 ms increase in QTc interval from baseline and/or a new absolute QTc interval $\geq$ 500 ms), and (2) a population-based mean increase in placebo-corrected peak or maximal QTc interval. Other parameters include QTc dispersion, time-averaged QTc intervals, and area under the QTc interval vs time curve (QTc–AUC). Also emerging is an interest in exploring the use of other supplementary parameters such as those indicative of spatial dispersion of repolarization (e.g., transmural dispersion in repolarization).

In North America, there appears to be a different emphasis on these indices. While the CPMP document is silent on the predictive utility of mean changes and recommends analysis only in terms of categorical responses, the preliminary concept paper from FDA–HC that was entered into the ICH process included a number of parameters with an emphasis on mean increases in QTc interval. Under the ICH recommendations when adopted the EU, Japan, and the United States will all assess the data, mainly on the basis of both categorical responses and mean placebo-corrected increases in peak QTc intervals ("central tendency"). However, it should be acknowledged that there is a clear need for more comparative, simultaneously gathered data on these three variables (ΔQTc $\geq$ 60 ms, a new absolute QTc interval $\geq$ 500 ms and/or a mean increase in placebo-corrected maximum or peak QTc interval) in order to reach a more informed consensus on which of them is the best predictor of TdP in the population at large as opposed to predicting the risk in a given individual. An integrated analysis of all the three variables, each appropriately weighted, might well prove to be necessary for optimal assessment of the risk.

CATEGORICAL RESPONSES

The categorical responses that are considered predictive of clinical risk (following administration of a drug that is found to prolong the QTc interval) are an increase in the QTc interval of 60 ms or more from baseline (ΔQTc $\geq$ 60 ms) and/or a new (that is not present at baseline) absolute QTc interval $\geq$ 500 ms. The latter is considered predictive of risk regardless of the magnitude of increase from baseline.

$\Delta QTc \geq 60$ ms

The need to set a threshold increase from baseline (before a potential risk can be attributed to a drug) arises from the spontaneous intra-individual variations in QTc interval. Because 40 ECGs were obtained while taking placebo in each participant (28 healthy volunteers with a mean age of 57 yr and 28 patients with stable cardiovascular disease with a mean age of 60 yr) in a double-blind, four-period crossover, dose escalation study of terfenadine, Pratt et al. *(38)* were able to determine the extent of spontaneous variability in QTc interval. It was calculated that the probability of a 50 ms increase being a result of chance was 0.0003 over 1 d and 0.002 over 6 d. From the observed placebo-induced variability in all participants, they calculated that an increase in (Bazett-corrected) QTc interval of 35 ms or more while receiving drug therapy is likely to represent a drug effect. Because placebo and the drug concerned (terfenadine) do not have an effect on heart rate, it is most likely that same probabilities also apply to Fridericia-corrected QTc intervals. It is important to recognize that ΔQTc $\geq$ 60 ms defines the risk of TdP at a population level and not necessarily in the individual subject in whom it occurred.

The CPMP strategy of risk assessment, and all others that have evolved since, is based on a Bazett-corrected ΔQTc > 60 ms, but some clinical investigators have recommended a ΔQTc >75 ms as an appropriate signal *(27,39)*. Using simulated data, it has been calculated that ΔQTc > 60 ms and ΔQTc $\geq$ 40 ms signals will have false-positive rates of about 1% and 5%, respectively *(40)*. Based on these calculations, it seems probable that ΔQTc > 75 ms will likely have an unacceptably high false-negative rate. Notwithstanding, in view of the distortions arising from changes in heart rate, a Fridericia-corrected ΔQTc $\geq$ 60 ms should be a more predictive categorical response than a Bazett-corrected ΔQTc $\geq$ 60 ms.

QTc Interval $\geq$ 500 ms

The risk of TdP usually begins when the QTc interval is about 500 ms and rises exponentially thereafter *(41,42)*. Regardless of the cause of QTc interval prolongation, the hazard ratio for a subsequent cardiac event including a potentially fatal arrhythmia is estimated to be 1.052^x where x is equal to (QTc interval minus 400) divided by 10 *(41)*. An absolute QTc interval, regardless of the post-dose increase from baseline, defines the risk of TdP in an individual subject, and therefore a new absolute QTc interval $\geq$ 500 ms following drug administration is a powerful categorical response by which to assess the clinical risk of TdP.

In 31 patients with documented quinidine-induced TdP, QTc intervals ranged from 390 to 580 (mean 470) ms off-therapy in 24 patients and from 390 to 630 (mean 510) ms on-therapy in 23 patients. Six (25%) of the 24 patients off-therapy and 15 (65%) of the 23 patients on-therapy had QTc interval $\geq$ 500 ms *(17)*. As stated previously, Makkar et al. *(29)* reported that 89.5% of the patients with TdP had a QTc interval > 500 ms. Yamaguchi et al. *(43)* reported on 27 patients with drug-induced prolongation of the QTc interval who were divided into two groups—12 with TdP and 15 without. The mean maximum QTc interval was 657 ms in those with and 505 ms in those without TdP. The corresponding mean minimum QTc interval values were 527 ms and 446 ms, respectively. Only one patient with TdP had a maximum QTc interval fractionally below 500 ms. These data support the predictive significance of a QTc interval of 500 ms as a proarrhythmic threshold.

The author has also analyzed data on cisapride ($n = 43$), terfenadine ($n = 17$), prenylamine ($n = 87$), terodiline ($n = 25$), and bepridil ($n = 27$)—all known to be potent torsadogens. The QT/QTc interval values were < 500 ms in 21 (12.4%) patients and $\geq$ 500 ms in the remaining 148 (87.6%) patients. Another analysis of 36 patients with prenylamine-induced ventricular tachycardia in whom QT/QTc intervals were known on therapy before the onset of arrhythmia and after prenylamine was discontinued strongly suggested 500 ms as a powerful predictive categorical response. Before the onset of arrhythmia, 33 of these 36 patients had QT/QTc intervals > 500 ms, and when the drug was discontinued the interval values were < 500 ms in 35 of these 36 patients. The remaining one patient was a 62-yr-old male who had an off-drug QT interval of 600 ms and an on-drug QT interval of 840 ms (heart rate 62 beats per minute). This patient had experienced TdP after only 6 d of treatment with prenylamine and probably had a congenital Long QT syndrome (LQTS).

A QTc interval ≥ 500 ms has also been identified as a major factor for high risk of cardiac events in patients with LQTS *(42)*. Although caution is usually advised, and may be necessary, when extrapolating observations from patients with congenital LQTS to patients with drug-induced QT interval prolongation, it has to be acknowledged that so far no major experimental or clinical peculiarity differentiating the two forms of LQT has emerged *(12)*. Just as drugs can inhibit one or more drug metabolizing enzymes to produce a phenocopy of a poor metabolizer, it follows that drugs can also inhibit one or more ion channels to produce a phenocopy of a congenital channelopathy.

Combined Assessment of Categorical Responses

It has been argued that such categorical signals as described earlier fail to take into account the tendency of QTc interval to regress towards a mean. Regression toward the mean refers to the tendency of subjects with high baseline values to have lower increases at later time points, whereas subjects with low baseline values tend to experience greater increases. Indeed, Makkar et al. (29) reported that in 154 patients with TdP (who had mean baseline QTc interval, ΔQTc and on-treatment QTc interval values of 440 ms, 150 ms and 590 ms, respectively), baseline QTc interval values of ≤ 410 ms, 420–460 ms and ≥ 470 ms were associated with on-treatment increases of 200 ms, 160 ms, and 70 ms, respectively. Funck-Brentano et al. *(44)* also reported that the change in QTc interval from baseline observed after 14 d of bepridil therapy was inversely proportional to the baseline QTc interval (r = –0.68; $p < 0.001$). The author has also observed an inverse correlation between percent increase in QTc interval and baseline QTc interval in 21 patients who had a QTc interval ≥ 500 ms while receiving sertindole, an atypical neuroleptic agent that is a potent inhibitor of I_{Kr} current.

However, the assessment of risk based on a combined evaluation of the two signals should compensate for the tendency of QTc interval changes to regress to a mean. As a broad generalization, an increase of QTc interval from 410 to 485 ms (ΔQTc = 75) appears to be less important than that from 450 to 500 ms (ΔQTc = 50) which in turn is less important than that from 490 to 530 ms (ΔQTc = 40). Expressed differently, since the risk of TdP depends on the duration of QTc interval and not on an increase from baseline, a new absolute QTc interval ≥ 500 ms in any subject is a better indicator of the risk than is a ΔQTc ≥ 60 ms. The CPMP is also of the view that while changes in QTc interval relative to baseline indicate a drug effect, an absolute QTc interval has greater prognostic significance.

It is worth investigating whether only those drugs that are associated, in an adequately powered study, with both the categorical responses in the same subject need be considered potent torsadogens. During treatment with prenylamine, a potent torsadogen in humans, 14 of the 26 patients experienced QTc interval prolongation of more than 40 ms, but 3 patients had to be withdrawn from the study as a result of marked prolongation *(45)*. Serial ECG data from 99 patients with advanced malignancies who received 170 courses of arsenic trioxide showed prolonged QT intervals in 38 patients (26 patients had intervals ≥ 500 ms). Compared with baseline, ΔQTc was 30–60 ms in 36.6% of treatment courses and > 60 ms in 35.4% of patients *(46)*. This is, however, an area that warrants further investigation. One way to compensate for any potential bias caused by the tendency of QTc interval to regress to a mean might be to examine the data stratified by baseline QTc interval into the following five subgroups: baseline QTc intervals of 371–390, 391–410, 411–430, 431–450, and 451–470 ms. However, for reasons just stated, it is questionable if this approach will prove to be any more helpful.

In the Pfizer study 054 *(2)* that compared the QT-prolonging potential of ziprasidone with five other neuroleptic agents, 2 of the 31 subjects on ziprasidone and 5 of the 30 subjects on thioridazine responded with $\Delta QTc \geq 60$ ms without anyone exceeding a QTc interval of 500 ms (corrected for heart rate by a study population-specific formula leading to a correction coefficient of 0.35 rather than 0.50 of the Bazett formula). These data might suggest that both these drugs have a comparable "QT-liability," but the study was not powered to detect differences in outliers. During clinical use thioridazine has been frequently reported to induce TdP, and despite extensive use over the last few years ziprasidone has not. The use of a $\Delta QTc > 75$ ms would have distinguished ziprasidone (0 subjects) from thioridazine (1 subject). Unless the incidence of TdP with thioridazine is very high, a study with 30 subjects is unlikely to identify anyone exceeding a QTc interval of 500 ms—it is probable that a larger cohort in both groups would have distinguished the two drugs even better. If the study were to be powered to detect differences in the number of outliers, each treatment arm would require very large sample sizes. Therefore, these categorical responses by ziprasidone and thioridazine are better interpreted together with their mean effects on QTc interval (placebo-uncorrected increases of 15.9 ms and 30.1 ms, respectively, from baseline).

One simulation study assessed the type I error rate and rank order of power for six different QTc-derived metrics using linear mixed-effect models *(47)*. These included maximal change in QTc interval from baseline, maximal QTc interval, area under the QTc interval-time curve (QTc–AUC), time-averaged QTc interval, maximal QTc interval with baseline QTc interval as covariate, and QTc–AUC with baseline QTc interval as covariate. The ability of the metrics to detect a drug effect was examined, assuming any drug effect followed either an Emax or linear model. All statistics had a type I error rate near the nominal value. It was concluded that when the IC_{50} was lower than or equal to the maximal plasma concentration of the drug, maximal change from baseline had a fairly good power. The power of maximal QTc interval was not as good. However, better than either of these was maximal QTc interval with baseline QTc interval as covariate.

MEAN INCREASE IN QTc INTERVAL

Mean increase in QTc interval discussed in this section refers to a mean increase in placebo-corrected maximum or peak QTc interval ("central tendency"). The maximal or peak mean change in the QTc interval and its timing should be reported. For analyses of central tendency, however, the effect of an investigational drug on the QTc interval is most commonly analyzed using time-matched QTc intervals (e.g., hourly). In this method, mean changes from baseline in the observed QTc interval are presented as time-matched control and treatment group values (e.g., hourly). However, there are inter-individual fluctuations on the same day, and intra-individual fluctuations on different days in QTc-time profile. These fluctuations raise serious concerns on the sensitivity and reliability of time-matched baseline subtraction method.

Analysis of placebo-corrected mean increases in QTc interval induced by a drug to assess its pro-arrhythmic safety continues to attract much discussion. The core of the issue is the magnitude of the mean increase at which a torsadogenic risk can confidently be attributed to a drug. Table 1 summarizes the mean increases in QTc interval following single and/or multiple oral doses of some drugs known to induce TdP.

A number of studies have been undertaken with cisapride, investigating various dosing regimens. Cisapride 20 mg twice a day for 7 d produced a mean increase in peak QTc interval of only 6.8 ms at 1.5 h and 10.9 ms at 3 h post-dose (2) (AstraZeneca, personal communication), whereas 5 mg thrice daily and 10 mg thrice daily for 1–4 wk produced changes of 7 and 13 ms, respectively, at steady-state (60). Diphenhydramine 50 mg and 100 mg to three volunteers each induced mean changes in maximum QTc interval of 11 ms and 32.3 ms, respectively (64). Although massive overdoses with diphenhydramine are often associated with reports of wide complex ventricular tachyarrhythmias, there is none of TdP.

Interpretation of QTc interval measurements made following repeated doses of drugs with class III activity over a few days is further complicated by a phenomenon of "pharmacodynamic tolerance." For a given concentration of a QTc-prolonging drug, QTc interval prolongation is greater after earlier doses than after subsequent repeated doses. This has been demonstrated for class III antiarrhythmic drugs such as racemic sotalol (65,66) and dofetilide (67). For example, following administration of dofetilide to 25 healthy volunteers, there was a linear relationship between plasma dofetilide concentration and the prolongation of the QTc interval. However, the slope of this relationship was significantly greater on d 1 (ranging from 12.9 to 14.2 ms.mL/ng) than on d 5 (ranging from 9.9 to 12. 8 ms.mL/ng) (67).

The difficulties in interpreting such heterogeneous data on mean increases from baseline, when comparing or evaluating drugs, are immediately apparent. Such heterogeneity of data arises from the frequency and quality of ECG assessments, population studied, sample size employed, and dose of the drug and the frequency of its administration. This constitutes a strong case (when warranted by nonclinical data) for a "standardized" clinical study dedicated to investigating the effect of an NCE on QTc interval.

Based on these considerations and other data on torsadogenic and nontorsadogenic drugs, the author has computed the likely prognostic significance of the effect of clinical doses on mean maximum or peak placebo-corrected QTc interval in humans (see Table 2). To put these mean increases in the context of categorical responses, it might be noted, for example, that the mean increase in QTc interval produced by 200 mg sparfloxacin in 813 patients amounted to only 11 ms (+ 2.9%), and yet the absolute QTc interval had exceeded 500 ms in 10 (1.23%) of these patients (62).

Data from more recently conducted studies appear to support this computation of risk. For example, Fridericia-corrected mean increases induced by single oral doses of 50 mg and 400 mg sildenafil were 6 ms and 9 ms, respectively (at 1 h post-dose) and 6 ms and 6 ms, respectively (at Tmax) (vardenafil study 10929). There were no outliers with signal categorical responses. Out of approx 58 million prescriptions to December 2002, there were only two cases of TdP/QT interval prolongation and/or polymorphic ventricular tachycardia reported in association with its use. One of the patients was taking sotalol and the other cisapride as co-medications. Therefore, these reports are almost certainly causally unrelated to sildenafil, especially since sildenafil has been shown to block I_{Kr} at concentrations (IC_{50} = 100 $m$mol/L) well exceeding those encountered therapeutically (1 $m$mol/L) (68). Even 30 $m$mol/L of sildenafil induces only a 15% inhibition of I_{Kr}, and therefore clinically significant effect on repolarization is clearly most unlikely during the therapeutic use of sildenafil (69,70). Single oral dose of 400 mg moxifloxacin, used as

Table 1
Mean Increases in QTc Interval (ms) Following
Single or Multiple Oral Doses of Some Drugs Known to Induce TdP

Drug	Increase (ms) during single dose studies	Increase (ms) during multiple doses studies	Reference(s)
Thioridazine			48
10 mg	9		
50 mg	22		
Terodiline			49
200 mg racemic	23		
100 mg R-terodiline	19		
100 mg S-terodiline	0		
Sparfloxacin			50–52
200 mg	10, 15	11	
400 mg	16, 14		
800 mg	29		
1200 mg	51		
1600 mg	60		
Moxifloxacin			
400 mg	15		53
800 mg	17		53
800 mg	16.34–17.83		54
Pimozide			
6 mg	13.3		55
10.7 mg		24	56
Halofantrine			
500 mg	17		57
500 mg	26		58
Cisapride			
10 mg	18		59
5 mg x 3		7	60
10 mg x 3		13	60
10 mg x 4		6	61
20 mg x 2		10.9	2
Erythromycin			62
500 mg x 3		13.8	
Arsenic trioxide		32.2	63
Bepridil		17	44
300–500 mg			
Prenylamine		33	45
180 mg			

a positive control in the same study, induced an increase of 8 ms and yet, in another study, it had induced an increase of 12.7 ms (alfuzosin study 5105). It is worth emphasizing that the vardenafil study was carried out in the United States, whereas the alfuzosin study was undertaken in Europe using different methodologies in respect of recording, measuring, and correcting the QT intervals. Out of 19 million prescriptions of moxifloxacin, there

Table 2
Likely Prognostic Significance of the
Effect of 1x Clinical Dose on Mean Maximum
or Peak Placebo-Corrected QTc Interval in Man

Mean maximum or peak placebo-corrected increase in QTc interval	Likely potential torsadogenic risk
≤ 5 ms	None
6–10 ms	Unlikely
11–15 ms	Possible
16–20 ms	Probable
21–25 ms	Almost definite
≥ 26 ms	Definite

were only 15 reports of TdP worldwide, almost all of which were confounded by the presence of known risk factors (age > 70 yr, cardiac disease, or concomitant drugs).

Although mean increases produced by the same dose of moxifloxacin (now frequently used as a positive control) were significantly different in the above two studies and in one published study (53), safety concerns regarding its inclusion as a "consistently performing positive control" are now alleviated. It has been shown in in vitro electrophysiological studies to block I_{Kr} in a dose-dependent manner, but the concentration-effect curve appears shallow. There is a 22-fold safety margin as determined from the IC_{50} value for I_{Kr} block relative to the plasma free drug concentration achieved following a therapeutic dose of 400 mg daily (11). Single oral doses of 400 mg moxifloxacin, tested over the last 24 mo in well over 20 specially designed studies in healthy volunteers that used standardized approaches and methods, have consistently produced mean increases in QTc interval ranging from 5 ms to 10 ms (J. Morganroth, 2004, personal communication).

Ziprasidone induces dose-dependent mean increases in QTc interval. In the Pfizer study 054, daily doses of 160 mg ziprasidone for 3 wk induced a Bazett-corrected, Fridericia-corrected, and baseline-corrected mean increases of 20.3 ms, 15.5 ms, and 15.9 ms, respectively (all uncorrected for placebo) (2). As stated earlier, 2 of the 31 subjects on ziprasidone and 5 of the 30 subjects on thioridazine responded with ΔQTc ≥ 60 ms without anyone exceeding a QTc interval of 500 ms. Although these findings may at first sight raise concerns on the safety of ziprasidone, there have been no reports of ziprasidone-induced TdP despite its very extensive clinical use. Indeed, the ECG of a man who had taken a ziprasidone overdose of 3120 mg showed a peak QTc interval of 490 ms at 4.5 h after the overdose and only nonspecific T wave flattening (71). At the FDA Psychopharmacological Drugs Advisory Committee meeting on July 19, 2000, the sponsor gave details of ten cases of ziprasidone overdoses (range of doses 240 mg to 4600 mg) with the highest QTc interval on drug being 478 ms (72). The complexity in using mean increases in QTc interval to evaluate the risk of proarrhythmia is exemplified by a comparison of sparfloxacin and ziprasidone. Although sparfloxacin produces a smaller mean increase in QTc interval (11 ms vs 15.9 ms), it has been reported to induce TdP whereas ziprasidone has not.

To return to the relative safety of oral haloperidol, it is interesting that in the Pfizer study 054 (2), daily oral doses of 15 mg haloperidol induced a (placebo-uncorrected) mean increase in QTc interval (corrected for heart rate by a study population-specific formula) of 7.1 ms at steady-state. However, another study reported a mean increase in QTc interval (corrected for heart rate by subject-specific formula) of 13.2 ms following a single 10 mg oral dose (73). Comparison of the data from these two studies is complicated by differences in study design and data analysis. There is probably no real difference between the two studies in terms of the effect of the drug—the author anticipates that a single oral dose of 10–15 mg haloperidol likely induces a mean placebo-corrected increase of 7 ms in the QTc interval, thus attesting to the relative cardiac safety of oral haloperidol.

DISPERSION IN REPOLARIZATION

Analysis of dispersion in repolarization, either as an individual categorical response or as a population mean change, is a controversial area in the assessment of risk of TdP. Relative to the epicardial and endocardial myocytes, the repolarizing I_{Ks} current is weak and the depolarizing sodium current (I_{Na}) more sustained in the midmyocardial M-cells. These result in a more prolonged action potential in M-cells. Not surprisingly, I_{Kr} blockers have profound effect in these cells, giving rise not only to prolongation of the QT interval but also to greater than normal transmural dispersion. Drugs that block I_{Kr} and I_{Ks} may be expected to prolong uniformly the action potential (and therefore, the QT interval) but have little or no effect on transmural dispersion.

As observed in numerous detailed laboratory studies such as those investigating tissue preparations (74) and those involving monophasic action potential mapping (75,76), intra-myocardial dispersion of refractoriness (that is the difference between APD in different regions of ventricular myocardium) plays an important role in both electrical stability of the ventricles and in arrhythmogenesis. Physiologically, there is a substantial degree of spatial dispersion in repolarization not only across the myocardial wall but also between the apex and base of ventricles, between the septum and free walls as well as between the right and left ventricles. To some extent, this anisotropy of APD is determined by differences in cellular electrophysiology, such as those between endocardial, midmyocardial (M-cells), and epicardial myocytes (77), as well as electrotonic interactions across gap junctions that lead to the excitation—repolarization equilibrium when, approximately, those cells that depolarize last repolarize first. It is easy to appreciate that the electrotonic equilibrium between excitation and repolarization is antiarrhythmic since it prevents creation of islands of excitable tissue surrounded by still repolarizing cells, which is the typical substrate of figure eight re-entry (78).

Whereas differences in APD occur along the apico-basal and antero-posterior axes in both epicardium and endocardium, transitions are usually gradual and readily tolerated. Therefore, from the point of view of arrhythmogenesis, the differences between APD in remote parts of the ventricles are of little consequence. On the other hand, closely coupled regions of myocardial tissue with substantial differences in their refractoriness can easily be pro-arrhythmic. When the regions are more or less anatomically determined or organized, such as in scarred tissue, dispersion in repolarization leads preferentially to ventricular tachycardia. However, ventricular fibrillation is more likely when the regions are less organized, such as in acute ischaemia.

While the mechanisms leading to drug-induced TdP are still not fully understood, it is likely that differential effects of the drug on different tissue types within the ventricles play an essential role. Recent experiments with myocardial wedge preparation suggest that those drugs that have differential effects on epicardial, midmyocardial (M-cells), and endocardial myocytes are particularly torsadogenic *(12)*. Whether similar differential drug effects exist between myocytes in the apex and the base or between myocytes in the left and right ventricles is not fully known, although it seems to be likely due to the different distribution of repolarization channels in the myocytes of these regions. Most likely, differential drug effects in closely coupled regions of the heart, such as in regions subjected to a different degree of ischaemia and fibrosis, is one of the major reasons for an increased incidence of drug-induced proarrhythmia in cardiac patients, especially those with CHF.

Against the above background, it is easier to discuss the regulatory perspective on the utility of dispersion in repolarization for risk assessment.

QT Dispersion

Drug-induced APD prolongation does not occur uniformly throughout the heart. These regional differences can lead to arrhythmogenic spatial dispersion of repolarization. The potential importance of myocardial spatial dispersion of refractoriness in arrhythmogenesis led to a number of attempts to assess it from the surface ECG. Perhaps the best known of these attempts was the concept of the so-called QT dispersion. This attempt was based on an unsubstantiated hypothesis that inter-ventricular and/or intra-ventricular differences in repolarization could be calculated by measuring inter-lead variability of QT interval in the standard 12-lead surface ECG *(79,80)*. QTc dispersion (QTd) was thus defined as the maximum inter-leads QTc interval range (maximum minus the minimum QTc intervals). The simplicity of the technique led to its widespread popularity with a substantial number of studies on the topic.

Earlier studies had suggested an association between QTd and clinical outcomes in conditions such as congenital LQTS *(81)* and myocardial infarction *(82)*. More recently, in the Strong Heart Study, which was a prospective study of cardiovascular disease in 1839 American Indians, prolonged QTc and increased QT dispersion were significant predictors of all-cause mortality and cardiovascular mortality. Analyses controlling for risk factors showed that QTc interval remained a strong predictor of all-cause mortality and a weaker predictor of cardiovascular mortality, whereas only QT dispersion remained a significant predictor of cardiovascular mortality *(83)*. Patients with LQTS not responding to β-adrenoreceptor blocking therapy were shown to have a significantly higher QTd than the responders; nonresponders, however, responded to left cardiac sympathetic denervation and remained asymptomatic thereafter *(84)*.

Because QTd was thought to reflect ventricular regional differences in repolarization, it was believed that it might have a potential utility in assessment of risk of drug-induced proarrhythmias *(85–87)*. A number of studies appeared to support this optimism. In a prospective study, patients developing TdP exhibited early during almokalant infusion a pronounced QT prolongation, increased QT dispersion, and marked morphological T wave changes *(87)*. Commensurate with its drug interaction potential, terfenadine 60 mg twice a day for 7 d increased QTd in six subjects from 5 ± 2.2 ms to 6.6 ± 11.8 ms only but to 63.3 ± 37.5 ms when co-administered with ketoconazole *(88)*. Treatment with halofantrine, a potent torsadogen, is followed by a significant increase in QTd at 9 h and 24 h. QTc interval, QT dispersion, and QT regression slopes were significantly correlated with halofantrine plasma concentrations *(89)*. In patients with CHF, β-adrenoreceptor blocking drugs are associated with reduction in both QTc interval and QT dispersion, raising the possibility that reduction in QT dispersion may be beneficial *(90)*. Of particular interest is the report that bisoprolol reduced QTd in patients with CHF, but the response of patients to bisoprolol was influenced by the aetiology of heart failure *(91)*. Bepridil is highly torsadogenic and in one study it significantly prolonged the QTc interval (420 ms to 500 ms), QTd (70 ms to 140 ms), and transmural dispersion. The addition of a β-adrenoreceptor blocking drug significantly decreased the QTc interval (500 ms to 470 ms), QTd (140 ms to 60 ms), and transmural dispersion. However, compared with the control, the combination therapy was associated with significantly prolonged QTc interval, but without any change in either QTd or transmural dispersion, and was effective in all patients with intractable atrial fibrillation. Given the pro-arrhythmic potential of bepridil, the safety of the combination therapy suggests that QTd and transmural dispersion might have a more specific predictive value for TdP in some instances *(92)*. However, the observations in this study might also be related solely to changes in transmural dispersion.

The CPMP document notes that the baseline QTd (defined as a maximal inter-lead variability) is generally estimated to be approx 40–60 ms. Although QT dispersion was thought to be investigational when the CPMP adopted their strategy, QTd greater than 100 ms and/or a change in dispersion of more than 100% from baseline induced by an NCE "in an individual subject" had been suggested as signals that should raise a concern about the potential of the NCE to induce arrhythmias including TdP.

Although the concept of QT dispersion is the best known and its application widely investigated, it has also proved to be the least successful. Inevitably, the CPMP guidance note led to numerous studies investigating the effect of drugs not only on the QTc interval but also on QT dispersion. Many studies attempted to correlate the two changes with clinical outcomes and determine which one of them might be a better predictor of risk. The assessment of QTd as a measure of pro-arrhythmic risk of a drug is still the subject of intense debate *(93,94)*. However, the available data have proved to be very disappointing, and the predictive value of this parameter (if it has any) has yet to be demonstrated. The literature arguing against the use of QT dispersion is now extensive but a few representative findings are summarized below.

Compared to 42 unmedicated patients, the ECGs of 111 patients taking neuroleptics showed frequent prolongations of the QTc interval but QTd was not significantly increased *(95)*. Terodiline, a drug indicated for urinary incontinence, was withdrawn from the market in 1991 because of its high torsadogenic potential. This potential resides in its (+)-(R)-isomer. Both racemic and (+)-(R)-terodiline significantly increased uncorrected QT interval and QTc interval without affecting QT dispersion *(49)*. However, an earlier study had reported a significant decrease in QTd from 76 ± 33 ms to 42 ± 17 ms ($p < 0.01$) on discontinuation of terodiline therapy in 15 asymptomatic elderly patients with urinary incontinence *(96)*. Their QTc interval decreased from 487 ± 41 ms to 434 ± 26 ms ($p < 0.05$). Although risperidone prolonged QT interval, it had no significant effect on QT dispersion in the elderly patients *(97)*. Similar disparities have been reported between the effects on QTc interval and QTd following administration of arsenic trioxide *(63)* and cisapride *(98)*. The odds of haloperidol-induced TdP have been computed to be higher in patients with QTc interval prolongation than in those with increased QT interval dispersion *(99)*. More strikingly, even a potent torsadogen like dofetilide prolongs the QTc interval but does not increase QTd *(100)*. In 463 patients with CHF, changes in QT dispersion following treatment with dofetilide did not predict all-cause or cardiac mortality.

Dofetilide-induced changes in QT dispersion were small and comparable to those seen in placebo-treated patients *(101)*. In 126 patients who had taken an overdose of diphenhydramine, the (Bazett-corrected) QTc interval was significantly longer but the QTd was significantly lower than in the control group *(102)*. The interpretation of these data is complicated by marked changes in heart rate induced by diphenhydramine. Analysis of one representative tracing in the publication suggests that Fridericia-corrected QTc interval does not appear to be significantly prolonged in these patients. In a study by Yamaguchi et al. *(43)*, rate-corrected QT dispersion was not as predictive of TdP as was transmural dispersion *(see* next section).

This approach for determining heterogeneity in ventricular repolarization has also been criticized on the basis of the lack of any credible link to the electrocardiographic lead theory that contradicts the notion of QT dispersion entirely *(103,104)*. It has also been observed from a very early period that the reproducibility of the measurement of QT dispersion is particularly poor, especially in ECGs showing some abnormality in T wave morphology *(105)*. More recently, it has become evident that the assessment of QT dispersion is actually based on a systematic bias in the errors of QT interval measurement. Briefly stated, the more abnormal repolarization patterns with notched and unusually shaped T waves (such as in congenital and acquired LQTS), the more difficult it is to measure the QT interval precisely in each lead of the ECG, thus creating greater errors in the measurement and hence observing an increased QT dispersion. In addition, QT dispersion is also substantially dependent on the projection of the three-dimensional T wave loop into individual ECG leads, and thus the more complicated the loop, the greater are the differences and errors in QT interval assessment in individual leads *(106,107)*. There is also another problem linked to the concept of QTd. Several studies showed that the QT (uncorrected) dispersion did not depend on heart rate, and thus did not need correcting for heart rate. Increased heart rate is a well-known risk factor on its own. Interestingly, it has been shown that even when taking data of absolutely no clinical relevance and correcting them for heart rate using the Bazett formula, significant differences in risk may be observed; for example, between "heart-rate corrected length of the surname" and high- and low-risk patients purely because of the heart rate difference *(108)*. Therefore, there is no legitimacy to the claims that the sheer number of studies with positive results establishes the value of QTd. There is little doubt that spatial heterogeneity of ventricular repolarization does exist and differs between different clinical groups. It is measurable in 12-lead resting ECGs but QT dispersion is not related to it.

In view of the technical flaws, limitations, and conflicting data, analysis of QTd may only supplement more standard analyses of QT/QTc interval duration. It is true that very marked prolongation of QT interval is frequently accompanied by substantial abnormalities of the T wave morphology which, when combined with simple measurement techniques, leads to increased QT dispersion. Nevertheless, from a regulatory as well as an academic perspective, QT dispersion as a technique of measuring intra-myocardial dispersion of repolarization has now been practically abandoned, and has been replaced by other scientific and more sophisticated analytical techniques.

Transmural Dispersion of Repolarization

More recently, another simple technique that measures the interval between the peak and the end of T wave in standard ECG leads is gaining popularity as previously enjoyed by QT dispersion. Because the ventricular wall is thin relative to ventricular surface area, relatively small transmural dispersions in repolarization (TDR) create significant gradients. Increase in TDR is now widely believed to be the principal substrate for induction of TdP and increase in TDR, rather that prolongation of QTc interval, induced by a drug probably predicts better the risk of TdP associated with its use. Experimental studies have shown that the interval from the peak to the end of T wave (T_{peak} to T_{end} or TPE) reflects TDR across the ventricular wall. This technique has been derived from a series of experiments with the ventricular wedge preparation where it is clearly capable of differentiating between drug effects on the different tissue types within the wedge, namely the endocardial, midmyocardial (M-cells), and epicardial myocytes. Because the M-cells are exquisitely responsive to pharmacological agents that block I_{Kr}, they often give rise to drug-induced changes in TDR. This is seen as prolongation of TPE on the surface ECG (109) and appears to correlate better with a potential for induction of TdP. In ventricular tissues from cardiac failure, electrical remodeling has been shown to result in much greater TDR, thus possibly explaining why patients with this condition are at a greater risk of drug-induced TdP.

This technique has been shown to provide reasonable results in some carefully conducted animal studies. In further support of the role of TDR in torsadogenesis, Di Diego et al. (110) demonstrated in the same isolated arterially perfused canine left ventricular preparation, the development of TdP by cisapride at a concentration that maximally increases TDR and the failure of TdP to develop after an increase in the concentration of cisapride that reduces TDR despite increasing QT interval. Studies with transmembrane action potentials of epicardial, midmyocardial, and endocardial cells, recorded simultaneously from such wedge preparations together with a transmural ECG, suggest that nicorandil (a potassium channel opener) may be capable of abbreviating the long QT interval, reducing TDR, and preventing spontaneous and stimulation-induced TdP in congenital or acquired LQTS caused by the inhibition of I_{Kr} or I_{Ks} (111). Similar studies have shown that amiodarone produces an important decrease in TDR, especially under conditions in which dispersion is exaggerated (112). Tissues from the ventricles of CHF patients receiving chronic amiodarone therapy displayed M-cell APD significantly shorter (404 ms) than that recorded in tissues from normal hearts (439 ms) or from CHF patients not treated with amiodarone (449 ms). Dispersion of ventricular repolarization in tissues from patients treated with amiodarone was considerably smaller than in the two other groups (113). These findings may partly explain the lower incidence of TdP observed with chronic amiodarone therapy as compared with other class III agents. Although sertindole prolongs the APD and QTc interval, it has no significant effect on TDR and does not induce EADs. Despite comparable QT prolongation, sertindole did not display the proarrhythmic profile typical of other blockers of I_{Kr} such as dl-sotalol (114).

A number of studies have also investigated TDR in patients with congenital LQTS. The median TPE interval has been reported to be greater in LQT2 patients (112 ms) than in LQT1 patients (91 ms) or unaffected patients (86 ms) (115). Because LQT1 results from mutations of I_{Ks} (a current activated by increased heart rate) and LQT2 from mutations of I_{Kr}, increase in heart rate, sympathetic stimulation, and exercise in LQT1 patients unmask deficiency of I_{Ks} function and produce much greater increase in TPE in LQT1 patients (115,116). Both QTc interval and TPE were significantly prolonged during exercise in LQT1 patients (from 510 to 599 ms and from 143 to 215 ms). In LQT2 patients, there were no significant changes in these parameters (from 520 to 502 ms and from 195 to 163 ms) (117). This may partially account for exercise-induced fatal cardiac events in LQT1 patients. Whereas syncope and sudden death in LQT1 are associated with sympathetic stimulation, LQT2 patients are more susceptible to arrhythmias during nonexertional states. Phenylephrine-induced bradycardia decreased TDR in symptomatic LQT1, but increased TDR in symptomatic LQT2 (118). These observations are consistent with the superior efficacy of β-adrenoreceptor blocking drugs in LQT1 and the increased arrhythmogenicity noted during nonexertional states in LQT2 (118,119).

Experimental model of LQT1 has indicated that a deficiency of I_{Ks} alone does not induce TdP but that the addition of β-adrenergic influence predisposes to the development of TdP by increasing TDR, most likely as a result of a large augmentation of residual I_{Ks} in epicardial and endocardial cells but not in M-cells, in which I_{Ks} is intrinsically weak (120). Propranolol prevented the ability of isoproterenol to increase TDR and to induce TdP. As stated earlier, bepridil is highly torsadogenic and in patients with intractable atrial fibrillation, it significantly prolonged the QTc interval, QTc dispersion, and TDR (100 ms to 160 ms) (92). The addition of a β-adrenoreceptor blocking drug significantly decreased the QTc interval, QTd, and TDR (160 ms to 110 ms). Compared with the control, the combination therapy was associated with significantly prolonged QTc interval without any changes in either the QTd or TDR. Given the pro-arrhythmic potential of bepridil, the safety and efficacy of the combination therapy in these patients might be a result of an antiarrhythmic prolongation of the QTc interval without any pro-arrhythmic changes in TDR.

Unfortunately, the relevance of TPE in drug-induced proarrhythmias has not been characterized as thoroughly in humans. The use of T_{peak} to T_{end} as a parameter of TDR will remain controversial until techniques for its measurement (e.g., which and how many leads) are refined and validated. Neither is it certain how local changes in TDR in a small area of ventricular myocardium will manifest on surface ECG. The relationship between TDR and changes in T wave (entire wave or terminal portion) also requires clarification. For example, sotalol preferentially prolongs APD in M-cells dose-dependently, leading to QT prolongation and an increase in TDR. However, sotalol-induced changes in repolarization are associated with morphological changes of T wave across the entire T wave segment. The ECG in humans integrates all the physiologic global differences in refractoriness (apex-base, left-right, septum-free wall, etc.), and the concept of TPE interval measured in a standard 12-lead ECG is likely to suffer from a weak link to the electrocardiographic lead theory that was the case with QT dispersion. It is also worth bearing in mind that in a number of normal ECGs and in a vast majority of recordings with repolarization abnormality, the TPE interval is very different from one lead to another. Large clinical studies suggest that there are problems with simple projections of the results from the wedge preparation to clinical recordings (121,122). Whereas the concept of TPE interval is certainly very valid and well documented in the myocardial wedge experiments, different and perhaps more complicated electrocardiographic analysis will be needed to find a realistic counterpart applicable to the clinical recordings.

In the study referred to earlier, Yamaguchi et al. (43) explored the value of a new index—the ratio of TPE to QT interval—that they term Tpe. Although maximum QTc interval was 657 ms in those with and 505 ms in those without TdP, this Tpe ratio (measured in lead V5) did not correlate with the maximum QTc interval, but it was found to be a reliable predictor for TdP. TPE was 185 ms in those with TdP and 84 ms in those without but the Tpe ratio was 0.337 in those with and 0.187 in those without TdP. Cumulative frequency distributions revealed that a Tpe ratio of 0.28 was a good cut-off point for risk of TdP. The sensitivity, specificity, and false-positive and false-negative predictive values for *Tpe* > 0.28 for predicting TdP were 0.80, 0.88, 0.80, and 0.88, respectively. The corresponding values for QTd were 0.70, 0.82, 0.70, and 0.82, respectively.

Unfortunately, the problem of heart rate correction also applies to these approaches. The TPE interval depends on heart rate in a different way than does the QT interval *(121)*, and thus the TPE to QT ratio changes with heart rate. Hence, without applying proper heart rate correction (i.e., different to QT correction) to both TPE and to the *Tpe* ratio, a reporting bias might again be introduced, as was the case with QTd. Nevertheless, there is fairly compelling evidence to show that agents that prolong the QT interval but do not induce EADs or ectopic beats and do not increase dispersion of repolarization are not capable of inducing TdP *(12,123)*. Therefore, it appears highly worthwhile gathering prospective data on new indices of drug-induced dispersion of repolarization from all trials, including the one dedicated to evaluating the effect of the NCE on QTc interval, and exploring further their predictive value.

Other Approaches to Analysis of Changes in Repolarization

The equilibrium between depolarization–repolarization processes has been appreciated from the very early days of electrocardiography, because of the similar polarity of the QRS complex and the T wave. As early as the 1930s, the concept of the so-called ventricular gradient, measuring the deviation between the principle direction of ventricular depolarization and repolarization waves, was proposed. Only recently, however, when substantial numbers of electronically recorded ECGs became routinely available was the concept of ventricular gradient evaluated in larger studies *(124)*. It has been observed that in both cardiac patients and in the overall elderly population, the increase of the vectorial difference between depolarization and repolarization is an important risk factor *(125,126)*. Substantial difference between healthy men and healthy women has also been found, which may partially explain the different incidence of both clinical and drug-induced arrhythmia between the two genders *(127)*. Unfortunately, experience with the use of ventricular gradient as a tool in assessing drug-induced repolarization abnormalities and the clinical risk is at present very limited.

Finally, most recently, the concept of measuring the so-called *nondipolar* components of the T wave has been proposed *(128,129)*. In principle, the repolarization differences that exist between different regions of the heart, especially those between closely coupled regions, cannot be explained within the three-dimensional loop of the T wave because this averages the repolarization process over the whole mass of both ventricles. QT dispersion that was thought to reflect spatial heterogeneity of ventricular refractoriness may be largely a result of the projections of the repolarization dipole rather than *nondipolar* signals. Consequently, it has been proposed to investigate and measure how much of the standard 12-lead ECG (considering only the eight truly independent leads) can be explained by a simple movement of a three-dimensional dipole, and what is the extent of the signal that cannot be explained by such a dipole and, which therefore must originate from differences in small neighboring regions. Whereas the extent of these nondipolar components is rather minute, it has been shown to constitute a powerful risk predictor both in patients with ischaemic heart disease and in the general population. Similar to the ventricular gradient, substantial differences between men and women have been found with women having a significantly increased nondipolar component of repolarization on the ECG *(130)*. Experience with drug-induced changes of the nondipolar components is also limited, although very initial indications suggest that this measure might be capable of differentiating between the drugs that lead to beneficial, i.e., antiarrhythmic QT interval prolongation (when the nondipolar components decrease) and the truly pro-arrhythmic and torsadogenic QT interval prolongation (when the nondipolar components increase on treatment) *(131)*.

OTHER QTc-DERIVED PARAMETERS

Other alternative parameters that have been proposed in assessing the QT-related risks are changes from baseline in time-averaged QTc intervals and in the QTc–AUC. These parameters too can be examined in terms of categorical increases in individual subjects or as increases in population-based mean values.

Time-Averaged QTc Intervals

Time-averaged QTc interval discussed in this subsection refers to the average of the sum of *all* QTc interval measurements made on an individual during the dosing/ECG measuring period. It is thus a measure of an average on-therapy QTc interval across the whole dosing or ECG measuring period. The mean population-based change in time-averaged QTc interval from baseline is derived from on-therapy changes in time-averaged QTc interval from baseline from all study participants. This parameter is suitable only for studies in which subjects are receiving a single dose or fixed dose treatment under steady-state conditions. Although this approach has the advantage of repeated measures being collapsed into a single summary value, there are significant disadvantages. The simulation study referred to earlier *(47)* concluded that mean time-averaged QTc interval had a poor power such that it should not be used. This is hardly surprising because the time-averaged value of QTc interval for each subject would depend on the number of ECG measurements made around Cmax and Cmin of the cardiotoxic drug-related species (parent drug or its metabolite)—more measurements around Cmax will increase, and the more around Cmin will decrease, the time-averaged QTc interval for each subject. This then influences the mean of time-averaged QTc intervals from all subjects. Importantly, time averaging of changes in the QTc intervals ignores the possible influence of concentration–effect relationships and circadian rhythm on intra-individual variation. Thus, changes in time-averaged QTc intervals will have a tendency to underestimate the magnitude of a drug effect.

Data on terfenadine illustrate the point. Mean increase in time-averaged QTc across the 12-h dosing interval with 60 mg dose was 6 ms. However, the mean increase in maximum QTc interval at any time point was 18 ms without a metabolic inhibitor *(132)*. In the presence of ketoconazole, a potent inhibitor of the metabolism of terfenadine, the mean increase in maximum QTc interval was up to 82 ms *(133)*.

It is acknowledged that time averaging provides yet another QTc-derived measure for evaluating a drug effect. Together with other QTc-derived parameters discussed earlier, it may be possible to use individual or population mean changes in time-averaged QTc intervals to further refine the assessment of clinical risk of TdP. Clearly, the study design would have to include a positive control as well as a placebo, and ensure that ECG sampling times and frequency are beyond reproach.

Area Under the QTc vs Time Curve

Just as with plasma drug concentrations over time (pharmacokinetic area under concentration time curve—AUC), it is possible to compute AUC of QTc interval by plotting QTc interval values against time following administration of a drug (pharmacodynamic

AUC). Clearly, the use of the QTc–AUC as a dependent variable requires the collection of multiple data points for each subject during the placebo and treatment phases.

One of the main problems with this approach is the point of reference for integration of individual values into a single QTc–AUC measure. For drug concentration-based AUC, this is straight forward—from a baseline concentration of 0 units. It is much less clear for effect-based AUC. Should the QTc–AUC be integrated from 0 ms or from QTc interval at baseline? Although this approach too has the advantage of repeated measures being collapsed into a single summary value, experience with this approach is limited. The summary values generated are large and interpretation is complicated by the lack of well-recognized criteria for distinguishing clinically relevant changes. For example, QTc–AUC$_{(0-12)}$ changes (with corresponding baseline values) induced by 7-d treatment with placebo, ebastine 60 mg and 100 mg and terfenadine 180 mg doses were 13.2 (4609), 49.9 (4613), 124.2 (4571), and 213.8 (4590) units, respectively (134). Compared to placebo (+ 0.3%), the changes induced by ebastine 100 mg (+ 2.7%) and terfenadine 180 mg (+ 4.7%) were statistically significant. The corresponding maximum increases in QTc interval were 0.7 ms, 2.2 ms, 8.2 ms, and 13.3 ms. However, in another study, a combination of a lower dose of 20 mg ebastine and placebo for 10 d increased QTc–AUC$_{(0-12)}$ by 96.6 (+ 2.1%) from a baseline of 4635 units (134).

Interestingly, the simulation study referred to earlier (47) also concluded that regardless of pharmacokinetic or pharmacodynamic model, QTc–AUC with baseline QTc interval as a covariate had the greatest power than any other metric examined for detecting a drug effect.

At present, the use of neither time-averaged QTc intervals nor QTc–AUC has any regulatory appeal because of lack of any experience with these parameters. Regulatory evaluation is based primarily on the number of subjects with categorical responses and population-based mean change from baseline in placebo-corrected maximum or peak QTc interval. Together with these "primary" endpoints of safety, it may become possible with experience to refine further the assessment of clinical risk of TdP by including other "secondary" endpoints of safety such as mean change in time-averaged QTc intervals or QTc–AUC.

MORPHOLOGICAL CHANGES IN REPOLARIZATION WAVEFORMS

Because QT interval prolongation and TdP are intricately linked to delayed repolarization of the action potential, it is not surprising that these repolarization abnormalities may also manifest as morphological changes in repolarization waves—changes in T wave morphology and the appearance of abnormal U waves. Critically timed, complex and frequent extrasystoles, and changes in T wave morphology have long been recognized as powerful precursors of TdP (14). Instability of the T wave frequently precedes TdP (87,135,136). Changes in T wave may be in terms of its diverse shapes (peaked, notched, widened, flattened, inverted, biphasic, or triphasic) and/or beat-to beat variation in amplitude and vector—the so-called T wave alternans. The following is a brief overview of a wealth of literature on morphological changes in repolarization waveforms

T Wave Alternans

T wave alternans (TWA) was first described in 1908. It is strongly associated with electrical instability in the heart, and is one of the established powerful markers of susceptibility to sudden cardiac death. Beat-to-beat variability in APD is not synchronized and this gives rise to TWA. Electrical alternans of the action potential develops when a series of short-long diastolic interval cycles generates a reciprocating long-short series of APDs *(137)*. It has been suggested that TWA observed at rapid rates under the settings of a prolonged QT interval is largely the result of alternation of the M-cell APD, leading to exaggeration of TDR during alternate beats and thus the potential for development of TdP *(138)*. Based on nonclinical studies with hERG-blocking drugs of varying torsadogenic potential, it has been suggested that the magnitude of effect on rate-dependent alternans may allow the differentiation of pro-arrhythmic and nonarrhythmic hERG blockers at clinically relevant concentrations *(137)*. Nonclinical studies in Langendorff-perfused guinea pig hearts and clinical observations in patients with LQTS or complete atrio-ventricular block have shown that nicorandil attenuates TDR and abolishes TWA, EADs, and TdP *(111,139–141)*. Armoundas et al. *(142,143)* have reviewed the current understanding of the pathophysiology of TWA, and suggest that repolarization alternans most likely results from diverse cellular and molecular changes that are associated with exaggerated regional repolarization heterogeneity. This then renders the heart susceptible to malignant arrhythmias.

T wave or TU wave alternans have long been reported in association with TdP in patients receiving chlorpromazine or pentamidine, and following arsenic poisoning or subarachnoid hemorrhage. T or U wave alternans in association with long QT interval and TdP is relatively uncommon. Zareba et al. *(135)* reviewed a total of 4656 ECG recordings in 2442 patients with LQTS for episodes of T wave alternans. T wave alternans was identified in 30 patients (25 of whom had a QTc interval > 500 ms). There was a strong association between QTc prolongation and TWA. However, careful statistical analyses with adjustment for age, gender, and QTc value revealed that TWA did not make a significant independent contribution to the risk of cardiac events. Other studies, however, have provided evidence to the contrary.

However, although overt TWA in the ECG recordings is not common, digital signal processing techniques capable of detecting subtle degrees of TWA (microvolt TWA) have shown that TWA may represent an important marker of vulnerability to ventricular tachyarrhythmias. In an analysis of TWA in 18 patients with LQTS, digital Holter ECG analysis showed macroscopic, true TWA in 3 of these 18 patients. Two of the identified patients with TWA experienced sudden cardiac death during follow-up *(144)*. In a patient on procainamide, TU alternans and TdP occurred at long cardiac cycles. In this patient, endocardial monophasic action potential recordings showed that TU alternans was associated with alternation of the duration of the plateau *(145)*. Interestingly, there is a reduction in TWA amplitude following the administration of β-adrenoreceptor blocking drugs *(146)*.

Changes in Repolarization Wave Morphology

Combined I_{Kr} and I_{Ks} block evidently gives rise to diverse morphologies of T wave resulting from a preferential prolongation of APD in different transmural layers, a dramatic increase in TDR, and a high incidence of EADs *(109,147)*. In nonclinical studies, when sotalol start generating EADs/TdP, widening and flattening of the T wave are observed *(114)*.

In an evaluation of 10 patients with LQTS and TdP, a flat and wide T wave and/or an abnormal increase in U wave amplitude close to the end or the peak of the T wave were observed. These changes were accentuated by pause or a sudden deceleration in ventricular rhythm *(148)*. There are other reports of genotype-specific patterns and changes in T wave morphologies before and during exercise in patients with LQTS *(117,149)*. Nakajima et al. *(150)* described an interesting case of a 35-yr-old woman who was hospitalized as a result of frequent attacks of syncope immediately after the ringing of a bell or alarm clock. She had a QTc interval of 560 ms with a bizarre T wave inversion in precordial leads. After admission, a total of nine events of syncope were observed. Malignant ventricular tachyarrhythmia (TdP, ventricular flutter, or fibrillation) was recorded during each episode. Auditory stimuli appeared to be involved in the initiation of malignant ventricular arrhythmia. Immediately after auditory stimuli, changes in the QT interval and T wave morphology resulted in ventricular premature beats, leading to ventricular tachycardia.

Widening and flattening of the T wave frequently precede clinical onset of TdP following torsadogenic agents *(14,87,146,151)*. In one study of 101 children administered cisapride, 12 were found to have a QTc > 440 ms and one other had a new prominent notched T wave in all leads *(152)*. During 43 episodes of TdP in seven patients with drug-induced QT interval prolongation, a notched T–U complex caused by a prominent U wave at the end of the T wave was noted in five patients immediately before the episodes of TdP. Prolongation of the preceding RR interval was directly related to the increase of the U wave amplitude *(25)*. The amplitude of EADs that trigger TdP is also cycle length dependent and there is a strong correlation between the preceding RR interval and the amplitude of EADs that follow *(153)*.

In view of the foregoing, it is not surprising that the CPMP strategy on investigating drug-induced QT interval prolongation emphasizes the need to report the effects of a drug on morphology of repolarization waveforms both during nonclinical and clinical studies *(3)*. According to CPMP *(3)*, "changes in the T wave morphology and/or the occurrence of U wave constitute important warning signs and they may precede the occurrence of TdP. Drug-induced changes in the T wave morphology and/or the occurrence of U waves must be attached the same significance as prolongation of the QT interval." These data are best presented in terms of the number and percentage of patients in each treatment group having changes from baseline that represent the appearance or worsening of the morphological abnormality, grouped by the nature of abnormality (that is, TWA, changes in T wave morphology, and appearance of U waves).

MODULATION OF RISK BY ANCILLARY PROPERTIES

Having determined that ventricular repolarization changes (e.g., prolongation of the QTc interval) induced by an NCE are clinically relevant, the next important task is to assess its potential for inducing TdP and other ventricular tachyarrhythmias during its routine clinical use. There are a number of factors that modulate the risk of TdP associated with a QT-prolonging drug *(2,154)*. Among the pharmacokinetic factors are the dose of the drug, presence of liver or kidney disease, and co-administration of drugs that might increase its concentration. As previously noted, common pharmacodynamic factors that predispose to the risk of TdP include electrolyte imbalance, bradycardia, pre-existing prolongation of the QTc interval, cardiac disease, and co-administration of another QT-prolonging drug(s). Presence of a clinically silent mutation in any one of the LQTS genes may also increase pharmacodynamic susceptibility in asymptomatic LQT patients with normal ECG phenotype *(8,154,155)*.

The dilemma of characterizing the clinical risk to patients from prolongation of QTc interval following studies in healthy volunteers is further aggravated by the fact that many noncardiac clinical conditions have now been unexpectedly found to be associated with increased pharmacodynamic susceptibility to QT interval prolongation and associated proarrhythmias. QTc interval prolongation is associated with, and has been identified as a risk factor for, malignant ventricular tachyarrhythmias in sudden deaths (usually labeled as sudden unexplained cardiac deaths) and a number of cardiovascular as well as noncardiovascular "natural" diseases. These include cardiomyopathy (156–158), cardiac failure (159,160), myocardial infarction (161), sudden infant death syndrome (162), hypoglycemia (163), cirrhosis (164, 165), and a number of other conditions associated with autonomic failure (166,167). A higher prevalence of QTc interval prolongation has also been reported in patients with human immunodeficiency virus infection compared to other hospitalized patients (28.6% vs 7%) (168). In this context, recent isolated reports of TdP associated with protease inhibitors are beginning to raise some concerns. However, these reports must be viewed with a careful perspective on risk–benefit of this therapy.

In retrospect, it is ironic that cisapride should have been indicated for the relief of symptoms of impaired gastric motility secondary to disturbed and delayed gastric emptying associated with diabetes and autonomic neuropathy. The prevalence of prolonged QTc interval in diabetic patients is significantly higher in comparison with the control group (8% vs 2%). Abnormality of the sympathetic nervous system is present in more than 50% of the case group, whereas the abnormality of the parasympathetic nervous system is even more common (169). One review (170) has estimated the prevalence of QT prolongation in type 1 and type 2 diabetic patients to be higher than 20%. Diabetic autonomic neuropathy is also associated with QTc interval prolongation (171–173). Autonomic failure in diabetes is reportedly 2.26 times more likely to be present in patients with, compared to patients without, QTc prolongation (172). In the subgroup with macroalbuminuria, maximum QTc interval was an independent risk factor for cardiovascular mortality (173). QTc interval prolongation was the only variable that showed a significant mortality odds ratio (24.6) in a multivariate analysis (171). In an informal analysis of 43 reports of cisapride-induced TdP by the author, 40% had diabetes. Not surprisingly, gastroparesis is disproportionately over represented in cisapride-induced TdP patients compared to normal cisapride users (16% vs 5%) (174). The use of erythromycin as a stimulant of gastrointestinal motility in diabetic gastroparesis further aggravates the proarrhythmic risks associated with the use of cisapride in these patients, because it is a powerful inhibitor of cisapride metabolism by CYP3A4 and is itself a potential hERG blocker. Not surprisingly, only 38 (11%) of the cases reported by Wysowski et al. (174) had no identifiable risk factors or contraindications. Another group of drugs with similar irony are the antipsychotic drugs that prolong the QTc interval. Schizophrenic patients during acute psychotic episode are reported to have agitation-induced hypokaelmia and consequently a prolonged QTc interval (175,176). In this context, reports of sudden death of some acutely psychotic patients following (rapid) parenteral administration of these drugs are a matter of concern. Issues such as these are central to understanding and assessing the clinical risk of TdP from QTc interval prolongation by non-antiarrhythmic drugs.

However, the two properties that deserve special consideration when assessing the clinical risks of TdP following QTc interval prolongation by an NCE are its autonomic or calcium channel blocking properties. Altered function of the ion channels involved in action potential by itself is not sufficient to induce TdP. Alterations in autonomic activity and abnormalities of ventricular repolarization are now considered to be the key features, both as triggers and as markers for vulnerability to TdP (177,178). Modulation of α-adrenoreceptor activity seems to have greater effect than that of β-adrenoreceptor activity *(178a)*. The literature on evidence, especially from nonclinical studies, is fairly extensive but the following discussion provides a brief representative overview.

β1-Adrenoreceptor activation inhibits I_{Kr} via cAMP/protein kinase A-dependent pathways *(179)*. Experimental evidence from studies in dogs has demonstrated that α-adrenoreceptor stimulation increases, whereas α-adrenoreceptor blockade decreases EADs and ventricular tachycardias *(180)*. Schwartz *(181)* has reviewed the implications of sympathetic nerve stimulation or isoproterenol administration for the antiarrhythmic and torsadogenic properties of potassium channel blockers.

Sertindole well illustrates the need for characterizing a drug for these ancillary pharmacological properties. The powerful α-adrenoreceptor blocking activity of sertindole requires its dose to be titrated upwards slowly over weeks to prevent postural hypotension. In Langendorff perfused rabbit hearts, despite comparable QT prolongation, sertindole did not display the pro-arrhythmic profile typical of other I_{Kr} blockers such as dl-sotalol *(114)*. Using patch clamp electrophysiology, sertindole has been shown to block hERG currents with an IC_{50} value of 14.0 n*M*—almost as powerful as the highly potent class III antiarrhythmic drug dofetilide (IC_{50} value of 9.5 n*M*) *(182)*. Neither the parent drug nor its hERG-active metabolites induce EADs *(183)*. In one nonclinical study, clinically relevant concentrations of sertindole blocked dofetilide-induced TdP *(184)*. Despite its high affinity antagonism of hERG and marked prolongation of the (Fridericia-corrected) QTc interval in many patients, there are hardly any well-documented reports of TdP associated with the use of sertindole. This dissociation between the "QT-liability" of sertindole and the absence of TdP associated with its use is attributable to its powerful α-adrenoreceptor blocking activity.

α-Adrenoreceptor blocking drugs such as prazosin, doxazosin, alfuzosin, terazosin, and tamulosin are potent hERG blockers, and yet there are hardly any reports of TdP associated with their use. For example, there were a total of 110 million prescriptions for doxazosin, terazosin, and tamulosin dispensed in the United States during the period 1998–2003, and yet there were only six reports of TdP in total. Since 1987, alfuzosin has been used in the EU, Australia, and Canada without any reports of TdP *(185)*. As of May 12, 2004, the Medicines and Healthcare products Regulatory Agency (MHRA) in the UK had received a total of 2944 reports of adverse drug reactions in association with these five drugs. These have included only one report of QT interval prolongation, one of TdP, one of ventricular tachycardia, and two of ventricular fibrillation.

Both epinephrine and dobutamine have also been reported in isolated cases to induce TdP in patients with LQTS *(186,187)*. Full β-blockade is effective in 75–80% of patients with LQTS. It is ineffective in the remaining 20–25% in whom addition of doxazosin shortened QTc interval in upright position before exercise from 523 ms to 483 ms *(188)*. A 7-yr-old boy with LQTS who began to experience recurrent syncopal attacks with TdP in spite of β-blockade illustrates the role of combined roles of α- and β-adrenoreceptors. Change of therapy to labetalol (a combined α1- and β-adrenoreceptors blocking drug) resulted in complete suppression of syncopal episodes *(189)*.

The effect of adrenergic stimulation is the basis of an epinephrine challenge test as a means of establishing an ECG diagnosis in silent LQT1 mutation carriers *(190)*.

The 12-lead ECG parameters before and after epinephrine infusion were compared among 19 mutation carriers with a baseline QTc interval $\geq$ 460 ms (group I), 15 mutation carriers with a QTc interval < 460 ms (group II), 12 nonmutation carriers (group III), and 15 controls (group IV). The mean QTc interval and T_{peak} to T_{end} before and after epinephrine were significantly greater in 15 symptomatic than in 19 asymptomatic mutation carriers in groups I and II. The mean QTc interval and T_{peak} to T_{end} interval before epinephrine were significantly greater in group I than in the other three groups. Epinephrine significantly increased these parameters in groups I and II, but not in groups III and IV. The sensitivity of the QTc interval to identify mutation carriers was improved from 59% before epinephrine to 91% after epinephrine, without adversely affecting specificity of 100%. Furthermore, infusion of epinephrine to patients with LQTS increases QTc interval in a genotype-specific manner *(191)*.

In contrast to the adverse effect of class III or class I antiarrhythmic drugs on mortality in patients with myocardial ischaemia, the survival benefits of amiodarone, β-adrenoreceptor blocking drugs, and calcium channel blockers are striking. As stated earlier, the class III activity of sotalol resides in both isomers whereas the β-adrenoreceptor blocking activity resides only in the (–)-(R)-isomer. Not surprisingly, whereas the racemic drug is predominantly antiarrhythmic, the (+)-(S)-isomer (d-sotalol) is predominantly pro-arrhythmic. The efficacy of β-adrenoreceptor blocking drugs in significantly decreasing the QTc interval and TDR in LQTS patients *(118,119)* and in patients receiving bepridil has already been referred to earlier *(92)*. Acute nonselective β-blockade reduced the duration of prolonged QTc interval from 460 ms to 440 ms in 17 cirrhotic patients *(192)*.

Calcium channel blockade also modulates torsadogenic risk following prolongation of the QTc interval. Apart from verapamil, there are other drugs that block the hERG channel or prolong the QTc interval but are relatively devoid of this risk. The relative rarity of TdP associated with amiodarone *(12,112,113)* is also a result of its other ancillary properties. These include its inhibitory effects on adenoreceptors, sodium and calcium currents, as well as I_{Ks}. Tolterodine, a structural analog of the highly torsadogenic drug terodiline, produces little QT prolongation clinically and there are no published reports of it inducing TdP. Yet, it blocks hERG (IC_{50} value 17 nM) with almost the same potency as dofetilide (IC_{50} value 11 nM, respectively), cisapride, terfenadine, and pimozide. This discrepancy is most likely caused by its low plasma therapeutic concentrations (total and free Cmax 12–16 nM and < 1 nM) and when the concentrations are higher, by its calcium channel blocking activity *(193)*. As of May 12, 2004, the UK adverse drug reactions database at MHRA included a total of 498 reports for tolterodine. There were only two reports of TdP, which were both confounded by other risk factors. Despite their hERG-blocking activity *(194)*, the torsadogenic potential of SSRIs, relative to neuroleptic drugs, is much lower. This is probably a result of their other pharmacological properties, such as calcium channel blocking activity *(195)*.

SB-237376, an investigational new drug, inhibits I_{Kr} with an IC_{50} of 0.42 mM and use-dependently blocks L-type calcium current at higher concentrations. It induces EADs in rabbits but not in dogs. This is probably caused by larger increases of APD, QT interval, and TDR in rabbits than dogs. These effects were self-limiting owing to the SB-237376-induced block of L-type calcium current at higher concentrations. This block of L-type calcium channel may also explain why pro-arrhythmic risk was found to be lower with SB-237376 than with dl-sotalol *(196)*.

CONCLUSIONS

Intuitively, it seems highly inappropriate to categorize drugs clinically as having an effect or no effect on QTc interval. Rather, there are three possible outcomes from the analysis of clinical QTc interval related data namely: (1) no effect, (2) a clinically insignificant effect, or (3) a clinically significant effect. This chapter provides an overview of how the clinical data from ECGs should be interpreted in (a) determining whether a drug produces clinically relevant QTc interval prolongation, and (b) assessing the clinical risk of TdP following administration of a drug that is deemed to prolong the QTc interval.

Provided the ECGs recorded are technically of high quality and the intervals are measured and corrected appropriately for changes in heart rate, a number of QTc-derived parameters may be used for assessment of risk. According to the author, the most reliable parameters among those easily derived are the categorical responses (a new absolute QTc interval $\geq$ 500 ms regardless of the magnitude of increase from baseline and/or ΔQTc $\geq$ 60 ms), and mean increase from baseline in placebo-corrected maximum or peak QTc interval. The former takes into account inter-individual differences in susceptibility whereas the latter provides information on response of the study population as a whole. Assessment based on the evaluation of both these parameters circumvents biases arising from the tendency of the QTc interval to regress towards a mean. Whereas QTd (defined as maximal inter-leads variability) has proved to be a disappointing tool, measurement of transmural dispersion appears a promising additional parameter by which to assess the torsadogenic potential of a drug.

Without dismissing any alternative proposals, the author's preferred hierarchical scheme for an integrated interpretation of drug-induced effects on ventricular repolarization and assessing the clinical risk of TdP associated with non-antiarrhythmic drugs is shown in Table 3. The term "diminished repolarization reserve" is intended in this scheme to include patients with mutations of I_{Kr}, as well as all those with pharmacodynamic risk factors that convert an otherwise benign inhibition of I_{Kr} into a clinically relevant inhibition. The application of the scheme requires a degree of pragmatism bearing in mind the greater importance of the clinical over the nonclinical data, and taking into consideration the proportion of trial population showing categorical responses, the mean placebo-corrected increase in QTc interval from baseline, the potencies (IC_{50} or EC_{50}) of the drug at the desired pharmacological target and potassium channels (I_{Kr}), and its ancillary pharmacological properties (autonomic and calcium channel modulating activities).

There are regional differences in the emphasis on safety, efficacy, and risk/benefit of a drug arising from local expectations, medical practice, and available alternatives. Inevitably, there will be differences in the way various regulatory authorities interpret or take account of the same set of data on repolarization changes. Vardenafil illustrates these important differences in terms of data requirements and labeling with regard to QTc interval. Its IC_{50} for the intended target enzyme (phosphodiesterase 5 inhibition) is 0.89 nM and for hERG is 84 mM. It was shown in in vivo studies in dogs to have no effect on QT interval. These results suggest a low potential for QT interval prolongation in humans *(197)* and, consequently, vardenafil was given a positive opinion by the CPMP in November 2002, and approved by the European Commission in March 2003 without any dedicated QTc study in healthy volunteers. In contrast, the FDA approved it in August 2003 subject to the sponsor committing to a post-marketing study to evaluate the impact on QT interval prolongation of combining vardenafil with another drug with a similar QT effect size. Although a single dedicated clinical trial showed that vardenafil had only a very modest effect on Fridericia-corrected QTc interval (+10 ms) even at eight times the recommended starting dose, the FDA contraindicated its use in patients who have pre-existing prolongation of the QT interval because of the possibility of producing an arrhythmia (despite the reassuring profile in the healthy volunteers study), whereas the CPMP

Table 3
Author's Preferred Hierarchical Scheme for Integrated Interpretation of Major Repolarization
Data and Assessing the Clinical Risk of TdP Associated With Non-Antiarrhythmic Drugs

1 The drug will likely prolong the QTc interval to clinically relevant magnitude if:

    1.1 nonclinical in vitro data show a safety margin (ratio of hERG IC_{50} to plasma Cmax) < 10;
        or

    1.2 unicellular APD studies show EADs;
        or

    1.3 nonclinical in vivo data show QTc interval prolongation

    Plus

    1.4 clinically, any (placebo corrected) categorical responders show: A new absolute QTc interval
        ≥ 500 ms and/or ΔQTc ≥ 60 ms;
        or

    1.5 clinically, mean placebo-corrected increase in QTc interval from baseline ≥ 11 ms;
        or

    1.6 the clinical target patient population is likely to have diminished repolarization reserve

2. Drug that prolongs the QTc interval to clinically relevant magnitude will likely be torsadogenic if:

    2.1 it lacks autonomic or calcium channel blocking activity;
        or

    2.2 it possesses sympathomimetic activity

    Plus

    2.3 it produces significant transmural dispersion;
        or

    2.4 it produces relevant morphological changes in repolarization waveforms;
        or

    2.5 the clinical target patient population is likely to have diminished repolarization reserve

See text for explanation.

were content to include only a descriptive narrative of the study and its results in the pharmacological properties section of the European labeling.

In the context of mean increases in QTc interval and categorical responses, the post-marketing safety of a fixed combination of piperaquine and dihydroartemisinin ("Artekin"), used in the treatment of malaria, will be of great interest. Compared with baseline, it prolonged the mean (placebo-uncorrected) QTc interval by 11 ms. While none of the 62 subjects showed a ΔQTc ≥ 60 ms; the maximal change observed was 53 ms in a female child *(198)*. Although the measured QT intervals were corrected by Bazett formula when the mean heart rate was just above 90 bpm, the observed mean effects are very much on the border line.

It should not, however, be assumed that drugs with a potential to prolong QTc interval will never be approved. They may be approved provided a carefully planned clinical development program has identified a population in whom the benefits of the drug can be shown to outweigh the small potential risk of proarrhythmias, or the drug can be shown to fulfil an unmet need.

Arsenic trioxide illustrates well how even a drug with very marked potential to prolong the QT interval and induce TdP may be approved with specific guidelines associated with its clinical use if it is shown to fulfil an unmet need. In clinical trials, QT prolongation with an interval > 500 ms in at least one ECG tracing was observed in 16 (40%) of 40 patients treated with arsenic trioxide *(199)*. Clinically, there is a delay of 2 h in maximum QTc following peaks in serum arsenic concentration *(63)*, suggesting a potential role for one of its metabolites in prolonging the QTc interval. In a multicenter study, QT prolongation following arsenic trioxide was common (63% of the 40 patients studied). One patient had an absolute QT interval of > 500 ms and experienced an asymptomatic episode of TdP *(200)*. In a Japanese study of arsenic trioxide in 14 patients, adverse events included 13 electrocardiogram abnormalities (including 13 QTc prolongations and four nonsustained ventricular tachycardia) *(201)*. Arsenic trioxide ("Trisenox") was approved in September 2000 in the United States and in October 2001 in the EU for its remarkable efficacy in induction of remission and consolidation in patients with a specific form of acute promyelocytic leukaemia who are refractory to, or have relapsed from, retinoid and anthracycline chemotherapy.

With respect to drug-induced TdP, there is also a more philosophical question of the definition of "clinical risk" and the level of risk that is unacceptable or tolerable. It seems inappropriate to categorize together a drug with an incidence of TdP of 1 in 500,000 patients with another with an incidence of 1 in 3000. As with other potentially fatal adverse drug reactions such as myelotoxicity, gastrointestinal hemorrhage, hepatotoxicity, or rhabdomyolysis, a level of risk may have to be tolerated. Whereas an incidence of a potentially fatal event at the rate of 1 in 3000 may be unacceptable, an incidence of 1 in 500,000 may be considered acceptable with a whole range in between. This perceived risk has to be seen in the context of benefit and available alternatives. The risk of not treating a disease is also an important component in risk assessment.

ACKNOWLEDGMENTS

I wish to express my sincere appreciation to Professor Charles Antzelevitch (Masonic Medical Research Laboratory, Utica, NY), Professor Christian Funck-Brentano (Saint-Antoine University Hospital, Paris, France), Professor Joel Morganroth (University of Pennsylvania, Philadelphia, PA), Professor Marek Malik (St. George's Hospital Medical School, London, UK), and Dr. Harry Witchel (Cardiovascular Research Laboratories, University of Bristol, UK) for their very helpful comments and constructive discussions during the preparation of this chapter. Any shortcomings, however, are entirely my own responsibility.

REFERENCES

1. Morganroth J. Relations of QTc prolongation on the electrocardiogram to torsades de pointes: definitions and mechanisms. Am J Cardiol 1993;72:10B–13B.
2. Shah RR. The significance of QT interval in drug development. Br J Clin Pharmacol 2002;54:188–202.
3. Committee for Proprietary Medicinal Products. Points to consider: The assessment of the potential for QT interval prolongation by non-cardiovascular medicinal products (CPMP/986/96) EMEA, 17 December 1997, London. http://www.emea.eu.int/pdfs/human/swp/098696en.pdf. (Accessed on 10 February 2004.)
4. US Food and Drug Administration/Health Canada The clinical evaluation of QT/QTc interval prolongation and pro-arrhythmic potential for non-antiarrhythmic drugs Preliminary Concept Paper (15 November 2002) http://www.fda.gov/ohrms/dockets/ac/03/briefing/pubs%5Cprelim.pdf. (Accessed on 10 February 2004.)
5. Sanguinetti MC, Jiang C, Curran ME, Keating MT. A mechanistic link between an inherited and an acquired cardiac arrhythmia: HERG encodes the I_{Kr} potassium channel. Cell 1995;81:299–307.
6. Mitcheson JS, Chen J, Lin M, Culberson C, Sanguinetti MC. A structural basis for drug-induced long QT syndrome. Proc Natl Acad Sci USA 2000;97:12329–12333.

7. Chachin M, Kurachi Y. Evaluation of pro-arrhythmic risk of drugs due to QT interval prolongation by the HERG expression system (Article in Japanese). Nippon Yakurigaku Zasshi 2002;119:345–351.

8. Roden DM. Drug-induced prolongation of the QT interval. N Engl J Med 2004;350:1013–1022.

9. Fermini B, Fossa AA. The impact of drug-induced QT interval prolongation on drug discovery and development. Nature Rev Drug Dis 2003;2:439–447.

10. Anon. Research and development costs: the great illusion. Prescrire Int 2004;13:32–36.

11. Kang J, Wang L, Chen XL, Triggle DJ, Rampe D. Interactions of a series of fluoroquinolone antibacterial drugs with the human cardiac K+ channel HERG. Mol Pharmacol 2001;59:122–126.

12. Belardinelli L, Antzelevitch C, Vos MA. Assessing predictors of drug-induced torsade de pointes. Trends Pharmacol Sci 2003;24:619–625.

13. Dessertenne F. La tachycardie ventriculaire á deux foyers opposes variable. Arch Mal Coeur Vaiss 1966;59:263–272.

14. Stratmann HG, Kennedy HL. Torsades de pointes associated with drugs and toxins: recognition and management. Am Heart J 1987;113:1470–1482.

15. Tzivoni D, Keren A, Banai S, Stern S. Terminology of torsades de pointes. Cardiovasc Drugs Ther 1991;5:505–507.

16. Passman R, Kadish A. Polymorphic ventricular tachycardia, long Q-T syndrome, and torsades de pointes. Med Clin North Am 2001;85:321–341.

17. Bauman JL, Bauernfeind RA, Hoff JV, Strasberg B, Swiryn S, Rosen KM. Torsade de pointes due to quinidine: observations in 31 patients. Am Heart J 1984;107:425–430.

18. Burket MW, Fraker TD, Temesy-Armos PN. Polymorphic ventricular tachycardia provoked by lidocaine. Am J Cardiol 1985;55:592–593.

19. Nguyen PT, Scheinman MM, Seger J. Polymorphous ventricular tachycardia: clinical characterization, therapy, and the QT interval. Circulation 1986;74:340–349.

20. Grogin HR, Scheinman M. Evaluation and management of patients with polymorphic ventricular tachycardia. Cardiol Clin 1993;11:39–54.

21. Eisenberg SJ, Scheinman MM, Dullet NK, et al. Sudden cardiac death and polymorphous ventricular tachycardia in patients with normal QT intervals and normal systolic cardiac function. Am J Cardiol 1995;75:687–692.

22. Brady WJ, DeBehnke DJ, Laundrie D. Prevalence, therapeutic response, and outcome of ventricular tachycardia in the out-of-hospital setting: a comparison of monomorphic ventricular tachycardia, polymorphic ventricular tachycardia, and torsades de pointes. Acad Emerg Med 1999;6:609–617.

23. Paltoo B, O'Donoghue S, Mousavi MS. Levofloxacin induced polymorphic ventricular tachycardia with normal QT interval. Pacing Clin Electrophysiol 2001;24:895–897.

24. Kusano KF, Hata Y, Yumoto A, Emori T, Sato T, Ohe T. Torsade de pointes with a normal QT interval associated with hypokalemia. Jpn Circ J 2001;65:757–760.

25. Takahashi N, Ito M, Inoue T, et al. Torsades de pointes associated with acquired long QT syndrome: observation of 7 cases. J Cardiol 1993;23:99–106.

26. Dota CD, Edvardsson N, Schutzer KM, et al. Inter- and intraday variability in major electrocardiogram intervals and amplitudes in healthy men and women. Pacing Clin Electrophysiol 2003;26(Pt 2):361–366.

27. Morganroth J, Brozovich FV, McDonald JT, Jacobs RA. Variability of the QT measurement in healthy men, with implications for selection of an abnormal QT value to predict drug toxicity and proarrhythmia. Am J Cardiol 1991;67:774–776.

28. Ganput MD, Williams P, Yogendran I, Keene ON, Maconochie JG. QTc, PR interval and heart rate variability in healthy volunteers–a review of 12-lead ECG data from clinical pharmacology studies. Br J Clin Pharmacol 1995;39:577P–578P.

29. Makkar RR, Fromm BS, Steinman RT, Meissner MD, Lehmann MH. Female gender as a risk factor for torsades de pointes associated with cardiovascular drugs. JAMA 1993;270:2590–2597.

30. Gussak I, Brugada P, Brugada J, et al. Idiopathic short QT interval: a new clinical syndrome. Cardiology 2000;94:99–102.

31. Gaita F, Giustetto C, Bianchi F, et al. Short QT syndrome: a familial cause of sudden death. Circulation 2003;108:965–970.

32. Schimpf R, Wolpert C, Bianchi F, et al. Congenital short QT syndrome and implantable cardioverter defibrillator treatment: inherent risk for inappropriate shock delivery. J Cardiovasc Electrophysiol 2003;14:1273–1277.

33. Makarov OM, Chuprova ON, Kiseleva OI. QT interval shortening in families with history of sudden death at young age (Article in Russian). Kardiologiia 2004;44:51–56.

34. Bezzina CR, Verkerk AO, Busjahn A, et al. A common polymorphism in KCNH2 (HERG) hastens cardiac repolarization. Cardiovasc Res 2003;59:27–36.

35. Pietila E, Fodstad H, Niskasaari E, et al. Association between HERG K897T polymorphism and QT interval prolongation in middle-aged Finnish women. J Am Coll Cardiol 2002;40:511–514.

36. Brugada R, Hong K, Dumaine R, et al. Sudden death associated with short-QT syndrome linked to mutations in HERG. Circulation 2004;109:30–35.

36a. Bellocq C, van Ginneken AC, Bezzina CR, et al. Mutation in the KCNQ1 gene leading to the short QT-interval syndrome. Circulation 2004;109:2394–2397.

37. DeSilvey DL, Moss AJ. Primidone in the treatment of the long QT syndrome: QT shortening and ventricular arrhythmia suppression. Ann Intern Med 1980;93:53–54.

38. Pratt CM, Ruberg S, Morganroth J, et al. Dose-response relation between terfenadine (Seldane) and the QTc interval on the scalar electrocardiogram: distinguishing a drug effect from spontaneous variability. Am Heart J 1996;131:472–480.

39. Garson A Jr. How to measure the QT interval - what is normal? Am J Cardiol 1993;72:14B–16B.

40. Bonate PL, Russell T. Assessment of QTc prolongations for noncardiac-related drugs from a drug development perspective. J Clin Pharmacol 1999;39:349–358.

41. Moss AJ. The QT interval and torsade de pointes. Drug Saf 1999;21(Suppl 1):5–10.

42. Priori SG, Schwartz PJ, Napolitano C, et al. Risk stratification in the long-QT syndrome. N Engl J Med 2003;348:1866–1874.

43. Yamaguchi M, Shimizu M, Ino H, et al. T wave peak-to-end interval and QT dispersion in acquired long QT syndrome: a new index for arrhythmogenicity. Clin Sci (Lond) 2003;105:671–676.

44. Funck-Brentano C, Coudray P, Planellas J, Motte G, Jaillon P. Effects of bepridil and diltiazem on ventricular repolarization in angina pectoris. Am J Cardiol 1990;66:812–817.

45. Oakley D, Jennings K, Puritz R, Krikler D, Chamberlain D. The effect of prenylamine on the QT interval of the resting electrocardiogram in patients with angina pectoris. Postgrad Med J 1980;56: 753–756.

46. Barbey JT, Pezzullo JC, Soignet SL. Effect of arsenic trioxide on QT interval in patients with advanced malignancies. J Clin Oncol 2003;21:3609–3615.

47. Bonate PL. Rank power of metrics used to assess QTc interval prolongation by clinical trial simulation. J Clin Pharmacol 2000;40:468–474.

48. Hartigan-Go K, Bateman DN, Nyberg G, Martensson E, Thomas SH. Concentration-related pharmacodynamic effects of thioridazine and its metabolites in humans. Clin Pharmacol Ther 1996;60:543–553.

49. Hartigan-Go K, Bateman ND, Daly AK, Thomas SHL. Stereoselective cardiotoxic effects of terodiline. Clin Pharmacol Ther 1996;60:89–98.

50. Démolis J-L, Charransol A, Funck-Brentano C, Jaillon P. Effects of a single oral dose of sparfloxacin on ventricular repolarization in healthy volunteers. Br J Clin Pharmacol 1996;41:499–503.

51. Morganroth J, Hunt T, Dorr MB, Magner D, Talbot GH. The cardiac pharmacodynamics of therapeutic doses of sparfloxacin. Clin Ther 1999;21:1171–1181.

52. Morganroth J, Talbot GH, Dorr MB, Johnson RD, Geary W, Magner D. Effect of single ascending supratherapeutic doses of sparfloxacin on cardiac repolarisation (QTc interval). Clin Ther 1999;21:818–828.

53. Démolis J-L, Kubitza D, Tennezé L, Funck-Brentano C. Effect of a single oral dose of moxifloxacin (400mg and 800mg) on ventricular repolarization in healthy subjects. Clin Pharmacol Ther 2000;68:658–666.

54. Noel GJ, Natarajan J, Chien S, Hunt TL, Goodman DB, Abels R. Effects of three fluoroquinolones on QT interval in healthy adults after single doses. Clin Pharmacol Ther 2003;73:292–303.

55. Desta Z, Kerbusch T, Flockhart DA. Effect of clarithromycin on the pharmacokinetics and pharmacodynamics of pimozide in healthy poor and extensive metabolizers of cytochrome P450 2D6 (CYP2D6). Clin Pharmacol Ther 1999;65:10–20.

56. Shapiro E, Shapiro AK, Fulop G, et al. Controlled study of haloperidol, pimozide and placebo for the treatment of Gilles de la Tourette's syndrome. Arch Gen Psychiatry 1989;46:722–730.

57. Charbit B, Becquemont L, Lepere B, Peytavin G, Funck-Brentano C. Pharmacokinetic and pharmacodynamic interaction between grapefruit juice and halofantrine. Clin Pharmacol Ther 2002;72:514–523.

58. Bindschedler M, Lefevre G, Degen P, Sioufi A. Comparison of the cardiac effects of the antimalarials co-artemether and halofantrine in healthy participants. Am J Trop Med Hyg 2002;66:293–298.

59. Kivisto KT, Lilja JJ, Backman JT, Neuvonen PJ. Repeated consumption of grapefruit juice considerably increases plasma concentrations of cisapride. Clin Pharmacol Ther 1999;66:448–453.

60. Wang SH, Lin CY, Huang TY, Wu WS, Chen CC, Tsai SH. QT interval effects of cisapride in the clinical setting. Int J Cardiol 2001;80:179–183.

61. van Haarst AD, van 't Klooster GA, van Gerven JM, et al. The influence of cisapride and clarithromycin on QT intervals in healthy volunteers. Clin Pharmacol Ther 1998;64:542–546.

62. Jaillon P, Morganroth J, Brumpt I, Talbot G and the Sparfloxacin Safety Group. Overview of electrocardiographic and cardiovascular safety data for sparfloxacin. J Antimicrob Chemotherap 1996;37(Supp A):161–167.

63. Zhou J, Meng R, Li X, Lu C, Fan S, Yang B. The effect of arsenic trioxide on QT interval prolongation during APL therapy. Chin Med J (Engl) 2003;116:1764–1766.

64. Khalifa M, Drolet B, Daleau P, et al. Block of potassium currents in guinea pig ventricular myocytes and lengthening of cardiac repolarization in man by the histamine H_1 receptor antagonist diphenhydramine. J Pharmacol Exp Ther 1999;288:858–865.

65. Le Coz F, Funck-Brentano C, Poirier JM, Kibleur Y, Mazoit FX, Jaillon P. Prediction of sotalol-induced maximum steady-state QTc prolongation from single-dose administration in healthy volunteers. Clin Pharmacol Ther 1992;52:417–426.

66. Padrini R, Gusella M, Al Bunni M, et al. Tolerance to the repolarization effects of rac-sotalol during long-term treatment. Br J Clin Pharmacol 1997;44:463–470.

67. Allen MJ, Nichols DJ, Oliver SD. The pharmacokinetics and pharmacodynamics of oral dofetilide after twice daily and three times daily dosing. Br J Clin Pharmacol 2000;50:247–253.

68. Geelen P, Drolet B, Rail J, Berube J, et al. Sildenafil (Viagra) prolongs cardiac repolarization by blocking the rapid component of the delayed rectifier potassium current. Circulation 2000;102: 275–277.

69. Sofowora G, Dishy V, Roden D, Wood AJJ, Stein CM. The effect of sildenafil on QT interval in healthy men. Clin Pharmacol Ther 2001;69:67.

70. Alpaslan M, Onrat E, Samli M, Dincel C. Sildenafil citrate does not affect QT intervals and QT dispersion: an important observation for drug safety. Ann Noninvasive Electrocardiol 2003;8:14–17.

71. Burton S, Heslop K, Harrison K, Barnes M. Ziprasidone overdose. Am J Psychiatry 2000;157:835. (See Erratum Am J Psychiatry 2000;157:1359.)

72. Ritrovato CA. Pfizer Briefing Document for Zeldox capsules FDA Psychopharmacological Drugs Advisory Committee http://www.fda.gov/ohrms/dockets/ac/00/backgrd/3619b1a.pdf. (Accessed on 10 February 2004.)

73. Desai M, Tanus-Santos JE, Li L, et al. Pharmacokinetics and QT interval pharmacodynamics of oral haloperidol in poor and extensive metabolizers of CYP2D6. Pharmacogenomics J 2003;3:105–113.

74. Antzelevitch C, Shimizu W, Yan GX, Sicouri S. Cellular basis for QT dispersion. J Electrocardiol 1998;30(Suppl):168–175.

75. Franz MR. Bridging the gap between basic and clinical electrophysiology: what can be learned from monophasic action potential recordings? J Cardiovasc Electrophysiol 1994;5:699–710.

76. Franz MR, Zabel M. Electrophysiological basis of QT dispersion measurements. Prog Cardiovasc Dis 2000;42:311–324.

77. Yan GX, Shimizu W, Antzelevitch C. Characteristics and distribution of M cells in arterially perfused canine left ventricular wedge preparations. Circulation 1998;98:1921–1927.

78. cl-Shcrif N. Electrophysiologic mcchanisms of vcntricular arrhythmias. Int J Card Imaging 1991;7:141–150.

79. Mirvis DM. Spatial variation of QT intervals in normal persons and patients with acute myocardial infarction. J Am Coll Cardiol 1985;5:625–631.

80. Cowan JC, Griffiths CJ, Hilton CJ, et al. Epicardial repolarization mapping in man. Eur Heart J 1987; 8:952–964.

81. Day CP, McComb JM, Campbell RW. QT dispersion: an indication of arrhythmia risk in patients with long QT intervals. Br Heart J 1990;63:342–344.

82. Higham PD, Furniss SS, Campbell RW. QT dispersion and components of the QT interval in ischaemia and infarction. Br Heart J 1995;73:32–36.

83. Okin PM, Devereux RB, Howard BV, Fabsitz RR, Lee ET, Welty TK. Assessment of QT interval and QT dispersion for prediction of all-cause and cardiovascular mortality in American Indians: The Strong Heart Study. Circulation 2000;101:61–66.

84. Priori SG, Napolitano C, Diehl L, Schwartz PJ. Dispersion of the QT interval. A marker of therapeutic efficacy in the idiopathic long QT syndrome. Circulation 1994;89:1681–1689.

85. Hii JT, Wyse DG, Gillis AM, Duff HJ, Solylo MA, Mitchell LB. Precordial QT interval dispersion as a marker of torsade de pointes. Disparate effects of class Ia antiarrhythmic drugs and amiodarone. Circulation 1992;86:1376–1382.

86. van de Loo A, Klingenheben T, Hohnloser SH. Amiodarone therapy after previous sotalol-induced torsade de pointes: Analysis of QT dispersion to predict proarrhythmia. J Cardiovasc Pharmacol Ther 1996;1:75–78.

87. Houltz B, Darpo B, Edvardsson N, et al. Electrocardiographic and clinical predictors of torsades de pointes induced by almokalant infusion in patients with chronic atrial fibrillation or flutter: a prospective study. Pacing Clin Electrophysiol 1998;21:1044–1057.

88. Cantelena LR, Honig PK. QT dispersion as a predictor of proarrhythmia in drug interactions with terfenadine. Clin Pharmacol Ther 1998;63:178.

89. Touze JE, Heno P, Fourcade L, et al. The effects of antimalarial drugs on ventricular repolarization. Am J Trop Med Hyg 2002;67:54–60.

90. Bonnar CE, Davie AP, Caruana L, et al. QT dispersion in patients with chronic heart failure: Beta blockers are associated with a reduction in QT dispersion. Heart 1999;81:297–302.

91. Peng DQ, Zhao SP, Chen Y, Li XP. Effect of bisoprolol on QT dispersion in patients with congestive heart failure—the etiology-dependent response. Int J Cardiol 2001;77:141–148.

92. Yoshiga Y, Shimizu A, Yamagata T, et al. Beta-blocker decreases the increase in QT dispersion and transmural dispersion of repolarization induced by bepridil. Circ J 2002;66:1024–1028.

93. Kautzner J, Malik M. QT interval dispersion and its clinical utility. Pacing Clin Electrophysiol 1997;20(Pt 2):2625–2640.

94. Gillis AM. Effects of antiarrhythmic drugs on QT interval dispersion—relationship to antiarrhythmic action and proarrhythmia. Prog Cardiovasc Dis 2000;42:385–396.

95. Warner JP, Barnes TR, Henry JA. Electrocardiographic changes in patients receiving neuroleptic medication. Acta Psychiatr Scand 1996;93:311–313.

96. Thomas SHL, Ford GA, Higham PD, Campbell RWF, Rawlins MD. Effects of terodiline on the QT interval and QT dispersion. Clin Pharmacol Ther 1993;53:136.

97. Yerrabolu M, Prabhudesai S, Tawam M, Winter L, Kamalesh M. Effect of risperidone on QT interval and QT dispersion in the elderly. Heart Dis 2000;2:10–12.

98. Tutar HE, Kansu A, Kalayci AG, Girgin N, Atalay S, Imamoglu A. Effects of cisapride on ventricular repolarization in children. Acta Paediatr 2000;89:820–823.

99. Tisdale JE, Rasty S, Padhi ID, Sharma ND, Rosman H. The effect of intravenous haloperidol on QT interval dispersion in critically ill patients: comparison with QT interval prolongation for assessment of risk of torsades de pointes. J Clin Pharmacol 2001;41:1310–1318.

100. Démolis JL, Funck-Brentano C, Ropers J, Ghadanfar M, Nichols DJ, Jaillon P. Influence of dofetilide on QT interval duration and dispersion at various heart rates during exercise in humans. Circulation 1996;94:1592–1599.

101. Brendorp B, Elming H, Jun L, Kober L, Torp-Pedersen C: DIAMOND Study Group. Danish Investigations Of Arrhythmia and Mortality On Dofetilide. Effect of dofetilide on QT dispersion and the prognostic implications of changes in QT dispersion for patients with congestive heart failure. Eur J Heart Fail 2002;4:201–206.

102. Zareba W, Moss AJ, Rosero SZ, Hajj-Ali R, Konecki J, Andrews M. Electrocardiographic findings in patients with diphenhydramine overdose. Am J Cardiol 1997;80:1168–1173.

103. Surawicz B. Will QT dispersion play a role in clinical decision-making? J Cardiovasc Electrophysiol 1996;7:777–784.

104. Rautaharju PM. Why did QT dispersion die? Card Electrophysiol Rev 2002;6:295–301.

105. Faber TS, Kautzner J, Zehender M, Camm AJ, Malik M. Impact of electrocardiogram recording format on QT interval measurement and QT dispersion assessment. Pacing Clin Electrophysiol 2001;24:1739–1747.

106. Malik M, Batchvarov VN. Measurement, interpretation and clinical potential of QT dispersion. J Am Coll Cardiol 2000;36:1749–1766.

107. Kors JA, van Herpen G, van Bemmel JH. QT dispersion as an attribute of T-loop morphology. Circulation 1999;99:1458–1463.

108. Malik M, Camm AJ. Mystery of QTc interval dispersion. Am J Cardiol 1997;79:785–787.

109. Yan GX, Antzelevitch C. Cellular basis for the normal T wave and the electrocardiographic manifestations of the long-QT syndrome. Circulation 1998;98:1928–1936.

110. Di Diego JM, Belardinelli L, Antzelevitch C. Cisapride-induced transmural dispersion of repolarization and torsade de pointes in the canine left ventricular wedge preparation during epicardial stimulation. Circulation 2003;108:1027–1033.

111. Shimizu W, Antzelevitch C. Effects of a K$^+$ channel opener to reduce transmural dispersion of repolarization and prevent torsade de pointes in LQT1, LQT2, and LQT3 models of the long-QT syndrome. Circulation 2000;102:706–712.

112. Sicouri S, Moro S, Litovsky S, Elizari MV, Antzelevitch C. Chronic amiodarone reduces transmural dispersion of repolarization in the canine heart. J Cardiovasc Electrophysiol 1997;8:1269–1279.

113. Drouin E, Lande G, Charpentier F. Amiodarone reduces transmural heterogeneity of repolarization in the human heart. J Am Coll Cardiol 1998;32:1063–1067.

114. Eckardt L, Breithardt G, Haverkamp W. Electrophysiologic characterization of the antipsychotic drug sertindole in a rabbit heart model of torsade de pointes: low torsadogenic potential despite QT prolongation. J Pharmacol Exp Ther 2002;300:64–71.

115. Viitasalo M, Oikarinen L, Swan H, et al. Ambulatory electrocardiographic evidence of transmural dispersion of repolarization in patients with long-QT syndrome type 1 and 2. Circulation 2002;106:2473–2478.

116. Tanabe Y, Inagaki M, Kurita T, et al. Sympathetic stimulation produces a greater increase in both transmural and spatial dispersion of repolarization in LQT1 than LQT2 forms of congenital long QT syndrome. J Am Coll Cardiol 2001;37:911–919.

117. Takenaka K, Ai T, Shimizu W, et al. Exercise stress test amplifies genotype-phenotype correlation in the LQT1 and LQT2 forms of the long-QT syndrome. Circulation 2003;107:838–844.

118. Khositseth A, Nemec J, Hejlik J, Shen WK, Ackerman MJ. Effect of phenylephrine provocation on dispersion of repolarization in congenital long QT syndrome. Ann Noninvasive Electrocardiol 2003;8:208–214.

119. Shimizu W, Tanabe Y, Aiba T, et al. Differential effects of beta-blockade on dispersion of repolarization in the absence and presence of sympathetic stimulation between the LQT1 and LQT2 forms of congenital long QT syndrome. J Am Coll Cardiol 2002;39:1984–1991.

120. Shimizu W, Antzelevitch C. Cellular basis for the ECG features of the LQT1 form of the long-QT syndrome: effects of beta-adrenergic agonists and antagonists and sodium channel blockers on transmural dispersion of repolarization and torsade de pointes. Circulation 1998;98:2314–2322.

121. Smetana P, Batchvarov V, Hnatkova K, Camm AJ, Malik M. Sex differences in the rate dependence of the T wave descending limb. Cardiovasc Res 2003;58:549–554.

122. Smetana P, Pueyo E, Hnatkova K, Batchvarov V, Camm AJ, Malik M. Effect of amiodarone on the descending limb of the T wave. Am J Cardiol 2003;92:742–746.

123. Antzelevitch C, Shimizu W. Cellular mechanisms underlying the long QT syndrome. Curr Opin Cardiol 2002;17:43–51.

124. Batchvarov V, Hnatkova K, Ghuran A, Poloniecki J, Camm AJ, Malik M. Ventricular gradient as a risk factor in survivors of acute myocardial infarction. Pacing Clin Electrophysiol 2003;26(Pt 2):373–376.

125. Zabel M, Malik M. Practical use of T wave morphology assessment. Card Electrophysiol Rev 2002;6:316–322.

126. Zabel M, Acar B, Klingenheben T, Franz MR, Hohnloser SH, Malik M. Analysis of 12-lead T-wave morphology for risk stratification after myocardial infarction. Circulation 2000;102:1252–1257.

127. Smetana P, Batchvarov VN, Hnatkova K, Camm AJ, Malik M. Sex differences in repolarization homogeneity and its circadian pattern. Am J Physiol Heart Circ Physiol. 2002;282:H1889–H1897.

128. Malik M, Acar B, Gang Y, Yap YG, Hnatkova K, Camm AJ. QT dispersion does not represent electrocardiographic interlead heterogeneity of ventricular repolarization. J Cardiovasc Electrophysiol 2000;11:835–843.

129. Zabel M, Malik M, Hnatkova K, et al. Analysis of T-wave morphology from the 12-lead electrocardiogram for prediction of long-term prognosis in male US veterans. Circulation 2002;105:1066–1070.

130. Smetana P, Batchvarov VN, Hnatkova K, Camm AJ, Malik M. Ventricular gradient and nondipolar repolarization components increase at higher heart rate. Am J Physiol Heart Circ Physiol 2004;286:H131–H136.

131. www.fda.gov/ohrms/dockets/ac/03/slides/4000S1_05_Malik_files/frame.htm. (Accessed 29 February 2004.)

132. Morganroth J, Brown AM, Critz S, et al. Variability of the QTc interval: impact on defining drug effect and low-frequency cardiac event. Am J Cardiol 1993;72:26B–32B.

133. Honig PK, Wortham DC, Zamani K, Conner DP, Mullin JC, Cantilena LR. Terfenadine-ketoconazole interaction. Pharmacokinetic and electrocardiographic consequences. JAMA 1993;269:1513–1518.

134. Moss AJ, Morganroth J. Cardiac effects of ebastine and other antihistamines in humans. Drug Saf 1999;21(Suppl 1):69–80.

135. Zareba W, Moss AJ, le Cessie S, Hall WJ. T wave alternans in idiopathic long QT syndrome. J Am Coll Cardiol 1994;23:1541–1546.

136. Kroll CR, Gettes LS. T wave alternans and torsades de pointes after the use of intravenous pentamidine. J Cardiovasc Electrophysiol 2002;13:936–938.

137. Fossa AA, Wisialowski T, Wolfgang E, et al. Differential effect of HERG blocking agents on cardiac electrical alternans in the guinea pig. Eur J Pharmacol 2004;486:209–221.

138. Shimizu W, Antzelevitch C. Cellular and ionic basis for T-wave alternans under long-QT conditions. Circulation 1999;99:1499–1507.

139. Watanabe O, Okumura T, Takeda H, et al. Nicorandil, a potassium channel opener, abolished torsades de pointes in a patient with complete atrioventricular block. Pacing Clin Electrophysiol 1999;22: 686–688.

140. Fujimoto Y, Kusano KF, Morita H, Hong K, Yamanari H, Ohe T. Nicorandil attenuates both temporal and spatial repolarization alternans. J Electrocardiol 2000;33:269–277.

141. Sato T, Hata Y, Yamamoto M, et al. Early afterdepolarization abolished by potassium channel opener in a patient with idiopathic long QT syndrome. J Cardiovasc Electrophysiol 1995;6:279–282.

142. Armoundas AA, Nanke T, Cohen RJ. Images in cardiovascular medicine. T-wave alternans preceding torsade de pointes ventricular tachycardia. Circulation 2000;101:2550.

143. Armoundas AA, Tomaselli GF, Esperer HD. Pathophysiological basis and clinical application of T-wave alternans. J Am Coll Cardiol 2002;40:207–217.

144. Brockmeier K, Aslan I, Hilbel T, Eberle T, Ulmer HE, Lux RL. T-wave alternans in LQTS: repolar-ization-rate dynamics from digital 12-lead Holter data. J Electrocardiol 2001;34(Suppl):93–96.

145. Habbab MA, el-Sherif N. TU alternans, long QTU, and torsade de pointes: clinical and experimental observations. Pacing Clin Electrophysiol 1992;15:916–931.

146. Klingenheben T, Gronefeld G, Li YG, Hohnloser SH. Effect of metoprolol and d,l-sotalol on micro-volt-level T-wave alternans. Results of a prospective, double-blind, randomized study. J Am Coll Cardiol 2001;38:2013–2019.

147. Emori T, Antzelevitch C. Cellular basis for complex T waves and arrhythmic activity following combined IKr and IKs block. J Cardiovasc Electrophysiol 2001;12:1369–1378.

148. Song YC. Clinical observation on pause-dependent long QT syndrome and torsade de pointes ventricu-lar tachycardia (Article in Chinese). Zhonghua Xin Xue Guan Bing Za Zhi 1992;20:349–351, 389.

149. Moss AJ. T-wave patterns associated with the hereditary long QT syndrome. Card Electrophysiol Rev 2002;6:311–315.

150. Nakajima T, Misu K, Iwasawa K, et al. Auditory stimuli as a major cause of syncope in a patient with idiopathic long QT syndrome. Jpn Circ J 1995;59:241–246.

151. White NJ, Looareesuwan S, Warrell DA. Quinine and quinidine: a comparison of EKG effects during the treatment of malaria. J Cardiovasc Pharmacol 1983;5:173–175.

152. Khongphatthanayothin A, Lane J, Thomas D, Yen L, Chang D, Bubolz B. Effects of cisapride on QT interval in children. J Pediatr 1998;133:51–56.

153. Shimizu W, Tanaka K, Suenaga K, Wakamoto A. Bradycardia-dependent early afterdepolarizations in a patient with QTU prolongation and torsade de pointes in association with marked bradycardia and hypokalemia. Pacing Clin Electrophysiol 1991;14:1105–1111.

154. Shah RR. Pharmacogenetic aspects of drug-induced torsade de pointes: Potential tool for improving clinical drug development and prescribing. Drug Saf 2004;27:145–172.

155. Paulussen AD, Gilissen RA, Armstrong M, et al. Genetic variations of KCNQ1, KCNH2, SCN5A, KCNE1, and KCNE2 in drug-induced long QT syndrome patients. J Mol Med 2004;82:182–188.

156. Gupta PR, Somani PN, Avasthey P, Singh VP. Prolonged QT and hypertrophic cardiomyopathy in two families with 10 sudden deaths. J Assoc Physicians India 1985;33:353–355.

157. Martin AB, Garson A Jr, Perry JC. Prolonged QT interval in hypertrophic and dilated cardiomyopathy in children. Am Heart J 1994;127:64–70.

158. Peters S, Rust H, Trummel M, Brattstrom A. Familial hypertrophic cardiomyopathy associated with prolongation of the QT interval. Z Kardiol 2000;89:624–629.

159. MacNeil DJ, Davies RO, Deitchman D. Clinical safety profile of sotalol in the treatment of arrhythmias. Am J Cardiol 1993;72:44A–50A.

160. Kaab S, Dixon J, Duc J, et al. Molecular basis of transient outward potassium current downregulation in human heart failure: a decrease in Kv4.3 mRNA correlates with a reduction in current density. Circulation 1998;98:1383–1393.

161. Schwartz PJ, Wolf S. QT interval prolongation as predictor of sudden death in patients with myocardial infarction. Circulation 1978;57:1074–1077.

162. Schwartz PJ, Stramba-Badiale M, Segantini A, et al. Prolongation of the QT interval and the sudden infant death syndrome. N Engl J Med 1998;338:1709–1714.

163. Marques JL, George E, Peacey SR, et al. Altered ventricular repolarization during hypoglycaemia in patients with diabetes. Diabet Med 1997;14:648–654.

164. Bernardi M, Calandra S, Colantoni A, et al. Q-T interval prolongation in cirrhosis: prevalence, relationship with severity, and etiology of the disease and possible pathogenetic factors. Hepatology 1998;27:28–34.

165. Bal JS, Thuluvath PJ. Prolongation of QTc interval: relationship with etiology and severity of liver disease, mortality and liver transplantation. Liver Int 2003;23:243–248.

166. Choy AM, Lang CC, Roden DM, et al. Abnormalities of the QT interval in primary disorders of autonomic failure. Am Heart J 1998;136:664–671.

167. Ishizaki F, Harada T, Yoshinaga H, Nakayama T, Yamamura Y, Nakamura S. Prolonged QTc intervals in Parkinson's disease—relation to sudden death and autonomic dysfunction (Article in Japanese). No To Shinkei 1996;48:443–448.

168. Kocheril AG, Bokhari SA, Batsford WP, Sinusas AJ. Long QTc and torsades de pointes in human immunodeficiency virus disease. Pacing Clin Electrophysiol 1997;20:2810–2816.

169. Pourmoghaddas A, Hekmatnia A. The relationship between QTc interval and cardiac autonomic neuropathy in diabetes mellitus. Mol Cell Biochem 2003;249:125–128.

170. Veglio M, Chinaglia A, Cavallo Perin P. The clinical utility of QT interval assessment in diabetes. Diabetes Nutr Metab 2000;13:356–365.

171. Veglio M, Sivieri R, Chinaglia A, Scaglione L, Cavallo-Perin P. QT interval prolongation and mortality in type 1 diabetic patients: A 5-year cohort prospective study. Neuropathy Study Group of the Italian Society of the Study of Diabetes, Piemonte Affiliate. Diabetes Care 2000;23:1381–1383.

172. Whitsel EA, Boyko EJ, Siscovick DS. Reassessing the role of QTc in the diagnosis of autonomic failure among patients with diabetes: a meta-analysis. Diabetes Care 2000;23:241–247.

173. Rossing P, Breum L, Major-Pedersen A, et al. Prolonged QTc interval predicts mortality in patients with Type 1 diabetes mellitus. Diabet Med 2001;18:199–205.

174. Wysowski DK, Corken A, Gallo-Torres H, Talarico L, Rodriguez EM. Postmarketing reports of QT prolongation and ventricular arrhythmia in association with cisapride and Food and Drug Administration regulatory actions. Am J Gastroenterol 2001;96:1698–1703.

175. Hatta K, Takahashi T, Nakamura H, Yamashiro H, Asukai N, Yonezawa Y. Hypokalemia and agitation in acute psychotic patients. Psychiatry Res 1999;86:85–88.

176. Hatta K, Takahashi T, Nakamura H, Yamashiro H, Yonezawa Y. Prolonged QT interval in acute psychotic patients. Psychiatry Res 2000;94:279–295.

177. Huikuri H. Dispersion of repolarisation and the autonomic system-can we predict torsade de pointes? Cardiovasc Drugs Ther 2002;16:93–99.

178. Antzelevitch C. Sympathetic modulation of the long QT syndrome. Eur Heart J 2002;23:1246–1252.

178a. Urao N, Shiraishi H, Ishibashi K, et al. Idiopathic long-QT syndrome with early after depolarizations induced by epinephrine. Circ J 2004;68:587–591.

179. Karle CA, Zitron E, Zhang W, Kathofer S, Schoels W, Kiehn J. Rapid component IKr of the guinea-pig cardiac delayed rectifier K^+ current is inhibited by $beta_1$-adrenoreceptor activation, via cAMP/protein kinase A-dependent pathways. Cardiovasc Res 2002;53:355–362.

180. Ben-David J, Zipes DP. Alpha-adrenoceptor stimulation and blockade modulates cesium-induced early afterdepolarizations and ventricular tachyarrhythmias in dogs. Circulation 1990;82:225–233.

181. Schwartz PJ. Do animal models have a clinical value? Am J Cardiol 1998;81(6A):14D–20D.

182. Rampe D, Murawsky MK, Grau J, Lewis EW. The antipsychotic agent sertindole is a high affinity antagonist of the human cardiac potassium channel HERG. J Pharmacol Exp Ther 1998;286:788–793.

183. Maginn M, Frederiksen K, Adamantidis MM, Bischoff U, Matz J. The effects of sertindole and its metabolites on cardiac ion channels and action potentials. J Physiol 2000;525:79P.

184. Thomsen MB, Volders PG, Stengl M, et al. Electrophysiological safety of sertindole in dogs with normal and remodeled hearts. J Pharmacol Exp Ther 2003;307:776–784.

185. Presentations at the FDA Cardiovascular and Renal Drugs Advisory Committee, 29 May 2003.

186. Richardson MG, Roark GL, Helfaer MA. Intraoperative epinephrine-induced torsades de pointes in a child with long QT syndrome. Anaesthesiology 1992;76:647–649.

187. Fujikawa H, Sato Y, Arakawa H, et al. Induction of torsades de pointes by dobutamine infusion in a patient with idiopathic long QT syndrome. Intern Med 1998;37:149–152.

188. Furushima H, Chinushi M, Washizuka T, Aizawa Y. Role of $alpha_1$-blockade in congenital long QT syndrome: investigation by exercise stress test. Jpn Circ J 2001;65:654–658.

189. Grubb BP. The use of oral labetalol in the treatment of arrhythmias associated with the long QT syndrome. Chest 1991;100:1724–1725.

190. Shimizu W, Noda T, Takaki H, et al. Epinephrine unmasks latent mutation carriers with LQT1 form of congenital long QT syndrome J Am Coll Cardiol 2003;41:633–642.

191. Noda T, Takaki H, Kurita T, et al. Gene-specific response of dynamic ventricular repolarization to sympathetic stimulation in LQT1, LQT2 and LQT3 forms of congenital long QT syndrome. Eur Heart J 2002;23:975–983.

192. Henriksen JH, Bendtsen F, Hansen EF, Moller S. Acute non-selective beta-adrenergic blockade reduces prolonged frequency-adjusted QT interval (QTc) in patients with cirrhosis. J Hepatol 2004; 40:239–246.

193. Kang J, Chen X-L, Wang H, et al. Cardiac ion channel effects of tolterodine. J Pharmacol Exp Ther 2004;308:935–940.

194. Thomas D, Gut B, Wendt-Nordahl G, Kiehn J. The antidepressant drug fluoxetine is an inhibitor of human ether-a-go-go-related gene (HERG) potassium channels. J Pharmacol Exp Ther 2002;300: 543–548.

195. Witchel HJ, Pabbathi VK, Hofmann G, Paul AA, Hancox JC. Inhibitory actions of the selective serotonin re-uptake inhibitor citalopram on HERG and ventricular L-type calcium currents. FEBS Lett 2002;512:59–66.

196. Xu X, Yan GX, Wu Y, Liu T, Kowey PR. Electrophysiologic effects of SB-237376: a new antiarrhythmic compound with dual potassium and calcium channel blocking action. J Cardiovasc Pharmacol 2003;41:414–421.

197. Committee for Proprietary Medicinal Products. European Public Assessment Report (EPAR) for Levitra (vardenafil) http://www.emea.eu.int/humandocs/Humans/EPAR/levitra/levitra.htm (Accessed on 2 February 2004.)

198. Karunajeewa H, Lim C, Hung T-Y, et al. Safety evaluation of fixed combination piperaquine plus dihydroartemisinin (Artekin) in Cambodian children and adults with malaria. Br J Clin Pharmacol 2004;57:93–99.

199. Rust DM, Soignet SL. Risk/benefit profile of arsenic trioxide. Oncologist 2001;6(Suppl 2):29–32.

200. Soignet SL, Frankel SR, Douer D, et al. United States multicenter study of arsenic trioxide in relapsed acute promyelocytic leukemia. J Clin Oncol 2001;19:3852–3860.

201. Ohnishi K, Yoshida H, Shigeno K, et al. Arsenic trioxide therapy for relapsed or refractory Japanese patients with acute promyelocytic leukemia: need for careful electrocardiogram monitoring. Leukemia 2002;16:617–622.

V   REGULATORY CONSIDERATIONS

16 The FDA's Digital ECG Initiative and Its Impact on Clinical Trials

Barry D. Brown

From: *Cardiac Safety of Noncardiac Drugs:*
Practical Guidelines for Clinical Research and Drug Development
Edited by: J. Morganroth and I. Gussak © Humana Press Inc., Totowa, NJ

INTRODUCTION

Cardiac safety of noncardiac drugs has become a major concern in recent years. Episodes of Torsade de Pointes (TdP) have been linked to QT prolongation from drugs such as the antihistamine terfenadine *(1)*. Regulators have responded by routinely requesting QT prolongation studies in human subjects to determine a drug's effects on cardiac safety. The recent QT concept paper put forth by the US Food and Drug Administration (FDA) and Health Canada November 2002 discusses definitive QT studies with a positive control and being able to detect a change in QT on the order of 5 ms *(2)*.

The FDA continues to take aggressive steps to ensure cardiac safety of new drugs. In November 2001, it held a public meeting announcing it would soon be requesting the electrocardiograms (ECGs) used in cardiac safety studies *(3)*. The FDA also made it clear it will not be accepting ECGs on paper. Rather, it wants digital ECGs that have been the state of the art in electrocardiography for the last two decades. The primary purpose for the digital ECGs is to allow regulators the ability to more carefully ensure that cardiac safety was effectively evaluated. Having the digital data gives flexibility in viewing the waveforms in as much detail as required. It is also conceivable that all the digital ECGs could potentially be used in secondary studies to further the development of cardiac safety evaluation methods.

After announcing its intention to request digital ECGs, the first hurdle the FDA had to overcome was to specify *how* the digital ECGs should be encoded. In the spring of 2002, the agency started working with an industry advisory panel to gather requirements and evaluate existing digital ECG standards. The advisory panel consisted of representatives from the pharmaceutical industry, contract research organizations, commercial and academic ECG core labs, ECG device manufacturers, and the CDISC *(4)* organization.

The advisory panel quickly put together a set of requirements for the digital ECG standard. The requirements showed that the FDA not only needed to have the waveforms for display, but also needed to see *how* the waveforms were used in the evaluation of cardiac safety. That is, it needed to see how the research was conducted using the waveforms. Because cardiac safety research can vary greatly from study to study and is continually evolving in sophistication, the digital ECG standard needed to be very flexible in the representation of the waveforms and any derivatives made from them. It also needed to have a rich mechanism for annotating the waveforms with any type of information relevant to how the waveforms were used in researching the cardiac safety.

The group concluded that existing ECG standards focused on encoding the waveforms directly collected by ECG devices along with standard clinical care demographic information. However, the existing standards lacked the features necessary to capture how the data was used in a clinical trial. There was not a good mechanism for capturing derivative data created from the original waveforms nor was there good support for rich annotations.

It was clear that a new ECG standard was needed to support the research requirements. The FDA was pushing for new electronic submission standards to be based on XML whenever possible. Also, Health and Human Services (HHS) had made a commitment to work with established Standards Development Organizations (SDOs) such as Health Level Seven (HL7). CDISC had been developing standards for clinical trials and was involved in the advisory panel but didn't have the same SDO status as HL7. So, there was already interest by CDISC membership and the FDA to move CDISC standards into HL7. Because HL7 was making use of XML in version 3 (V3), and FDA and CDSIC were moving new standards development efforts into HL7, the panel decided that HL7 would

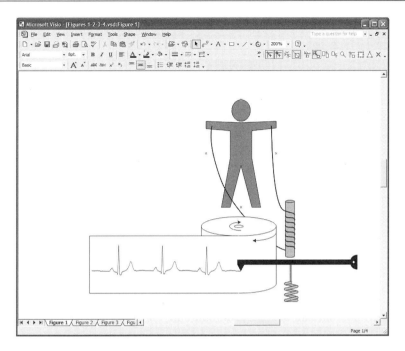

Fig. 1. Single channel electrocardiograph with deflecting stylus on paper.

be a good place to develop the new ECG standard. Hence, the HL7 V3 annotated ECG (aECG) standard was developed and fully approved by HL7 membership in January 2004.

Before the HL7 aECG standard is discussed later in this chapter, an understanding of what a digital ECG is and how it changes the collection and analysis of ECG data during a typical cardiac safety trial is necessary. The key differences between processing paper ECGs and digital ECGs are presented. Next is a discussion about what kinds of ECG data the FDA will most likely want to review. Finally, the aECG standard is presented at a high level. Detailed information about the aECG standard itself, including the XML schema is not presented here. Those details are found in the standards published by the HL7 organization.

THE TRADITIONAL PAPER ELECTROCARDIOGRAM

The heart is a major source of electrical activity in the human body. The currents running through the heart tissue during each beat can be detected by electrical sensors attached to the skin. When amplified sufficiently, these currents can be run through an electromagnet that can be used to deflect a stylus. The basic principal behind the early ECG was to deflect a stylus back and forth with such an electromagnet, while a continuous roll of paper was dragged underneath the stylus (*see* Fig. 1). The stylus left a tracing on the paper that could be interpreted by a cardiologist.

If multiple styluses and electromagnets are employed simultaneously side-by-side, multiple tracings can be made on the paper. The early multichannel devices typically had three. A switch was used to change the waveforms fed to the three styluses until 12 separate leads were recorded on the paper. The first 2.5 s of leads I, II, and III were traced on the paper. Then 2.5 s of leads aVR, aVL, and aVF were traced, followed by leads V1,

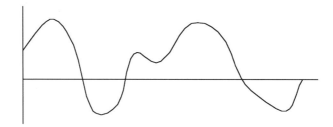

Fig. 2. Diagram of a continuous waveform.

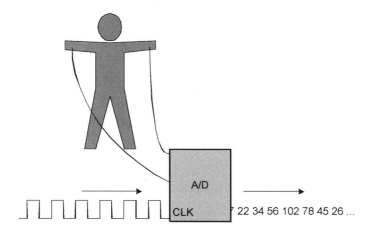

Fig. 3. A/D converter in an electrocardiograph gives sequence of voltage measurements.

V2, and V3, and finally leads V4, V5, and V6. Cardiologists started to recognize disease as patterns in the waveforms presented in this format. This 3 x 4 12-lead format is still the standard presentation that most cardiologists want to see.

The waveform tracings left on the paper by the styluses are considered "continuous" waveform recordings. The paper is always moving, the styluses are always in contact with the paper, and the waveforms from the skin are always fed to the electromagnets. There is no interruption of the waveforms being recorded on the paper. Figure 2 shows a diagram of a continuous waveform.

THE DIGITAL ELECTROCARDIOGRAM

Modern-day microcontroller based ECGs make use of analog-to-digital (A/D) converters. The A/D converters are connected to the same electrodes as the electromagnets in the paper ECG example. The A/D converters are fed a clock signal that drives the conversions. On every clock cycle, each A/D converter measures the voltage it senses from the electrodes and gives a number representing the voltage it measured. Each A/D converter is triggered by the clock and gives a sequence of numbers that represent the ECG waveform (*see* Fig. 3).

This means the continuous signal is now represented by a sequence of discrete numbers shown as vertical bars in Fig. 4. The width of each bar represents the amount of time between each clock cycle that triggered an A/D conversion. The height of each bar

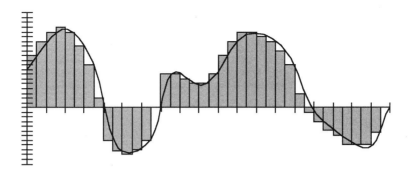

Fig. 4. Digitized waveform.

Table 1
12-Lead ECG as Table of Voltage Sequences

Time (ms)	Lead I (μV)	Lead II (μV)	Lead III (μV)	Other 7 leads	Lead V5 (μV)	Lead V6 (μV)
0	215	−61	−276	...	373	507
2	201	−97	−298	...	329	467
4	187	−133	−320	...	285	427
6	173	−169	−342	...	241	387
8	157	−205	−362	...	193	343
10	136	−236	−372	...	134	289
12	118	−249	−367	...	76	240
14	98	−263	−361	...	15	189
16	83	−268	−351	...	−46	132
18	71	−267	−338	...	−108	62
20	62	−262	−324	...	−152	5
22	54	−254	−308	...	−183	−50
24	46	−246	−292	...	−194	−83

represents the value the A/D converter measured. Note that the bar heights have discrete steps and only approximate the true signal. The step size is known as the A/D converter's *resolution*. If the resolution is 2 μV, for example, the voltage of 45.3 μV will be reported as 46 μV, the closer value of 44 and 46. Modern-day electrocardiographs have sufficient resolution to encode the diagnostic information contained in an ECG waveform, and the resolution is therefore not usually a concern.

A simple way to think about collecting a traditional 12-lead ECG digitally is to think of 12 A/D converters operating simultaneously. (Note, usually only 8 A/D converters are used to collect a 12-lead ECG, but that detail is not important to understand here.) All the converters are fed the same clock, which causes all the converters to make a voltage measurement at the same time. The resulting digital 12-lead ECG, then, can be represented as a table of numbers (*see* Table 1). The first column on the left shows the time points at which the A/D conversions were triggered. The other 12 columns show the voltages measured by the 12 A/D converters when they were triggered.

PAPER ELECTROCARDIOGRAMS
FROM DIGITAL ELECTROCARDIOGRAPHS

Even though today's ECGs use A/D converters and not a stylus moving over paper, ECGs with built-in printers are still able to make paper ECGs. They convert the sequence of numbers representing the digital ECG waveforms into pixels and arrange them into a digital image. The resulting digital image of the ECG is printed onto the paper as tiny dots, also known as pixels. This is no different than a word processing application printing an electronic document's image on a laser printer.

THE SCANNED ELECTROCARDIOGRAM

Many ECG trials still collect and analyze the ECGs on paper even though most ECGs in use today collect the waveforms digitally. Naturally, the question comes up about the FDA accepting scanned paper ECGs. It is true that a scanned ECG is digital, but it is a digital *image* of a *paper* ECG. It is not a digital ECG. During the requirements gathering period, the FDA made it clear to the advisory panel that it wanted digital ECGs, not digital images of paper ECGs.

To understand why, it is important to realize the type of information encoded in a digital ECG is time and voltage information for each lead. This *waveform* information can be used and manipulated by computers and algorithms as *waveform* data. For example, the waveforms can be displayed in a variety of ways including different zoom factors, with or without a grid, with or without the annotations, leads displayed superimposed, waveforms from multiple trial time points displayed simultaneously to facilitate serial comparison, etc. On the other hand, the information encoded in a digital image of a paper ECG is the color of each pixel. Little can be done with a digital image except to view it on a computer screen and print it on paper.

CONVERTING A SCANNED ELECTROCARDIOGRAM
INTO A DIGITAL ELECTROCARDIOGRAM

Because paper ECGs have been widely used in trials, some have considered converting the paper ECGs into digital ECGs. Under ideal conditions, it may be possible to do a crude conversion. The conversion process starts with a scanned digital image of the paper ECG. A sophisticated image-processing algorithm is run over the digital image to detect the ECG waveforms. With the help of human training, the algorithm detects which pixels represent the leads of the ECG and converts the relative pixel positions into units of time and voltage. Human training is usually necessary to indicate where on the paper each ECG lead is and how many pixels in the digital image represent a unit of time and a unit of voltage.

As you can imagine, there are a number of variables in this image-to-waveform conversion process that potentially introduce inaccuracies in the resulting digital waveforms. The first variable is the resolution of the waveforms originally printed on the paper. The traditional resolution of a resting 10 s 12-lead ECG is to use 10 mm in the vertical direction to represent 1 mV and 25 mm in the horizontal direction to represent 1 s. This resolution gives a good balance between showing detail about the contour of each beat while showing all 10 s on a standard sheet of paper. There is not enough room, however, to show all 10 s of all 12 leads at this resolution. The 12 waveforms would start to overlap when laid out across a sheet of paper in the landscape orientation. Either the amplitude

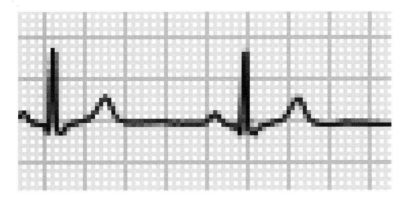

Fig. 5. Digitized image of a waveform.

of the waveforms would need to be reduced, or two sheets of paper would need to be used. Something would have to be sacrificed: only part of each lead can be printed, or the leads must be printed at reduced amplitude, or the conversion algorithm has to "stitch" images of multiple sheets of paper together and precisely correlate the timing of each lead.

To give better resolution, the waveforms should be printed using a large gain and a fast paper speed. This just makes the problem worse and necessitates the need for multiple sheets of paper. Again, the algorithm will need a level of sophistication for precisely aligning the waveforms in time.

Another factor impacting the accuracy of the digitization process is the physical paper on which the original ECG was printed. This paper can shrink and expand owing to environmental factors such as heat and humidity. And, the change in physical character-istics can be nonhomogenous; that is, the shrinkage could vary across the sheet of paper and could be different in the horizontal and vertical directions. If a photocopy or facsimile is used instead of the original from the ECG device, the accuracy of those devices to faithfully reproduce the image contributes to the problem.

Next, the accuracy of the scanning device comes into question. If the scanner uses a movable mirror or array of sensors, any imprecision of the mechanics will directly distort the scanned image of the paper ECG.

Finally, there is the ability of the digital image-processing algorithm to find and accurately trace the waveform. If the waveform is several pixels wide, it will have to "guess" the center of the waveform. If there is any noise in the image, a grid, or any other markings, it will have to successfully ignore these nonwaveform artifacts so it does not start tracing the wrong information. The blown up image shown in Fig. 5 (without any noise) gives an idea of what challenges a conversion algorithm might face. Can a conver-sion from an image to waveforms be accurate and reliable enough for finding QT prolon-gation signals of 5 ms?

HOW THE ELECTROCARDIOGRAM TRIAL CHANGES

It is clear that the FDA's digital ECG waveform initiative is best met by directly saving the digital waveforms collected by digital ECGs. Any other indirect method of obtaining digital ECG waveforms potentially introduces inaccuracies and greater variance in the ECG measurements made from the data.

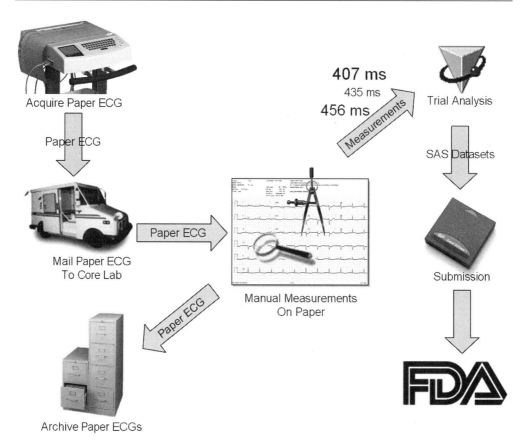

Fig. 6. Paper ECG trial process.

Besides having the digital ECG waveforms to review, the FDA is asking for annotations to be placed on the waveforms to indicate *how* the data was used to make the measurements. Regardless of how the digital waveforms are obtained, the digital data *must* be used to make the ECG measurements. For example, if a QT measurement is made on the second beat in lead II, the FDA will expect to see a QRS onset and a T offset annotation on that beat. The only way to accurately associate these annotations with the digital waveforms is to use ECG analysis software that displays the waveforms onscreen and allows onscreen calipers to be placed on them.

The digital ECG initiative impacts many aspects of a cardiac safety trial that collects, analyzes, and submits ECG data. Before the FDA's digital ECG initiative, a trial could use paper ECGs from any electrocardiographs that produced them (*see* Fig. 6). The paper ECGs were collected by the sites and mailed to an ECG core lab for consistent analysis. Because the paper ECGs were considered source documents, the paper ECGs were archived along with other papers collected during the trial, like case report forms (CRFs). A small group of trained technicians or cardiologists would use calipers, rulers, digitization pads, and other techniques to make measurements directly from the paper ECGs. The measurements were entered into a statistical analysis package where the drug effects were quantified. Finally, the analysis datasets were submitted to the FDA.

To supply the FDA with the annotated digital ECGs they are requesting, the process needs to start with the collection of digital ECG waveforms by using a digital electrocar-

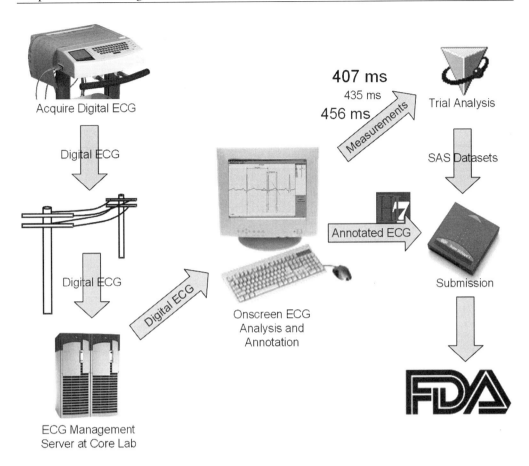

Fig. 7. Digital ECG trial process.

diograph (*see* Fig. 7). Instead of sending paper ECGs from the sites to the ECG core lab, the digital ECG devices transmit the ECGs to a central ECG management system at the core lab via modem or network. The central ECG management system becomes the archival mechanism for the *source* ECGs in the trial. A trained technician or cardiologist at the core lab uses ECG measurement software to display the digital ECG waveforms onscreen and place virtual calipers on the waveforms to make the necessary measurements. The measurement software then exports the digital ECG waveforms and annotations corresponding to the measurements made. The waveforms and annotations are exported in the HL7 aECG format and eventually made available to the FDA for review. The measurement tool is also responsible for exporting the measurement values to the statistical analysis system for the quantification of the drug's cardiac effects.

ANALYSIS OF DIGITAL ELECTROCARDIOGRAMS

Analysis of digital ECGs with the help of software applications opens the door to new and interesting analysis techniques. Computer algorithms for the analysis of ECG waveforms have been around about as long as digital ECGs. These algorithms vary in sophistication, but generally are able to detect beats, classify them, and identify the component waves of each beat (e.g., P, QRS, T waves). These algorithms tend to do a reasonably good job on normal, low-noise waveforms. However, in the presence of noise or abnormal ECG rhythms, the algorithms can sometimes be inaccurate.

Onscreen ECG analysis can generally be done three different ways. The *manual* process uses no computer algorithm assistance. The reviewer simply zooms in on a beat and places the calipers wherever he determines is the right place. This is the same technique used with paper, and some ECG trial experts argue this is the best approach for assessments unbiased by computer algorithms.

Another way is the *automatic* analysis of the digital ECGs with computer algorithms alone. The algorithms have gotten more sophisticated over the years and are able to deal with more noise and strange rhythms. Also, algorithms give a very repeatable, consistent measurement. However, some would argue that the algorithms are not perfect yet and must always be verified by a cardiologist.

The third way to analyze digital ECGs is to combine both the manual and automatic methods. This *semi-automatic* method initially positions the calipers on the waveforms by using ECG analysis algorithms. However, a cardiologist is required to review the placement of the calipers and adjusts them if the algorithm failed in some way. This method has the advantage of providing consistent, repeatable algorithm-based measurements while allowing a cardiologist to catch and fix cases where the algorithm failed for some reason.

REPRESENTATIVE BEATS

Most ECG algorithms will form a representative beat (a.k.a. median beat) for analysis. The representative beat is formed by combining all the dominant, normally conducted beats together. This compositional beat is considered a good representation of the cardiac cycle during that time window. This technique has the advantage of reducing the noise and smoothing out small beat-to-beat variances. Some electrocardiographs are able to export this representative beat. Therefore, the onscreen ECG analysis software may have the option of displaying the representative beat and allowing ECG measurements to be made on it. If measurements are made on it, the aECG file exported for FDA review will need to include the representative beat with its corresponding annotations.

HOW MUCH WAVEFORM DATA
DOES THE FDA WANT TO REVIEW?

At the time of this writing, there has been no final guidance published by the FDA stating exactly what it will want to review. The November 2002 QT concept paper clearly stated that the FDA intends to review the ECGs collected during intensive QT prolongation studies *(5)*. It also stated they will accept any ECG data a sponsor wants to submit. It is not clear, however, if ECG data from other types of trials will be systematically requested by the agency. As usual, a sponsor should consult with the FDA prior to starting a trial if there is any question about what data the agency might want to review from the trial.

Holter recorders are increasingly being used for the collection of ECG data, and they elicit more questions. These devices can record continuous 12-lead ECG data for 24 h. Will the FDA want to review the 24-h recordings in their entirety? It is not clear, but at the very least it makes sense to review the relevant waveform data that directly contributed to the study of cardiac effects. Since 10 s 12-lead resting ECGs have been the standard tool for studying cardiac effects, it can be a guide for how much waveform data is relevant for a given time point. For example, if the QT is assessed at a time point 30 min post-dose by measuring QT in three consecutive beats in lead II, then the 12-lead wave-forms for the three relevant beats plus several beats surrounding them for a total of 10 s seems about right. Waveform data 5 min before and after the three measured beats does not have much relevance and probably does not need to be reviewed. On the other hand, if an advanced QT correction method is used where the RR history from the prior 5 min is used to correct the three QT measurements, then the waveforms from prior 5 min has relevance and needs to be included along with the corresponding RR annotations.

HOW MANY ANNOTATIONS DOES THE FDA WANT TO REVIEW?

Reviewing only ECG waveforms is of marginal value. The FDA needs to see *how* the ECG waveforms were used to study the cardiac effects. The way to show how the ECG waveforms were used is to place annotations on those waveforms.

The term "annotation" can mean a lot of different things, and the aECG standard allows just about anything to be associated with the waveforms. So, clarification is needed about what annotations are and how to decide which ones are needed under which conditions.

Technically, the aECG HL7 standard defines an annotation as an observation made upon the waveform data. An HL7 observation can be anything. It can be an uncoded natural language statement like "this spike in the waveform was due to the subject sneez-ing." It can be a coded period of time calling out "ST elevation," or it can be a coded point in time calling out "R-wave peak." Just about any type of observation you can imagine making on the waveform data can be made an annotation in an aECG message.

VOCABULARIES

Before discussing particular annotation examples for common ECG measurements, it is important to understand what a coded and uncoded observation is. A coded observation uses a code from a recognized vocabulary (a.k.a. dictionary, nomenclature, etc.). Examples of some well-known vocabularies are SNOMED *(6)*, LOINC *(7)*, CPT *(8)*, and ICD *(9)*. Each vocabulary has a focus and defines the meaning of a set of related codes that can be processed by computers. For example, LOINC is a large vocabulary that includes terms for observations and defines the code 10001-6 as "R WAVE DURATION in LEAD I." If the R-wave duration in Lead I is 60 ms and needs to be reported in an HL7 message, the observation in the message would encode three pieces of information: the observed value of 60 ms, the observation code of 10001-6, and a reference to the LOINC vocabulary using the HL7 assigned id 2.16.840.1.113883.6.1.

To make the ECG annotations that will be submitted to the FDA useful, a vocabulary of ECG codes is required. The IEEE 1073 Medical Device Communication (MDC) standards organization *(10)* has compiled a comprehensive list of ECG codes that can be used in aECG messages. It includes codes for naming ECG leads; waveform components such as P, Q, R, S, T; beat types; pacemaker artifacts; rhythms; noise levels; contours; measurements; and control variables. HL7 has named this vocabulary MDC and assigned it the id 2.16.840.1.113883.6.24.

WHAT TO ANNOTATE

The trial protocol or other trial procedural documentation will declare the types of ECG assessments to be made at the various time points in the trial. There will also be a specification of how those findings will be derived from measurements taken directly from the ECG waveforms. For example, the protocol may specify that a QTc finding be derived from an ECG by measuring QT and RR on three consecutive beats in Lead II. It will also specify the derivation method, like using the Bazett's correction formula for each QT/RR pair and then averaging the three QTc's together. The ECG reviewed by the FDA in this example would therefore need to have annotations placed on the waveform to show the three RR and three QT measurements made. There would be a total of six R-peak fiducial markings, three QRS-onset fiducial markings, and three T-offset fiducial markings.

The following examples discuss annotations for some common ECG measurements.

PR INTERVAL

The PR interval measures time between the start of the atrial contraction and the start of ventricular contraction. The start of atrial contraction is shown with a fiducial marking at the onset of the P-wave. The start of ventricular contraction is shown with a fiducial marking at the beginning of the QRS-complex. Therefore, the annotations placed on the waveforms for FDA review when making a PR interval measurement are P-onset and QRS-onset (*see* Fig. 8).

ST LEVEL

The ST level of a particular beat is the amplitude of the beat's ST segment relative to the beat's isoelectric level. Fiducial markings for the ST measurement can either be annotated in the time domain (vertical lines marking time points) or in the amplitude domain (horizontal lines marking voltage levels) or both. Isoelectric is normally defined as the voltage level between the P-wave and QRS complex. The isoelectric level can be marked as a time point defining the isoelectric measurement location on the waveform, or a voltage level (that does not even have to intersect the waveform).

The ST fiducial marking can either be a horizontal annotation showing the voltage level measured, or it can be a vertical annotation showing the point at which the ST level was measured on the waveform. If the ST measurement point is established by first finding the J-point and measuring a fixed time delay from it, marking the J-point as well as the ST measurement point would be appropriate.

Figure 9 shows both voltage (horizontal) and time (vertical) annotations. Horizontal annotations show the isoelectric and ST voltage levels. Vertical annotations show where the J-point was established and where the ST level was measured (J + 60 ms). This is just one example of annotating a ST level. Other methods of showing the ST level may be appropriate depending on the measurement method used.

R-PEAK AMPLITUDE

The R-peak amplitude of a particular beat is the amplitude of the beat's R-peak relative to the beat's isoelectric level. Fiducial markings for the R-peak amplitude measurement can either be annotated in the time domain (vertical lines marking timepoints) or in the amplitude domain (horizontal lines marking voltage levels) or both. Isoelectric is normally defined as the voltage level between the P-wave and QRS complex. The isoelectric level can be marked as a time point defining the isoelectric measurement location on the waveform, or a voltage level (which does not even have to intersect the waveform).

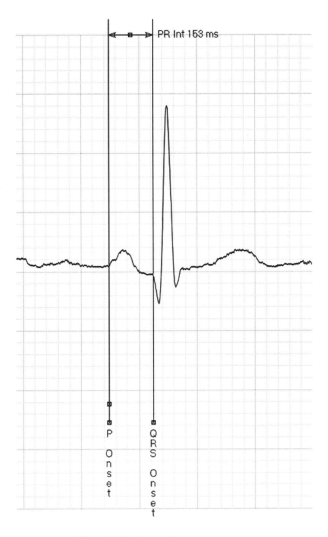

Fig. 8. PR interval measurement.

The R-peak fiducial marking can either be a horizontal annotation showing the voltage level measured, or it can be a vertical annotation showing where the R-peak level was measured on the waveform.

Figure 10 shows the voltage (horizontal) type annotations. There are horizontal annotations showing the isoelectric and R-peak voltage levels. This is just one example of annotating a R-peak amplitude. Other methods of showing the R-peak amplitude may be appropriate depending on the measurement method used.

QT AND QTc DURATIONS

The QT duration measures the time between the start of the ventricular contraction and the end of ventricular repolarization. The start of ventricular contraction is shown as a fiducial marking at the onset of the QRS-complex. The end of ventricular repolarization

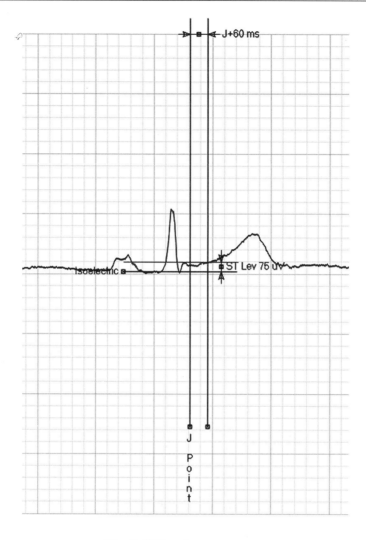

Fig. 9. ST level measurement.

is shown as a fiducial marking at the end of the T wave. Therefore, the annotations placed on the waveforms for FDA review when making a QT duration measurement are QRS-onset and T-offset.

The QT duration changes with heart rate and is therefore difficult to compare from one time point to the next if heart rates are different. Therefore, the QT duration is often corrected (normalized) for the heart rate when looking for QT changes in a clinical trial. Some popular correction methods use the RR interval between the beat being measured for QT and the preceding one. In this case, the reviewer would expect to see not only the annotations related to the QT measurement, but also the annotations related to measuring the RR interval. For example, if the RR interval was determined by finding the R-peaks of the two beats, two R-peak annotations would be expected. Figure 11 shows annotations for the two R-peaks, the QRS-onset, and the T-offset.

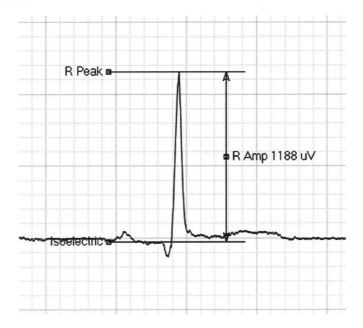

Fig. 10. R-Peak level measurement.

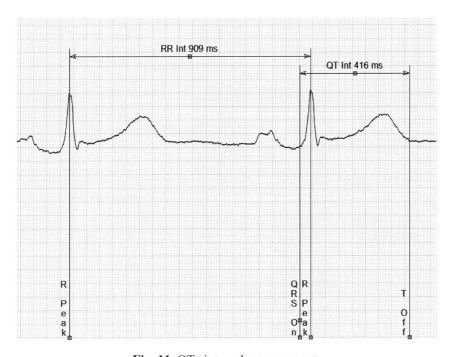

Fig. 11. QTc interval measurement.

USING MULTIPLE LEADS FOR A SINGLE MEASUREMENT

Some ECG measurements like R-peak amplitude and ST level can only be made in one lead at a time. Other measurements like QT, RR, PR, etc. can be made in a single lead or by using multiple leads. Some researchers think a more global approach using several or all the available leads is better for determining time intervals. The aECG standard allows annotations to be placed on any number of leads. So, if several leads were used to determine the QT interval, the QRS-onset and T-offset annotations must reference all the leads used.

QT ON THE REPRESENTATIVE BEAT

An example of using all the leads to determine a QT interval is shown in Fig. 12. In this example, all the leads of the representative beat are superimposed to help the researcher find the "global" QRS-onset and T-offset. The resulting aECG file, therefore, would have a single QRS-onset and T-offset annotation referencing all the leads of the representative beat.

HEALTH LEVEL SEVEN

Section 12(d) of United States Public Law 104-113, the "National Technology Transfer and Advancement Act of 1995" (NTTAA) directs "federal agencies to focus upon increasing their use of [voluntary consensus] standards whenever possible." The Act gives the agencies discretion to use other standards in lieu of voluntary consensus standards where use of the latter would be "inconsistent with applicable law or otherwise impractical." However, in such cases, the head of an agency or department must send to the Office of Management and Budget (OMB), through National Institute of Standards and Technology (NIST), "an explanation of the reasons for using such standards" (11).

HL7 is such a voluntary consensus standards development organization. It is an ANSI ASD creating information exchange standards in the healthcare arena. The HL7 standards allow for the interchange of clinical as well as administrative information between organizations, information systems, devices, and such. HL7 is a nonprofit organization composed of member organizations and individuals coming from all aspects of healthcare including healthcare providers, payers, consultants, government bodies, pharmaceutical, device manufacturers, and others. The standards are developed by its members on a voluntary basis. HL7 adheres to a strict and well-defined set of operating procedures that ensure consensus, openness, and balance of interest between all interested parties.

The United States department of Health and Human Services is committed to working with established standards development organizations like HL7 to develop healthcare standards needed by the government. An FDA representative co-chairs the Regulated Clinical Research Information Management (RCRIM) HL7 technical committee (TC) within HL7. The RCRIM TC develops standards needed for the research and regulatory evaluation of the safety and efficacy of therapeutic products or procedures (12).

The HL7 version 2 (V2) messaging standards are the most widely used healthcare information exchange standards today. They enable disparate healthcare applications to exchange key sets of clinical and administrative data.

For several years HL7 has been working on version 3 (V3) of its messaging standard. V3 has the advantage of using the well-established object oriented (OO) design approach. The information models are described in a graphical language following the principals of the popular Unified Modeling Language (UML) (13).

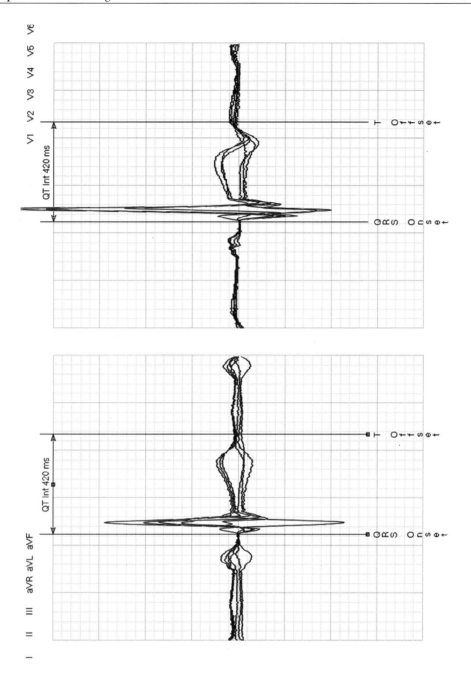

Fig. 12. Global QT interval measurement on representative beat.

STORYBOARD

V3 message development starts with a storyboard that gives a narrative describing a set of actions that give the message its context. Figure 13 shows the storyboard for aECG *(14)*.

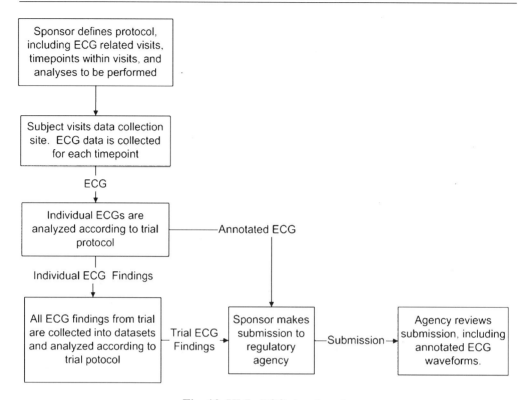

Fig. 13. HL7 aECG storyboard.

Preparing Annotated Electrocardiograms

The story starts when the sponsor decides to study the effects of a new drug on a population's cardiac electrophysiology. The sponsor decides the effects to be studied can be seen in ECG data, or information derived from ECG data. The sponsor designs a protocol specifying the population to be studied, the data to be collected, the equipment to be used for gathering the ECG data, the analysis tools to use, and how any effects will be studied using the ECG data and analysis tools.

The sponsor (or a contract research organization [CRO] engaged by the sponsor) hires investigators to collect the data, and the investigators in turn enroll subjects in the trial. The subject visits the collection site. During the subject's visit, equipment is connected to the subject. The equipment records the subject's ECG along with other physiologic parameters, if appropriate. Trial and subject identifying information is associated with the ECG data, such as subject id, gender, date of birth, investigator and site id's, protocol id, etc. After the individual ECGs are collected from the subject for that visit, it is transferred to a central ECG lab for analysis.

The ECG waveforms can be loaded into an analysis tool for making findings (measurements) and possibly deriving other data according to the trial protocol. The findings are oftentimes in the form of time and amplitude values for the parts of the cardiac process being studied. The analysis produces two types of information: findings to be used for further statistical analysis on the entire population enrolled in the trial, and annotated ECG waveforms with trial specific fiducial markings, etc., indicating key features used for obtaining the findings.

Submitting Annotated Electrocardiograms

The supporting annotated ECG waveforms become part of the sponsor's submission to the regulatory agency. The communication of the annotated ECG waveforms from the sponsor to the regulatory agency is the primary focus of this standard.

During the regulatory agency's review of a submission, the agency may come across a conclusion drawn from a statistical analysis of ECG findings it wishes to investigate further. The reviewer may review the ECG analysis protocol and the analysis dataset. The reviewer may question an ECG finding in the dataset and review the annotated ECG waveforms. The reviewer may be satisfied with what he sees or may investigate further the ECG measurement protocol and its consistent application during the trial.

In addition to the storyboard above, the aECG standard discusses the following information model that was used as input requirements during the development of the V3 aECG message.

Data Describing the Clinical Trial Context of the Annotated Electrocardiogram

The annotated ECG waveforms are the focus of this message. For each annotated ECG, information is included describing the trial conditions under which the ECG was recorded. At a minimum, the unique identifiers for the ECG, trial subject, the trial itself are required. In addition to the required identifiers, the message must contain the time of the ECG data collection. This is the minimal set of data considered necessary to properly identify an ECG within a regulatory submission.

These requirements are illustrated in Fig. 14, which shows the annotated ECG itself as a category of data to be included in the message. Other trial context categories are also shown, along with the relationships among the categories. All of the individual trial context data items that can be communicated using the HL7 annotated ECG message are listed and categorized on the diagram, with an indication of whether they are optional or required. Some entity-relationship (ER) constructs and conventions have been used in this diagram, as described in the key, but this is not intended to be a formal ER diagram.

Data Describing the Annotations and Waveforms

Figure 15 shows how the waveforms and annotations are organized relative to the main annotated ECG object from the previous diagram. Starting from the bottom of the diagram, each lead and the time associated with the samples is represented as a sequence—a sequence of values. Each sequence has a type (lead name or time type) and the list of values.

Sequences that were recorded simultaneously are grouped as sequence sets. A modern ECG can represent a 12-lead ECG as a single sequence set. A three-channel ECG would typically use four sequence sets for a 12-lead ECG (e.g., set 1 having leads I, II, III; set 2 having leads aVR, aVF, aVL; set 3 having leads V1, V2, V3; and set 4 having leads V4, V5, V5).

A series contains all the sequence sets that share a common frame of reference. Typically, the series will contain the data collected from a single device with a single time reference. If a representative beat is algorithmically derived from the rhythm data, it will form another series (derived from the rhythm data series).

A number of annotation sets can be attached to the series. The annotation sets contain an arbitrary nesting of annotations. The nesting of annotations allows parent/child

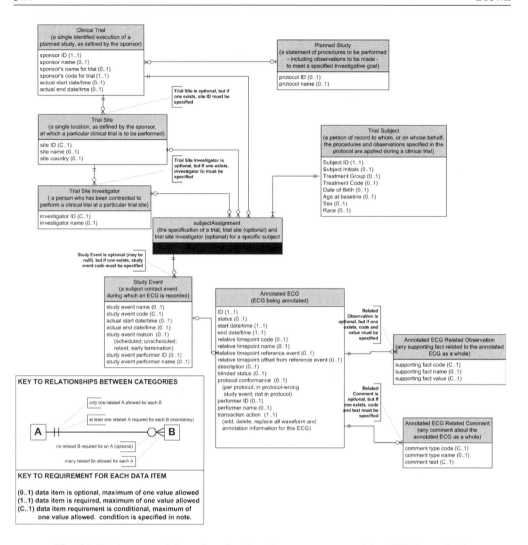

Fig. 14. Business model used to develop the context part of the aECG standard.

relationships to be communicated. For example, a beat annotation can be the parent of wave component annotations (P wave, QRS wave, T wave, etc.).

If an annotation has a location within the series, it is associated with a region of interest (ROI). The ROI specifies the leads and time period for the annotation. A fully specified ROI contains a boundary for each lead and/or time dimension within it. A partially specified ROI will contain a boundary for each lead and/or time that is not wholly in it. For example, if a global QRS onset is to be specified, a partially specified ROI will only have a boundary for the time dimension. It is assumed that all the other dimensions (leads) are wholly in the ROI.

REFERENCE INFORMATION MODEL

Information models for V3 messages are derived from the reference information model (RIM). The RIM provides a unified framework for, and a comprehensive source of, all information used in an HL7 specification. The RIM has two main concepts called act and

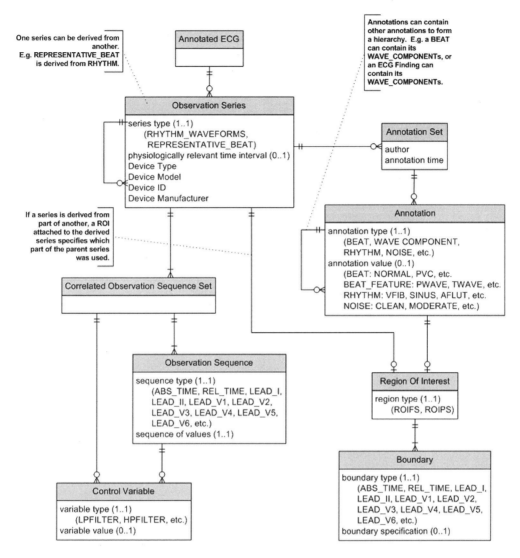

One series can be derived from another. E.g. REPRESENTATIVE_BEAT is derived from RHYTHM.

Annotations can contain other annotations to form a hierarchy. E.g. a BEAT can contain its WAVE_COMPONENTs, or an ECG Finding can contain its WAVE_COMPONENTs.

If a series is derived from part of another, a ROI attached to the derived series specifies which part of the parent series was used.

Fig. 15. Business model used to develop the waveform part of the aECG standard.

entity. There are three concepts that connect act and entity; they are participation, role, and act relationship. Figure 16 shows the core RIM concepts.

REFINED MESSAGE INFORMATION MODEL

The first step in developing a V3 message is to model the information contained in the message. A refined message information model (R-MIM) is developed using the graphical language shown in Fig. 17. Each object in the graphical language corresponds to a concept from the RIM. As each information object is placed into the R-MIM, it is declared to be an instance of a concept from the RIM. For example, the top-level object in the aECG message is the annotated ECG and is modeled as an instance of an observation, a special kind of act. The subject of the ECG in the aECG message is modeled as a person, a special kind of entity.

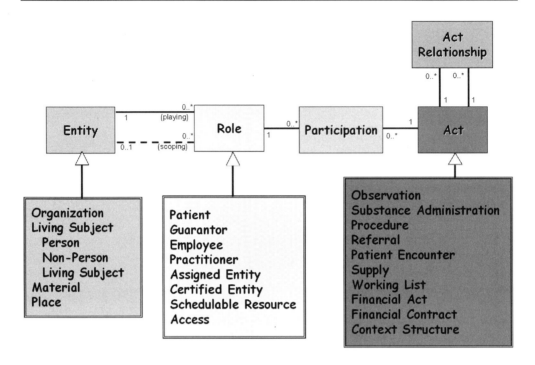

Fig. 16. Core HL7 RIM concepts.

THE ANNOTATED ELECTROCARDIOGRAM REFINED MESSAGE INFORMATION MODEL

Figure 18 shows the entire aECG R-MIM. It is a graphical representation of the information contained within an aECG message. Please refer to the standard published by HL7 for a scalable copy.

The model has an upper half and a lower half. The upper half represents the contextual information for the aECG. It contains information about the protocol, trial, sponsor, investigator, subject, and time point. The lower half represents the waveforms and annotations. It contains the sequences of voltage numbers representing the digital waveforms, information about the device that collected the digital waveforms, and the annotations made on the waveforms.

HEALTH LEVEL SEVEN WAVEFORM REPRESENTATION

Details about how all the information is represented in the aECG message can be found in the standards published by HL7. However, since the digital waveforms are one of the more interesting parts of the aECG message, those will be discussed in a little more detail.

Referring back to the digital ECG discussion in this chapter, the digital ECG can be thought of as a table of numbers. The first column contains a sequence of numbers representing the time points at which the A/D converters measured the voltages, and the other columns represent the sequence of numbers representing the voltages measured by the A/D converters. HL7 V3 messages represent digital waveforms in the same way, as sequences of numbers. Each sequence in the table becomes a sequence in the aECG

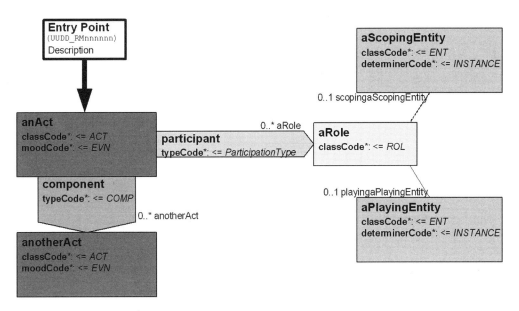

Fig. 17. HL7 R–MIM modeling language.

message. A 12-lead ECG has 13 columns in the table and is therefore represented as 13 sequences in the aECG message.

Quite often the sequence of time points is a regular pattern. This is because most devices measure the voltages at regular intervals (called the sampling frequency). Because the sequence is a regular pattern, a special HL7 datatype called the generated list (GLIST) can be used. This datatype allows the specification of a starting value and an increment. So, for the digital ECG example earlier in the chapter, the starting time point would be specified as 0 ms, and the increment would be specified as 2 ms. If, on the other hand, the time points were not regular, the sequence of time points could be explicitly enumerated in the aECG message using the sampled list (SLIST) datatype described next.

The SLIST is appropriate for encoding the sequence of A/D values. A/D converters produce integer information that must be scaled when converting to a physical quantity like voltage. SLIST allows for the efficient encoding of the raw integer values from the A/D converter along with the specification of the scale factor for converting the integers into physical quantities. For example, if each step of an A/D converter represents 2.5 µV, then the SLIST scale factor would be specified as 2.5 µV and the raw A/D values would be encoded.

HL7 V3 groups the related sequences together as sequence sets. The sequences contained within a sequence set must all be the same length and the values in sequence must be related to the values in the other sequences based on index. For example, the fifth value in the time sequence should be the time point at which the fifth value in each voltage sequence was obtained.

Most of today's digital ECGs record the 12 leads during the entire 10 s of a standard ECG. The waveforms from such a device can be encoded in a single sequence set. There would be 13 sequences each running the duration of the entire ECG. On the other hand, older three channel ECGs will collect the waveform data in four periods. The first period will collect leads I, II, and III for 2.5 s; the second period will collect leads aVR, aVL,

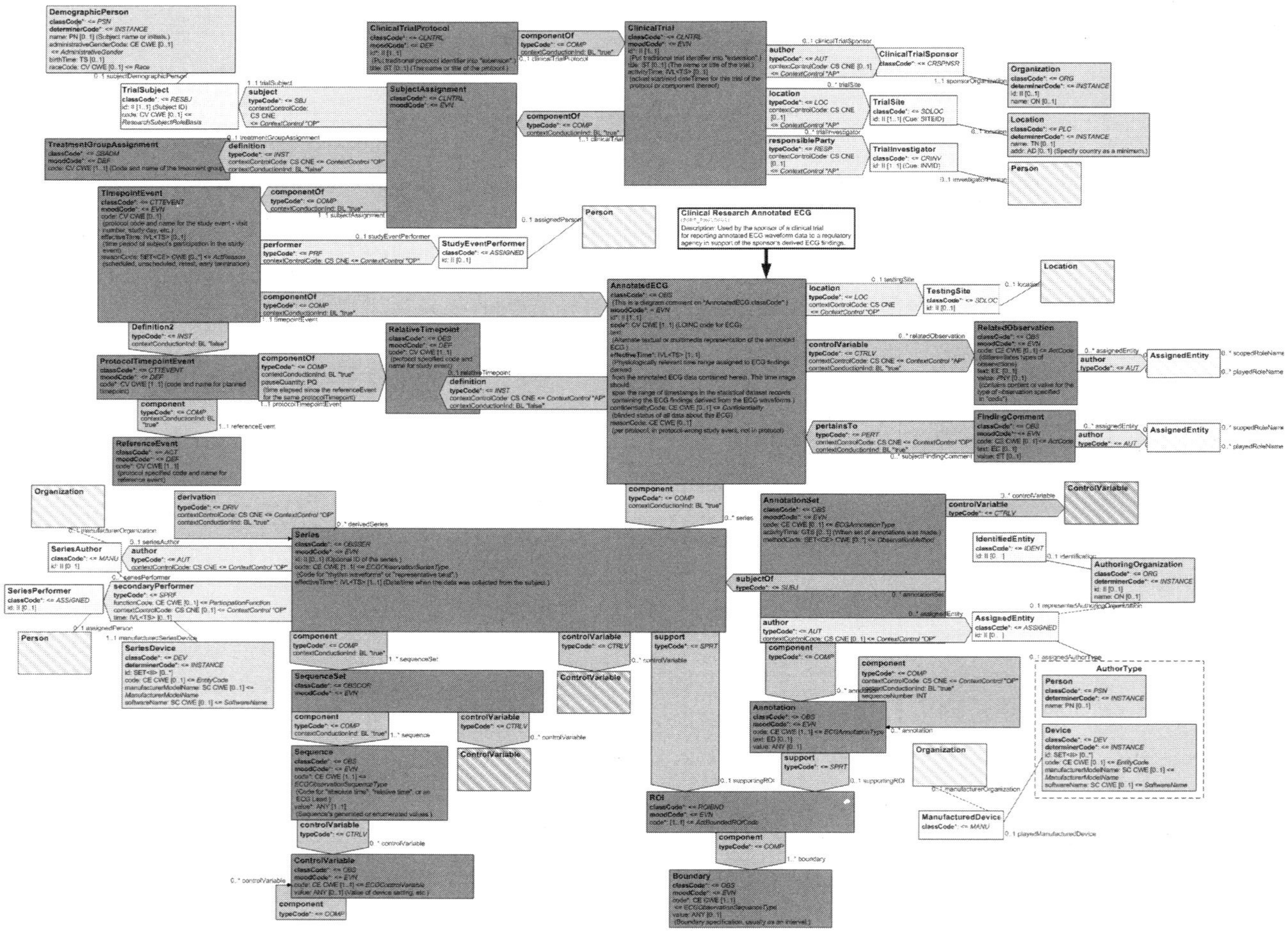

Fig. 18. HL7 R–MIM for aECG.

324

and aVF for 2.5 s; and so on. In the three-channel case, the ECG will need to be encoded as four sequence sets, one for each period. The first sequence set would have a time sequence for the first 2.5 s of time points along with sequences for the three leads I, II, and III. The second sequence set would have a time sequence for the second 2.5 s of time points along with sequences for the three leads aVR, aVL, aVF, and so on.

HL7 V3 groups sequence sets into series. The series defines a fixed frame of reference. For ECGs, the frame of reference has to do with time and electrode placement. If all the time sequences are using relative time points and are contained within a single series, then all the relative time points are relative to the same fixed point in time. Therefore, in the previous three-channel ECG example, the time sequence in the second sequence set will start at 2.5 s if the sequence sets were contained within the same series.

Another frame of reference concept for ECGs is electrode placement. If the electrodes are replaced or moved, the leads have technically moved and are not exactly the same as they were before. Therefore, a new series should be used when electrodes are moved. If there is anything else that might change the data (e.g., patient position, different waveform filter, etc.), a new series should be used as well.

HEALTH LEVEL SEVEN ANNOTATION REPRESENTATION

The aECG Annotation is just a general HL7 observation. An observation contains a *code* that indicates the type of observation being made. For example, if a rhythm is observed in an ECG, the MDC code MDC_ECG_RHY would be used. An observation also contains a *value* that indicates the specific observation made. For example, if the observed rhythm is sinus bradycardia, the value would be the MDC code MDC_ECG_RHY_BRADY. Likewise, if a QT duration of 453 ms is observed, the observation code would be MDC_ECG_TIME_PD_QT and the value would be 453 ms.

The main type of annotation the FDA will want to review is fiducial markings indicating key measurement points in the ECG like the QRS-onset and T-offset. The MDC nomenclature calls these types of ECG observations *waveform components*. The MDC code for these fiducial-type annotations is MDC_ECG_WAVC, and the values are MDC_ECG_WAVC_QRSWAVE, MDC_ECG_WAVC_TWAVE, etc. There are other sets of MDC codes for beats, rhythms, pacemaker artifacts, noise, measurements, and contours. Refer to the IEEE 1073 MDC standards for the complete list of available codes.

The aECG standard allows the annotations to be organized into a hierarchy. This hierarchy is useful for communicating multiple levels of detail and grouping related annotations together. For example, if a sponsor wants to group all of the fiducial markings for a given beat together so it is clear that they belong to the same beat, a parent MDC_ECG_BEAT annotation can contain the children MDC_ECG_WAVC annotations. Likewise, if a sponsor wishes to group all the fiducial markings together for a given measurement like QT, a parent MDC_ECG_TIME_PD_QT annotation can contain children MDC_ECG_WAVC annotations for MDC_ECG_WAVC_QRSWAVE and MDC_ECG_WAVC_TWAVE. Arranging the annotations in appropriate hierarchies will enhance the reviewer's ability to review related annotations together.

Each annotation can be associated with a ROI. The ROI specifies exactly where in the waveforms the observation was made (i.e., where the annotation is located). The ROI is specified by one or more boundaries. A boundary names one of the sequence types in the series (e.g., the time sequence) and specifies how the ROI is bounded in that sequence. For example, if a QRS-onset is located 4.327 ms into the ECG, the time boundary for the

QRS-wave annotation ROI would be a time interval starting at 4.327 ms (with an unspecified ending). If this QRS-wave was observed in lead II, another boundary would specify lead II (without specifying any voltage interval). Another example to help illustrate an annotation could be an isoelectric voltage level for a beat in lead II starting around 3.023 ms and ending 3.855 ms. The ROI's time boundary would be specified as an interval starting at 3.023 ms and ending 3.855 ms. The ROI's lead II boundary would specify the voltage level at which the beat's isoelectric level was set, for example, 0.12 mV.

For more details about the aECG standard, please refer to the standards published by HL7.

WHAT IS NOT IN AN ANNOTATED ELECTROCARDIOGRAM

It is important to remember that the FDA will still receive the analysis datasets in the usual way. The ECG assessments made at the various time points are included in those datasets. The aECGs should not repeat the numerical assessments already in those datasets, because there would be a potential consistency problem and confusion about what decisions were made from each instance. The aECGs are meant to *support* the assessments found in the analysis datasets. They show the waveforms and fiducial markings used in the derivation of the assessments. They do not, however, include information about how the analysis dataset assessments were derived. The derivation methods are documented in the trial protocols and standard operating procedures.

CONCLUSION

The FDA's request to review annotated, digital ECG waveforms has some impact on the way cardiac safety trials are performed. Digital ECG devices should be used for the collection of the ECG data. The digital waveforms from those devices should be electronically managed in some way. Measurements taken from the ECG waveforms should be made using onscreen tools, and those tools should export the waveforms and related annotations in the HL7 aECG standard. Finally, the annotated ECGs should be made available to the FDA for review. If sponsors do not do these things, they may find it increasingly difficult in the future to convince the FDA that their drug does not have cardiac safety issues.

REFERENCES

1. Monahan BP, Ferguson CL, Killeavy ES, Lloyd BK, Troy J, Cantilena LR. Torsades de pointes occurring in association with terfenadine use. JAMA 1990;264:2788-2790.
2. The Clinical Evaluation of QT/QTc Interval Prolongation and Proarrhythmic Potential for Non-Antiarrhythmic Drugs, Preliminary Concept Paper, November 15, 2002, FDA and Health Canada.
3. Federal Register: October 24, 2001 (Volume 66, Number 206), Department of Health and Human Services, Food and Drug Administration, [Docket No. 01N-0476], Electronic Interchange Standard for Digital ECG and Similar Data; Public Meeting.
4. Clinical Data Interchange Standards Consortium; www.cdisc.org.
5. The Clinical Evaluation of QT/QTc Interval Prolongation and Proarrhythmic Potential for Non-Antiarrhythmic Drugs, Preliminary Concept Paper, November 15, 2002, FDA and Health Canada.
6. Systematized Nomenclature of Medicine Clinical Terms (SNOMED CT) published by College of American Pathologists, http://www.snomed.org/, contains codes for clinical findings, procedures, interventions, organisms, substances, pharmaceutical products, specimens, events, etc.
7. Logical Observation Identifiers Names and Codes (LOINC) published by the Regenstrief Institute, http://www.loinc.org/, contains codes for identifying individual laboratory and clinical results.

8. Current Procedural Terminology (CPT) published by the American Medical Association, http://www.ama-assn.org/ama/pub/category/3113.html, contains codes for reporting procedures and services.
9. International Classification of Diseases (ICD) published by the World Health Organization, http://www.who.int/en/, contains codes for classifying diseases and related health problems.
10. Institute of Electrical and Electronics Engineers (IEEE) 1073 Medical Device Communications standards development organization, http://www.ieee1073.org.
11. OMB Circular A-119; Federal Participation in the Development and Use of Voluntary Consensus Standards and in Conformity Assessment Activities, Federal Register / Vol. 63, No. 33 / Thursday, February 19, 1998 / Notices, http://ts.nist.gov/ts/htdocs/210/sccg/ir6412omb.pdf.
12. From the Mission statement of the HL7 RCRIM TC http://www.hl7.org/Special/committees/rcrim/rcrim.htm.
13. HL7 Version 3 Statement of Principles, Revised 1/22/98, http://www.hl7.org/Library/data-model/SOP_980123_final.zip.
14. HL7 V3 Ballot, http://www.hl7.org/v3ballot/html/index.htm.

17 Quality Control and Quality Assurance for Core ECG Laboratories

Amy M. Annand-Furlong

CONTENTS

INTRODUCTION

Recent regulatory guidances for electrocardiograph (ECG) analysis have caused new considerations and challenges for sponsors when designing new drug development programs. As part of these initiatives, the role of the ECG core laboratory has been redefined as a "trusted third party" for the generation, management, and delivery of digital ECG files. As a result, mandatory quality programs for the ECG core laboratory have expanded from assuring the accuracy and precision of key ECG endpoints to now including a complex combination of evolving technology, process, and data verification in the collection, evaluation, and management of digital data files. The successful collection of quality ECG data in the digital era is highly dependent upon superior technology and user training based on predefined processes to properly collect, identify, and process ECGs.

To this end, there are several logistical, equipment, data, and record management issues that the ECG core laboratory must realize, in addition to the clinical ECG analysis methodology itself. There are a number of technology solutions, ECG analyses, evaluation methodologies, and data management decisions to be made. In the definition of adequate and well-controlled ECG studies, a balance of these factors must be defined to determine the approach that best suits each protocol. The ECG core laboratory should have the flexibility and experience to make these decisions in a validated and controlled environment.

This chapter will provide an overview of the key issues to consider during the evaluation of a ECG core laboratory to ensure adequate quality management systems are in place:

- equipment selection and system validation
- site training and management

From: *Cardiac Safety of Noncardiac Drugs:*
Practical Guidelines for Clinical Research and Drug Development
Edited by: J. Morganroth and I. Gussak © Humana Press Inc., Totowa, NJ

- quality control and quality assurance of ECG endpoints
- record management and archiving

The quality management system required to support digital ECG collection and processing must be supported by thorough standard operating procedures that clearly define the responsibilities and deliverables associated with each aspect of the ECG process, from study initiation through database lock. These processes should allow for flexibility of protocol specific requirements. The following key topics should be defined within controlled standard operating procedures at the ECG core laboratory:

- standard operating procedures management
- training of personnel
- training of clinical sites
- study start up
- study database verifications
- ECG receipt, analysis, and reporting
- query resolution
- quality control and quality assurance
- equipment testing and management
- data management (including database transfers, programming, database lock)
- contingency planning
- data back up and recovery
- security
- system validation
- configuration management

EQUIPMENT SELECTION AND SYSTEM VALIDATION

The selection of ECG equipment to meet the specific study and site requirements is essential to ensure the acquisition of quality ECGs that provide the necessary endpoints for evaluation. Factors that influence the ECG acquisition system include: number of study subjects, number and frequency of ECG collection, and site experience with ECG acquisition. There are a variety of ECG acquisition devices available in the healthcare industry including static 12-lead ECG machines with paper print out, hand-held ECG devices, and Holter recording devices. However, not all of these devices are acceptable for clinical research purposes based on regulatory requirements, including FDA Title 21 CFR Part 11 and predicate good clinical practice (GCP) requirements for complete and accurate research data collection.

The traditional use of the ECG machines and corresponding receiving stations has been developed specifically for healthcare. A receiving station is a proprietary software system which receives the digital ECG file from the electrocaardiograph at the clinical site. The vendor supplied receiving stations were not developed to support data management activities inherent to the clinical research process, such as patient indexing and query resolution. Based on the type of ECG machine utilized, some areas of noncompliance may be addressed by procedural work-arounds or specific ECG recorder configurations. Thorough knowledge and evaluation of the ECG machine is required to assess regulatory compliance. It should be noted that some ECG equipment providers have produced "pharmaceutical" versions of their systems to better comply with research requirements. Until these complete solutions are available, operational procedures and/

or integrated systems are required to maintain quality data in compliance with regulatory requirements.

Vendor testing of these systems, in most cases, is not equivalent to that expected by the drug development industry and regulatory agencies with regard to both documentation and testing strategies. Because these systems were not specifically designed for clinical research use, the testing for intended use and exception testing based on data types would not be considered during vendor testing. Vendor audits, an essential element of the quality system, are beneficial to the ECG core laboratory to understand the application and evaluate product support, quality, and future development efforts, but should not be the sole element of the validation process. In addition to ensuring the appropriate regulatory certifications have been granted for such equipment (e.g., FDA 510K and CE Mark), the ECG core laboratory must provide detailed validation documentation to demonstrate appropriate functionality for intended use in the regulated clinical research environment and compliance with FDA Title 21 CFR Part 11 requirements. This validation activity should be documented by approved and version controlled deliverables supporting a system development life cycle including: user/ functional requirements, risk assessment, test plans, test scripts, test output, deviation forms, and summary reports. The validation activities should include not only functional testing, but also validation of the clinical methodology for ECG analysis incorporating verification of all cardiac safety calculations (e.g., corrected QT formulas provide the correct result). For example, if digital ECG images are utilized as the primary source record and paper ECGs scanned to digital files are utilized when transmission failures occur, a validation of the compatibility of these sources must be analyzed and documented. This same requirement extends to the utilization of different acquisition equipment or methodology within or across protocols for a specific program. Whereas the best practice is to maintain a single ECG equipment type and analysis methodology, where this cannot be accommodated as a result of site constraints, documented validation of the mixed methods should be available. Security verification of data transfers and verification of data integrity upon receipt is critical. All electronic activities should be supported by audit trails that are verified as part of the test effort. This includes the transmission of data from the investigator site to the core laboratory through transmission to the sponsor study database.

Where automated algorithms are utilized as the primary ECG endpoints, thorough validation of the algorithms from both functional and clinical methodology studies is essential. As a result of the variance in algorithms across ECG machines and even across versions of a specific ECG machine type, one single version of an ECG machine should be utilized for the duration of a study.

Figure 1 displays the key elements to a validated system clinical system. The four components:

1. Standard operating procedures (SOPs): defined procedures for how systems are developed, implemented, maintained, and used.
2. System documentation: includes all documents that define the system architecture, functionality, test records, user manuals, maintenance records, contingency plans, and change control.
3. Training: for validated systems, all persons that develop, maintain, or utilize the system must have documented training based on their roles.

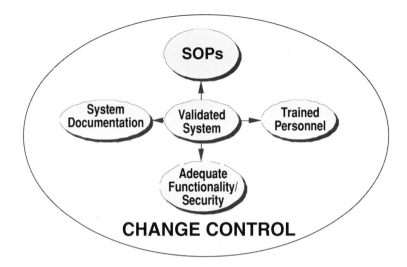

Fig. 1. Key elements to a validated system clinical system.

4. Adequate functionality: the application utilized whether for ECG acquisition and/or ECG analysis must have adequate functionality to support business requirements, GCP requirements, and electronic record regulations (e.g., FDA Title 21 CFR Part 11).

Change Control

If one of the four components is deficient, the system is not in a validated state. For example, all system functionality may be present, documented by SOPs and system documents, but if the end users are not trained on these procedures and proper system use, the data integrity is in jeopardy.

Each of the four components is subject to change at various stages of the application life cycle in response to business and/or regulatory requirements. The maintenance of each item in a compliant state is achieved through a stable well-controlled change management process. Careful consideration needs to be given to the introduction of equipment/systems that may have modified algorithms during the course of the trial. A risk assessment should be prepared and documented when upgrades are implemented during a trial to determine the impact to data integrity and consistency. The ECG core laboratory is responsible for ensuring a validated computer system to maintain the integrity of the data throughout the course of the trial. The stringent change control procedures allow the ECG core laboratory to meet evolving regulatory and business requirements while maintaining the data quality for specific trials.

SITE TRAINING AND MANAGEMENT

Upon selection of appropriate and validated equipment, the site needs to be trained. Lack of training leads to incorrect source data that may not be retrievable. Examples include deleted ECGs, misidentified ECGs, or incorrectly formatted ECGs. The equipment should provide sufficient controls to limit human error.

The collection of quality ECG data initiates at the clinical site with the acquisition of adequate ECG waveforms that are properly identified with subject, visit, and study information. Training programs are essential to digital collection of ECGs, not just for proper patient hook up but also for data collection and transmission. ECGs that are not properly identified may cause delays in the reporting of key safety information. Appropriate ECG analysis cannot be performed when key ECG information is missing (e.g., age/gender ranges may not be applied or ECG comparison cannot be performed). The implementation of a solid training program serves to ensure good quality data and reduce missing data points caused by site error. Because of the criticality of site training for the overall data quality, the ECG core laboratory should be equipped with adequate resources and training alternatives to address various study requirements.

Based on the type of study and experience of the site personnel, training may be conducted through various methods including, but not limited to, instructor-led training with hands-on workshop, self-directed training via web courses/videos, and teleconferences. The use of digital equipment requires more training beyond an investigator meeting presentation that may occur several months prior the study initiation. The most effective training method includes hands-on use by study personnel that is conducted as close as possible to the study start. One method to reinforce training is to perform a "test" ECG prior to the first patient visit to confirm proper lead hook up, equipment use, and successful transmission (in the case of digital acquisition) to the ECG core laboratory. Periodic reminders or retraining should be considered for long-term studies. Where more than one person is approved to capture ECGs, each technician should be qualified. Use of equipment should be supported by clearly defined manuals specific to site requirements, and should identify proper steps for action as well as warnings for flags of improper use. Consideration should also be given to "certifying" sponsor monitors that routinely visit the site. This is particularly useful for international studies where access to some sites may be restrictive.

Most ECG machines are self-calibrating and require little or no maintenance, but should be periodically checked for proper function. The instructions for proper use and storage, based on vendor instructions, should be documented in site materials and reviewed during the training process. The ECG core laboratory, or other facility procuring the equipment for the site, is responsible for the retaining all equipment records related to distribution, fault resolution, preventative maintenance, and testing. These records are the responsibility of the ECG core laboratory but may be made available to the site and/or sponsor as required.

Although the ECG core laboratory has no regulatory responsibility for the monitoring or site management, the laboratory can provide tools to flag consistent site errors and unresponsive sites to query resolution or other requests. These flags are raised through the number and type of queries generated to clarify ECG identification, as well as identification of poor quality tracings that impact the collection of interval durations measurements and morphology assessment. Communication of these issues through periodic reports, which should be available through secured web access systems, can facilitate the identification and resolution of issues proactively throughout the trial.

QUALITY CONTROL AND QUALITY ASSURANCE OF ECG ENDPOINTS

Training of ECG core laboratory personnel for internal duration measurement (IDM) collection needs to be documented with consistent review of procedures and methodology. For manual evaluations, consistency in measurements is maintained through intensive ongoing training, detailed and global standard operating procedures, and where applicable, through technological enhancements.

In accordance with the FDA Concept Paper "The Clinical Evaluation of QT/QTc Interval Prolongation and Proarrhythmic Potential for Nonantiarrhythmic Drugs," *(1)* manual measurement of ECG is the preferred method based on the current status of the algorithms available. Consistency of the ECG measurements and evaluation is achieved through defined evaluation standards, training programs, ongoing quality control reviews, and inter- and intra–reader analysis. As recommended in the FDA Concept Paper *(1)*, the use of a few cardiologists and technical staff may reduce the amount of variability. However, given the ECG core laboratory has maintained well-defined evaluation criteria that is effectively communicated to all staff and facilitated by technology-aids as appropriate, the use of two or more readers may have little impact.

The types of quality programs implemented and expected inter/intra- reader variability is dependent upon the methodology selected. The traditional paper methodology using "eyeball" technique may vary up to 40 ms based on the use of grid paper and manual calipers *(2)*. More advanced technologies incorporating the use of digital waveforms and onscreen annotation of waveforms have enhanced the quality control (QC) review of the manual method by identifying incorrect measurements within 1 ms, based on the sampling rate of the received digital file. Ongoing quality control reviews of the ECG results prior to reporting should be implemented based on the parameters defined by the core ECG laboratory related to methodology variance and clinical considerations. For example, perhaps all "alert" values are reviewed and a random sampling of remaining results. This QC review should include the confirmation of the annotation placement. While in ECG evaluation mode, whether interval duration measurements are performed by trained technical specialists or automated algorithms, the cardiologist performing the morphology evaluation also reviews the annotation placement. During the cardiologist review, confirmation of the annotations is primarily evaluated based on the cardiologist's view of the ECG. Prior to the cardiologist review, a quality control review by technical personnel allows for precision-focused evaluation of caliper placement that should be based on defined company standards.

The reproducibility of data collected by manual methods is monitored through inter- and intra- observer programs. These programs may be executed in a number of conditions based on the ECG analysis method employed. For digital annotation studies, the over reader should be blinded to the original annotations. Whereas this process may introduce some variance based on the beats selected (specifically RR interval), it avoids bias by the over reader and allows for evaluation of the complete process including lead and beat selection. The QC/QA programs at the core ECG laboratory should be performed and analyzed on a study specific basis. There is value in reviewing pooled data by the core ECG laboratory based on standard QA programs that cross multiple protocols. This information displays reproducibility of results over time and across all resources and provides a baseline for the evaluation of protocol specific programs, so long as the conditions are consistent.

In defining the statistical analysis of over read programs consideration must be given not only to the sample size and power required for adequate analysis, but also all external factors that may impact the results. For example, in the manual method of defining interval durations, the expected variance is not limited solely to the operator. The sampling rate of the digital file impacts the variance in placement of the annotation. For

Table 1
Blinded Inter-Observer Over Read

Interval	N	Original mean (ms)	Over read mean (ms)	Original—over read mean difference (ms)	Original—over read min/max difference (ms)	Original—over 95% confidence interval difference
QT	976	380.6	379.8	0.8	−58/37	0.2/1.3
RR	976	894.7	893.3	1.4	−243/789	−1.0/3.9

digital annotation, the distance between pixels determines in part the precision of the ECG measurement. Depending on the sampling rate of the ECG acquisition device, the distance between pixels for any given interval measurement may vary from 1 to 4 ms. The quality of the ECG tracing or morphology also effects the precision of measurements. The expected variance under specific conditions should be defined as part of the over read program. Once the appropriate acceptable limits have bee established ongoing analysis of results may include the usually defined central tendency descriptive statistics including mean, standard deviation, minimum and maximum of original, and over read results. Categorization of results based on acceptable limits should be performed based on the limitations of the methodology implemented, considering the factors defined earlier. Bland–Altman plots may also be utilized to visualize the uniformity of results *(3)*. These analyses should be performed independently for each interval duration measurement (PR, QRS, QT, and RR).

Table 1 and Fig. 2 display the type of information from a routine inter-observer program used by one core ECG laboratory (eResearchTechnology, Inc. Philadelphia, PA), and include data from multiple protocols and sponsors. All over reads of the ECG were performed using manual digital method on ECGs collected from various ECG acquisition devices.

For studies utilizing automated algorithms for interval duration measurements and interpretation, intensive validation of the algorithms should be documented in both functional testing as well as clinical methodology tests. Machine generated ECG algorithms are often based on complex derived measurements using "mean" or "global" beat patterns. The accuracy of results under specific conditions, such as low T wave amplitude or presence of U waves, should be documented and will factor into the design of the quality control/quality assurance program for this method. Based on the proprietary nature of each algorithm, various factors need to be considered for each ECG algorithm type. Where automated interpretations are also being utilized, a defined mapping of all possible machine terms to standard evaluation criteria must also be defined and validated. The terminology provided by the ECG machine is for diagnostic purposes and cannot be used for statistical analysis and standardized reporting. The core ECG laboratory should have defined standards to map the ECG machine interpretations into standard terminology for consistent reporting and evaluation purposes. The mapping of these terms should be flexible to meet study sponsor requirements.

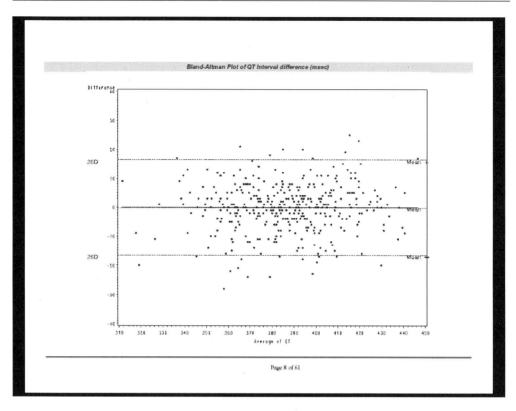

Fig. 2. Bland–Altman plot—blinded inter-observer over read of QT results.

RECORD MANAGEMENT AND ARCHIVING

In the digital initiative, the core ECG laboratory has become the "trusted third party" of the ECG source documents. While a paper tracing, in most systems is printed at the site, it is the digital file that is utilized for all ECG evaluations. The source ECG file is maintained in a proprietary format specific to each ECG machine vendor (e.g., GE Marquette, Mortara Instruments, etc.). To view the proprietary file in the format in which it was received, the study sponsor would be required to maintain the necessary vendor systems themselves. The cost and validation to maintain these systems may be prohibitive, leaving this responsibility to the core ECG laboratory. To provide a digital file to the study sponsor and ultimately regulatory authorities, standard output extensible mark up language (XML) files can be generated for viewing in both human readable form and through systems. The core ECG laboratory should have validated procedures and a standard format for the creation and storing of the XML consistent with regulatory requirements *(4)*. The XML file should display subject information, waveform, and annotations, as well as interval duration values. There are various applications freely available to view these XML files, and some proprietary systems that allow for the movement of calipers to confirm annotations as well as organize the tens of thousands of the XMLs that will be accumulated in a drug development program.

The organization and retention of these XML files in accordance with regulatory requirements is a substantial endeavor and should be a long-term commitment of the ECG core laboratory. Standard nomenclature for files should be defined by the sponsor to assure consistency across protocols, and allow for easy compilation of files across protocols for regulatory submissions. The capabilities of the core ECG laboratory to ensure the retention and ready retrieval of both source files and XML files to meet regulatory requirements (e.g., two years following approval by Food and Drug Administration for U.S. studies) should be thoroughly evaluated prior to contractual obligations for record retention responsibilities.

As outlined in this chapter, the quality programs for the core ECG laboratory must address the wide spectrum of issues related to digital ECG collection, processing, and management. The use of an core ECG laboratory with validated technology solutions, scientifically proven methodologies, and strong processes driven by a solid quality management system, provides study sponsors with an effective solution to collect and maintain quality cardiac safety data that meet regulatory requirements.

REFERENCES

1. Food and Drug Administration and Health Canada. The clinical evaluation of QT/QTc interval prolongation and proarrhythmic potential for non-antiarrhythmic drugs. Preliminary Concept paper, November 15, 2002.
2. Morganroth J, Silber SS. How to obtain and analyze electrocardiograms in clinical trials: Focus on issues in measuring and interpreting changes in the QTc interval duration. A N E 1999;4:425–433.
3. Bland JM, Altman DG. Measuring agreement in method comparison studies. Stat Meth Clin Res 1999;8:135–160.
4. FDA XML Data Format Requirements Specification. DRAFT – Revision B. March 21, 2002.

18 ECG Digital Communities and Electronic Reporting of Cardiac Safety Data

New Technologies for Reporting Digital ECG Data in Clinical Research Settings

Scott Grisanti and Robert Brown

CONTENTS

INTRODUCTION

Since 1996, worldwide regulatory authorities have been providing guidance on cardiac safety as assessed by the standard 12-lead electrocardiogram (ECG), with the European Union's Committee for Proprietary Medicinal Products (CPMP) document ("Points to Consider") for the evaluation of the potential for QT prolongation with noncardiovascular medicinal products in both preclinical and clinical studies. The initiative gained momentum with Health Canada's March 2001 draft guidance document entitled "Assessment of the QT Prolongation Potential of Non-Antiarrhythmic Drugs," and continued to evolve with the November 2002 joint FDA-Health Canada concept paper entitled, "The Clinical Evaluation of QT/QTc Interval Prolongation and Proarrhythmic Potential for Non-Antiarrhythmic Drugs" (see http://www.fda.gov/cder/guidance/index.htm for details). Since 2002, an accelerating focus on cardiac safety in new drug development has been observed throughout the international clinical research industry. Throughout 2003 and 2004, cardiac safety guidance advanced from discussions held as part of the International Conference on Harmonization process, with strong input from research industry and regulatory authorities in Europe and Japan.

A key practical implication of this global ECG regulatory interest has been the evolution of the "digital ECG in clinical research initiative." This has manifested as a move from a predominantly paper-based process of collecting ECGs in clinical trials to an environment characterized by the digital collection, interpretation, management, and

From: *Cardiac Safety of Noncardiac Drugs:*
Practical Guidelines for Clinical Research and Drug Development
Edited by: J. Morganroth and I. Gussak © Humana Press Inc., Totowa, NJ

distribution of ECG safety data. The digital ECG evolution has brought a unique set of challenges and opportunities. There is increased reliance on clinical trial sites to effectively operate specially programmed digital ECG equipment. These new site activities include the electronic capture of demographic data that enable proper identification of a discrete ECG transaction at the trial, site, patient, visit, and time point levels. When conducted with appropriate planning, comprehensive support, and attentive execution, a clinical trial using digital ECGs delivers superior levels of accuracy and efficiency about cardiac safety to the clinical research process.

Digital ECGs enable enhanced collaboration and communication between all participants in the clinical trial process. These constituencies include researchers and staff, sponsor personnel, safety monitoring boards, and associated parties such as development partners, thought leaders, and even regulators. Electronic reporting and distribution of cardiac safety data creates an information platform that can be supplemented by related data (such as enrollment metrics), distance learning curricula to support site personnel engaged in cardiac safety data collection activities, and a variety of communications capabilities. These may include frequently asked questions (FAQ) databases, moderated discussion groups, and other trial specific documents and resources. Overall, these information assets can be deployed as a critical component in an e-clinical strategy. Such "digital communities" can even form the nexus from clinical research to clinical care, as the network of researchers expands to include the larger population of physicians and caregivers.

To be useful, digital communities need to deliver information that is scientifically valuable through an approach that is both technically feasible and compliant with applicable regulations. The following presents eResearchTechnology's (eRT) (Philadelphia, PA) Digital ECG Community as a case study outlining deployment of a collaborative web-based resource that leverages the information and communications opportunities presented by the digital ECG age. eRT is a leading provider of technology and services that facilitate the collection, analysis, and distribution of cardiac safety and clinical data. The company has been making the Digital ECG Community available for several years to sponsors that have contracted with eRT to provide ECG core laboratory services.

DIGITAL ELECTROCARDIOGRAM COMMUNITY

The Digital ECG Community is an *Internet-based web portal* that provides ready access to key study metrics related to cardiac safety. The Digital ECG Community allows participants in the clinical trial to follow the progress and conduct of a study based on frequently updated data. Some of the many features this hosted service offers are secured, user profile-based access to the following:

- Analyses and comprehensive reports supporting proactive decision-making based on ECG findings and other key study metrics and visit tracking reports, across the protocol by patient and site.
- The ability to organize and publish a variety of study-related information such as newsletters, industry resources, study documentation sets, discussion groups, and FAQ databases.
- A range of valuable tools and resources to support all dimensions of clinical research, including eRT's eHealth Education web-based training (WBT) and distance learning

programs, designed to support geographically disperse study personnel with varied clinical and technical backgrounds.
- eRT's end-to-end clinical research applications, as well as other clinical systems and databases.

Digital Electrocardiogram Cardiac Safety Dashboard

A central component of the Digital ECG Community is eRT's Digital ECG Cardiac Safety Dashboard reporting network. The Dashboard aggregates, integrates, migrates, and disseminates cardiac safety and clinical data from its original source. Because these data are updated continuously, users have the flexibility to make near real-time decisions concerning their study initiatives and, as appropriate, take corrective action on a proactive basis. Based on the user's privileges, the Dashboard displays a variety of critical information including enrollment, data collection, data quality, and analysis of specific outlier data points. Viewing of this information is further refined by the ability of the Dashboard to present the information at multiple study levels: program, protocol, investigation site/center, and patient. The Dashboard is ideal for global research activities because of its ability to compile, analyze, and disseminate cardiac safety data to study personnel, regardless of geographic location. This feature not only allows for efficient study monitoring, but also promotes greater communication between sponsors, sites, contract research organizations, and other parties.

The Digital ECG Community is designed to enable near real-time access to decision-grade study data to support early analysis and proactive decision-making. Among its key features are the following:

- Protocol List
- Protocol Dashboard
- Protocol ECG Analysis Report
- Center ECG Analysis Dashboard
- Patient ECG Analysis Report
- Enrollment Dashboard
- Links for Site Instruction
- Optional Drill-Down Capabilities
- QTcF Report
- QTcB Report
- QTcF change from baseline report
- QTcB change from baseline report
- eReporting

One of the Digital ECG Community's most powerful capabilities is its optional Insight analytic tool. Insight provides the ability to reconfigure existing standard reports, develop new reports, and create pivot tables using its drill-down/drill-anywhere functionality. This offers users virtually unlimited views and analyses of their cardiac safety data.

Protocol List

The Protocol List displays the protocol status as "active" (ongoing) or "completed" (Fig. 1). If access to unblinded data is permitted, completed protocols can contain detailed treatment group information. Trial results from completed protocols can be presented in a regulatory grade format within a few days of the last patient visit to facilitate early

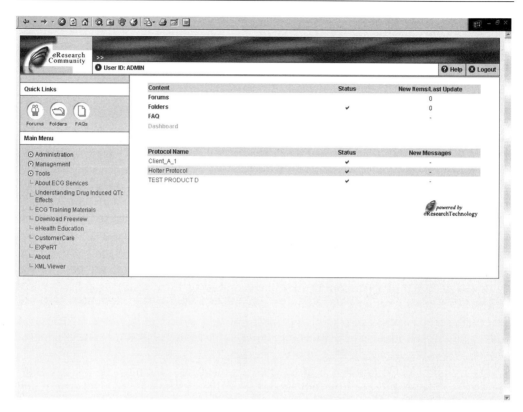

Fig. 1. Protocol list.

decision-making and rapid study closure. Additionally, data from multiple protocols may be rolled into a single program level database for an integrated analysis.

Protocol Dashboard

The Protocol Dashboard reports the incidence of ECG abnormalities while a trial is blinded, which allows for prompt identification of any disproportionate occurrences of adverse effects (Fig. 2). Possible implications might include cardiac safety issues if there is a higher than expected number of ECG abnormalities, or study methodology flaws in the event a lower than expected number of abnormalities is reported. The Protocol Dashboard presents the user with a high level overview of the key metrics of the ECG data that has been collected. These include the total number of ECGs analyzed, and the percentage of patients that displayed abnormalities in the following categories: rhythms, conduction, morphology, myocardial infarction, ST segment, T waves, and U waves. Additionally, the number of centers and number of patients enrolled are presented.

Protocol Electrocardiogram Analysis Report

The Protocol ECG Analysis Report compares the incidence of ECG findings within patients, across visits, and/or between different treatment groups (Fig. 3). This information can be used to determine whether immediate re-evaluation of a patient's ECG status should occur. Furthermore, the findings from this report can be used in the study's medical summary report to explain the observed ECG changes. Contained within the

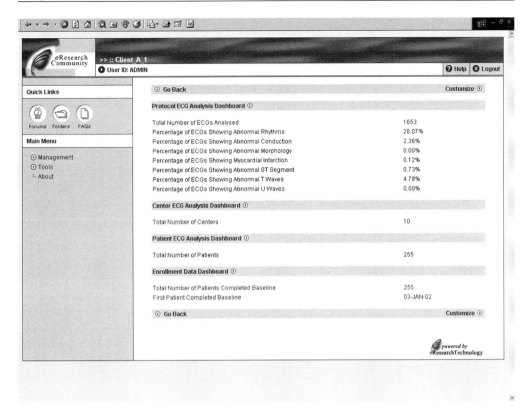

Fig. 2. Protocol dashboard.

Protocol ECG Analysis Report is the detailed breakdown of the percentages of abnormalities from the Protocol Dashboard. The detailed breakdown contains patient counts for abnormalities in: rhythms, conduction, morphology, myocardial infarction, ST segment, T waves, and U waves. The data is presented for the entire protocol with the user given the ability to drill-down to individual sites and patients.

This capability enables comparison of cardiac safety findings between centers based on selected variables such as geography (e.g., European centers vs US centers), or a specific set of assigned sites to allow for rapid and easy identification of inconsistencies or outliers in study findings (Fig. 4). The standard prebuilt reports include: heart rate, PR, QRS, QT, QTcB, QTcB change > 60 ms, QTcF, QTcF change > 60 ms, and the center ECG analysis report.

Patient Electrocardiogram Analysis Report

The Patient ECG Analysis Report provides both sponsors and investigators access to their own patients' data to effectively monitor their progress over the course of the study (Fig. 5). Access to this information allows investigators to ensure patient safety and to respond to questions from study monitors should they arise. The report breaks out all of the interval duration measurements: HR, PR, QRS, QT, QTcB and QTcF, and all other findings: rhythm, conduction, morphology, myocardial infarction, ST segment, T waves, and U waves for each patient's ECGs over time/visit. The report automatically highlights abnormalities for ease of identification.

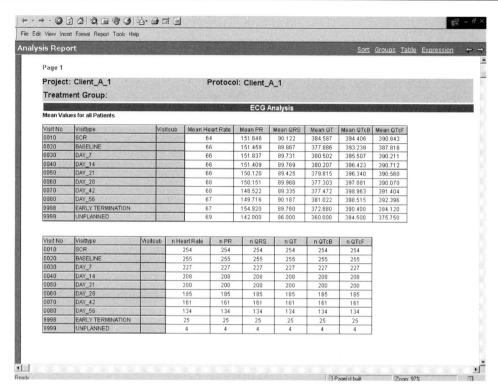

Fig. 3. Protocol ECG analysis report.

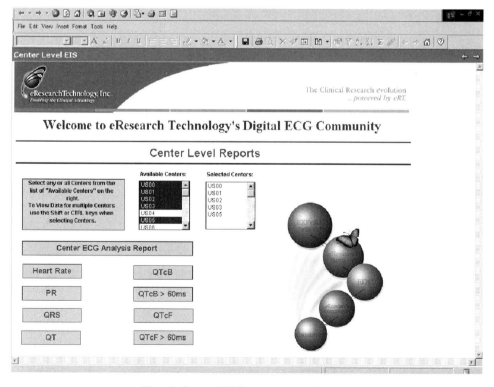

Fig. 4. Center ECG analysis dashboard.

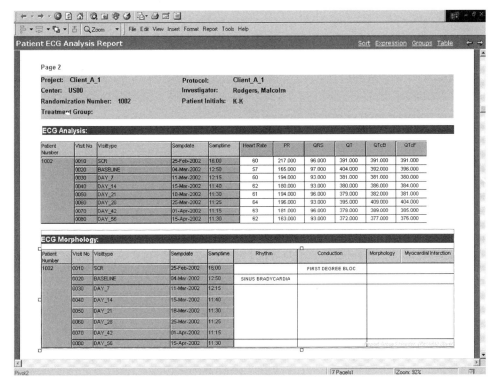

Fig. 5. Patient ECG analysis report

Enrollment Dashboard

The Enrollment Dashboard provides analyses of critical enrollment and demographic information to facilitate prompt identification of sites that may need assistance with study conduct activities, such as patient recruitment or verification of adequate patient documentation (Fig. 6). Access to both the overall enrollment activity as well as individual sites enrollment are available.

Users may also configure a patient visit schedule to track individual patients visits, missed visits, unscheduled visits, and terminated patients/subjects through the course of the trial (Fig. 7). All data may be viewed in table or graphic format, and the ability to export data off of the web is also available.

Links for Site Instructions

This section provides access to supporting documentation, study guides, and other relevant materials to ensure that sites have access to the necessary resources to perform safety tests in a uniform manner (Fig. 8). Users may store documents in various formats including, but not limited to Microsoft Word, Excel, and pdf.

Analytical Capabilities

The Digital ECG Community provides optional analytic functionality, Insight, to drill-down into the community database to perform more complex analyses based on any available data variables. This function permits easy identification of cardiac safety outliers or changes from baseline. With this function a user may begin their analysis with one

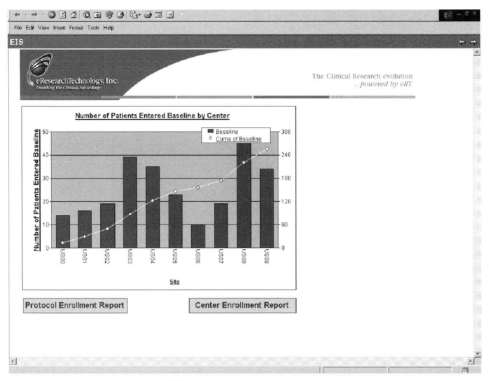

Fig. 6. Enrollment dashboard

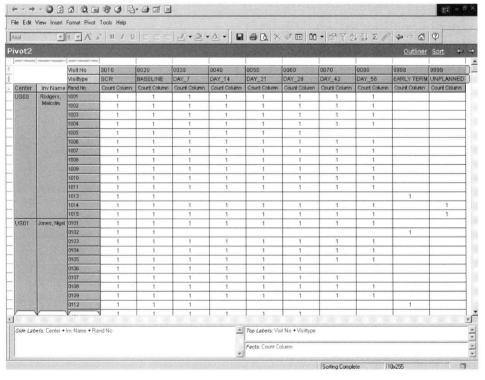

Fig. 7. Patient visit schedule.

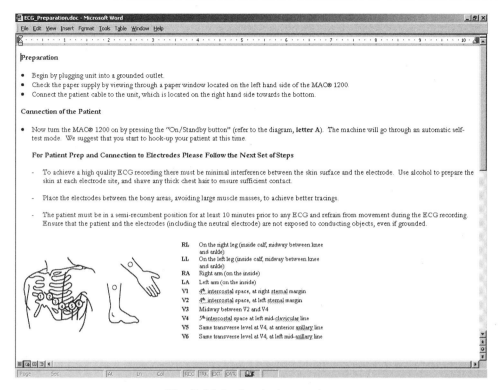

Fig. 8. Links for site instruction.

of the prebuilt Protocol, Center, Patient, or Enrollment reports (e.g., change from baseline in QTcF). From that report the user may then drill-down into the underlying database to access additional variables to add to the existing report (e.g., add to the report any abnormal T waves reported for that subject, and if a myocardial infarction was present at the time the ECG was taken) (Fig. 9).

Contained within Insight is a conditional formatting tool, Spotlighter (Fig. 10). The Spotlighter permits users to highlight any values within a table for ease of viewing (e.g., users could highlight all change from baseline values in QTcB between 30 and 60 ms). Multiple values may be highlighted from multiple fields.

QTcF and QTcB Reports

Once the treatment code information is added, reports can be readily generated to determine if a drug effects cardiac repolarization as evidenced by changes from baseline, or by the number of outliers identified in placebo and for each drug dose (Fig. 11). (For example, any patient that experiences a change from baseline of more than 60 ms would be considered an outlier.) Prior to unblinding, the Digital ECG Community provides the same information across the entire study that can be reviewed by site, country, or other demographic variables contained in the database. The data contained in the prebuilt QTcF and QTcB reports is displayed both graphically and in tabular format. In addition to the export capability defined earlier, users may also copy and paste the graphical elements of the reports for inclusion in Word documents or PowerPoint presentations.

Separate reports for outliers are standard for both QTcF and QTcB change from baseline greater than 60 ms (Fig. 12).

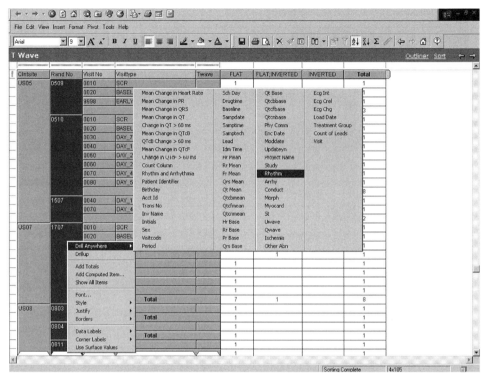

Fig. 9. Optional drill-down capabilities.

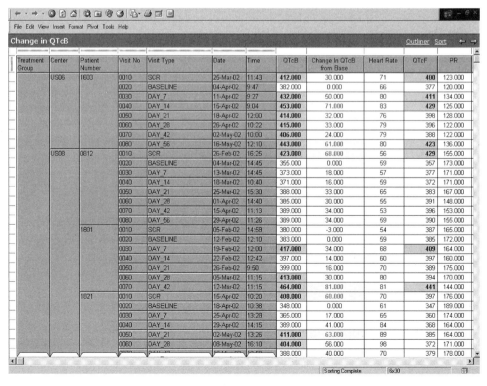

Fig. 10. Spotlighter.

Visit No	Visittype	Treatment Group Visitsub	n	Mean QTcB	Mean Change from Base	Change > 60 ms
0010	SCR		254	394.406	1.231	1
0020	BASELINE		255	393.239	0.063	
0030	DAY_7		227	395.507	2.462	
0040	DAY_14		208	396.423	3.098	2
0050	DAY_21		200	396.340	2.874	1

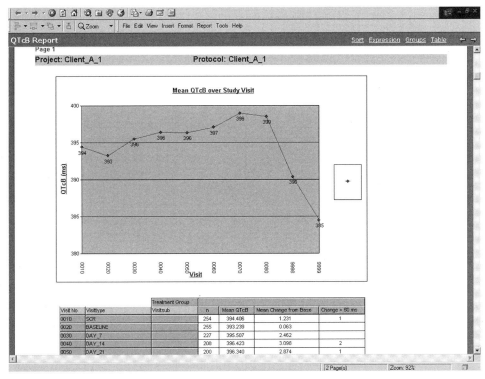

Fig. 11. QTcF and QTcB reports.

Treatment Group	Center	Patient Number	Visit No	Visit Type	Date	Time	QTcB	Change In QTcB from Base	Heart Rate	PR	QRS
	US06	1603	0010	SCR	25-Mar-02	11:43	412.000	30.000	71	123.000	86.000
			0020	BASELINE	04-Apr-02	9:47	382.000	0.000	66	120.000	89.000
			0030	DAY_7	11-Apr-02	9:27	432.000	50.000	80	134.000	81.000
			0040	DAY_14	15-Apr-02	9:04	453.000	71.000	83	125.000	87.000
			0050	DAY_21	18-Apr-02	12:00	414.000	32.000	76	128.000	85.000
			0060	DAY_28	26-Apr-02	10:22	415.000	33.000	79	122.000	87.000
			0070	DAY_42	02-May-02	10:00	406.000	24.000	79	122.000	85.000
			0080	DAY_56	16-May-02	12:10	443.000	61.000	80	136.000	87.000
	US08	0812	0010	SCR	26-Feb-02	16:25	423.000	68.000	56	155.000	89.000
			0020	BASELINE	04-Mar-02	14:45	355.000	0.000	59	173.000	87.000
			0030	DAY_7	13-Mar-02	14:45	373.000	18.000	57	171.000	93.000
			0040	DAY_14	18-Mar-02	10:40	371.000	16.000	59	171.000	88.000
			0050	DAY_21	25-Mar-02	15:30	388.000	33.000	65	167.000	85.000
			0060	DAY_28	01-Apr-02	14:40	385.000	30.000	55	148.000	89.000
			0070	DAY_42	15-Apr-02	11:13	389.000	34.000	53	153.000	93.000
			0080	DAY_56	29-Apr-02	11:26	389.000	34.000	59	155.000	84.000
		1801	0010	SCR	05-Feb-02	14:58	380.000	-3.000	54	165.000	94.000
			0020	BASELINE	12-Feb-02	12:10	383.000	0.000	59	172.000	90.000
			0030	DAY_7	19-Feb-02	12:00	417.000	34.000	68	164.000	84.000
			0040	DAY_14	22-Feb-02	12:42	397.000	14.000	60	160.000	87.000
			0050	DAY_21	26-Feb-02	9:50	399.000	16.000	70	175.000	95.000
			0060	DAY_28	05-Mar-02	11:15	413.000	30.000	80	170.000	95.000
			0070	DAY_42	12-Mar-02	11:15	464.000	81.000	81	144.000	85.000
		1821	0010	SCR	15-Apr-02	10:20	408.000	60.000	70	176.000	89.000
			0020	BASELINE	18-Apr-02	10:38	348.000	0.000	61	109.000	91.000

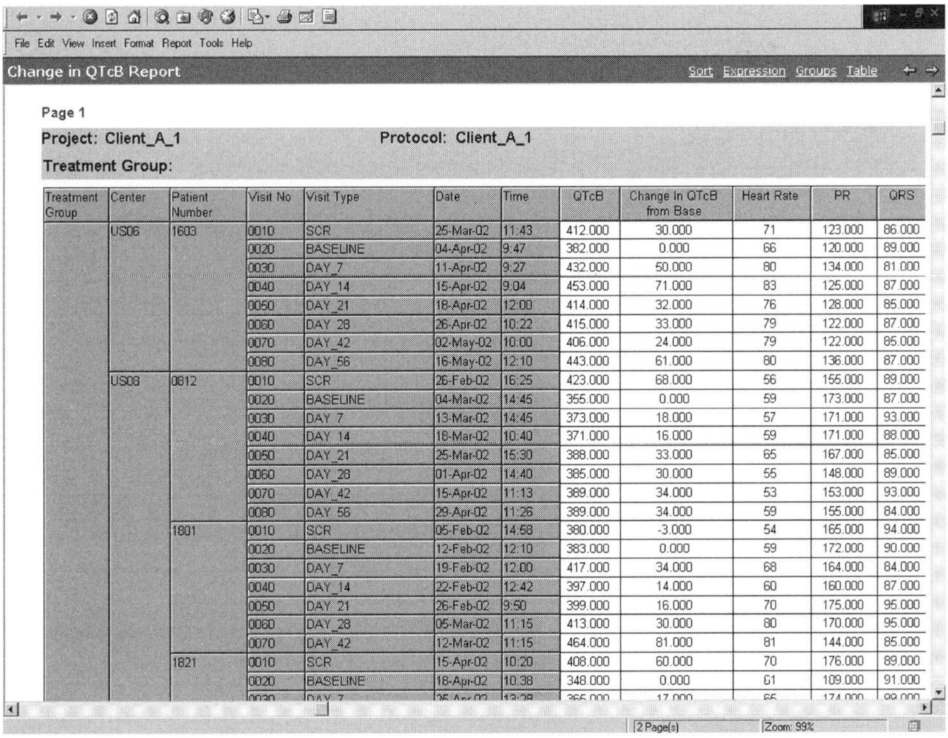

Fig. 12. QTcF and QTcB change from baseline reports.

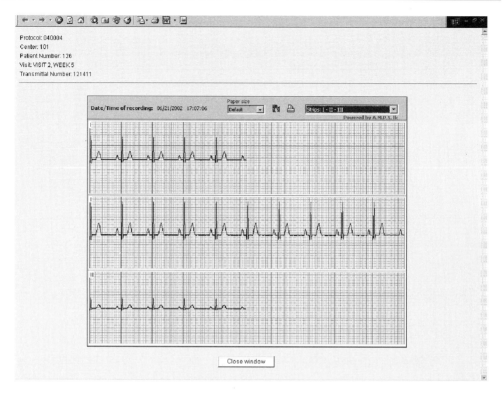

Fig. 13. Patient ECG analysis dashboard.

Digital Electrocardiogram Waveform Display and Management

Upon analysis of any of the prebuilt patient reports, sponsors or investigators may desire to access the individual waveform for any given ECG. From the Patient ECG Analysis Dashboard users may choose a specific patient and visit time point and click to display the waveform (Fig. 13). The annotated waveform for the specific ECG and time point will be displayed in a separate window. Users then have various display options that include median beats, superimposed median beats, rhythm strips for all 12-leads, rhythm strips for select leads, or rhythm strips for groupings of limb leads or precordial leads. Users may not alter any annotations on the waveform itself, but are given the ability to print off a hardcopy of the waveform.

eReporting

The eReporting functionality brings to the user a set of prebuilt reports. In the Digital ECG Community scenario, these reports are auto-generated from eRT's EXPeRT® system. EXPeRT is eRT's cardiac safety database management, communication, and reporting system. The prebuilt reports are stored in an on-line folder in pdf format. These reports are read-only and may be printed to the user's local printer.

The *Unsolved Query Report* that displays all of the unresolved queries currently in the EXPeRT system (Fig. 14). These include but are not limited to missing visits, demographic inconsistencies, missing data, etc.

The *Visit Tracking Report* tracks by patient and time point the collection date and time, date received, and date reported (Fig. 15).

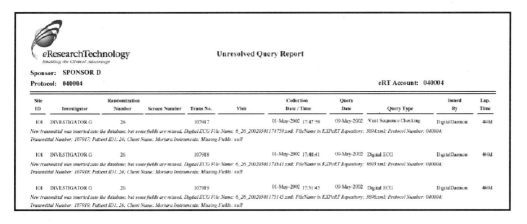

Fig. 14. Unsolved query report.

Fig. 15. Visit tracking report.

The *Abnormal ECG Report* displays by patient within site all of the ECGs that displayed an abnormal finding (Fig. 16). In addition to the abnormal findings being detailed, the reviewer of the ECG is identified and a change from comparison variable time point may be displayed.

The *Study Tracking Report* tracks by patient and time point within site the collection date and time, data entry date, analysis date, review date, and date reported (Fig. 17).

The *Summary of QTc Results* displays the total number of ECGs processed to date for the selected protocol (Fig. 18).

Number of ECGs with abnormal QTcB results for the protocol:

    Number of screening ECGs with a QTcB of > 480 ms but < 500 ms
    Number of screening ECGs with a QTcB of > 500 ms
    Number of baseline ECGs with a QTcB of > 480 ms but < 500 ms
    Number of baseline ECGs with a QTcB of >500 ms
    Number of treatment ECGs with a QTcB of > 480 ms but < 500 ms

eResearchTechnology
Enabling the Clinical Advantage

Abnormal ECGs

Sponsor: SPONSOR D

Protocol: 040004 **eRT Account: 040004**

Site ID	Investigator	Randomization Number	Screen Number	Trans. No.	Visit	Collection Date / Time	Reviewer	Change from Comparison	Finding(s)
101	INVESTIGATOR G	25111117		107907	2W5	02-May-2002 17:34:00	Terry Filbert		Rhythm : Sinus Bradycardia
101	INVESTIGATOR G	00000144		120411		21-Jun-2002 18:10:20	Joel Morganroth, M.D.		Conduction: Intraventricular Conduction Defect
101	Doctor F	00000062	201	137141	2W5	21-Feb-2003 15:39:50	L Frasca		Rhythm : Sinus Bradycardia

Number of Abnormal Transmittals for Account 040004: 3

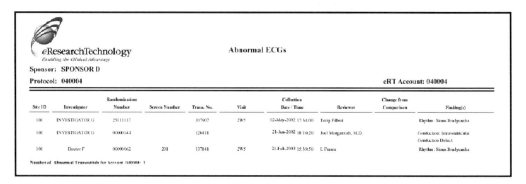

Fig. 16. Abnormal ECG report.

eResearchTechnology
Enabling the Clinical Advantage

Study Tracking Report

Sponsor: SPONSOR D

Protocol: 040004 **eRT Account: 040004**

SiteID	Investigator	Initials	Randomization Number	Screen Number	Trans. No.	Visit	Collection Date / Time	Data Entry Date	Analysis Date	Review Date	Report Date
101	Doctor F	EPR	00000056	1	136941	IB	21-FEB-2003 15:21:10	06-Jun-2003	06-Jun-2003	09-Jun-2003	09-Jun-2003
		EPR	00000056	1	136951	3W10	21-FEB-2003 15:23:05	06-Jun-2003	06-Jun-2003	09-Jun-2003	09-Jun-2003
		EPR	00000056	1	136961	2W5	21-FEB-2003 15:23:57	06-Jun-2003	06-Jun-2003	09-Jun-2003	09-Jun-2003
		ESR	00000056	56	136971	2W5	21-FEB-2003 15:34:35	06-Jun-2003	06-Jun-2003	09-Jun-2003	09-Jun-2003
		ETR	00000057		142161 *	2W5	21-FEB-2003 15:26:05				
		ETR	00000057	2	136981	IB	21-FEB-2003 15:25:17	06-Jun-2003	06-Jun-2003	09-Jun-2003	09-Jun-2003
		ETR	00000057	2	136991	2W5	21-FEB-2003 15:26:05	06-Jun-2003	06-Jun-2003	09-Jun-2003	09-Jun-2003
		EVR	00000058	23	137011	IB	21-FEB-2003 15:28:20	06-Jun-2003	06-Jun-2003	09-Jun-2003	09-Jun-2003

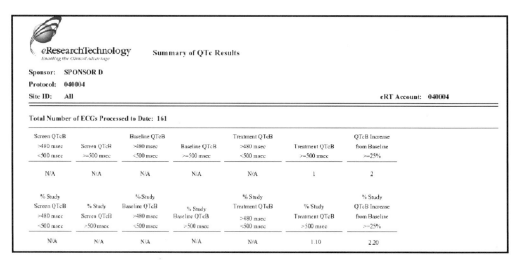

Fig. 17. Study tracking report.

eResearchTechnology
Enabling the Clinical Advantage

Summary of QTc Results

Sponsor: SPONSOR D

Protocol: 040004

Site ID: All **eRT Account: 040004**

Total Number of ECGs Processed to Date: 161

Screen QTcB >480 msec <500 msec	Screen QTcB >=500 msec	Baseline QTcB >480 msec <500 msec	Baseline QTcB >=500 msec	Treatment QTcB >480 msec <500 msec	Treatment QTcB >=500 msec	QTcB Increase from Baseline >=25%
N/A	N/A	N/A	N/A	N/A	1	2

% Study Screen QTcB >480 msec <500 msec	% Study Screen QTcB >500msec	% Study Baseline QTcB >480 msec <500 msec	% Study Baseline QTcB >500 msec	% Study Treatment QTcB >480 msec <500 msec	% Study Treatment QTcB >500 msec	% Study QTcB Increase from Baseline >=25%
N/A	N/A	N/A	N/A	N/A	1.10	2.20

Fig. 18. Summary of QTc results.

Number of treatment ECGs with a QTcB of > 500 ms

Number of treatment ECGs where QTcB increased from baseline > 25%

Percentage of ECGs with abnormal QTcB results for the protocol:

Percentage of screening ECGs with a QTcB of > 480 ms but < 500 ms

Percentage of screening ECGs with a QTcB of > 500 ms

Percentage of baseline ECGs with a QTcB of > 480 ms but < 500 ms

Percentage of baseline ECGs with a QTcB of > 500 ms

Percentage of treatment ECGs with a QTcB of > 480 ms but < 500 ms

Percentage of treatment ECGs with a QTcB of > 500 ms

Percentage of treatment ECGs where QTcB increased from baseline > 25%

Additional Digital Community Services

The Digital ECG Community offers a broad array of services to enhance content and enable communication. Among the Community's many attributes are its ability to support knowledge transfer, and to serve as a vehicle for cultivating and maintaining investigator relationships.

Another key feature of the Digital ECG Community is the access it provides to targeted educational curricula, known as eHealth Education. eHealth Education provides access to a series of sophisticated, interactive WBT programs that are designed not only to optimize the user's comprehension of clinical research processes and procedures, but to effect long-term retention of this information. Quality WBT courses are developed in accordance with established Instructional Systems Design methodology, with course content developed using scenario-based training principles to ensure that theory can be seen in its practical context.

eHealth Education is offered as a service through the Digital ECG Community. The courses are targeted toward ensuring effective knowledge transfer for the skills necessary to effectively execute a digital ECG trial. When deployed through the Digital ECG Community, eHealth Education provides users an ideal environment to accelerate their clinical research efforts. eHealth Education courses have been designed using a highly flexible format that allows users to choose how they want to learn. Specifically, users can allow the system to determine their learning path based on their performance on a certification test, or users can simply select their own topics for study. Either way, users benefit from a series of interactive demonstrations that visually reinforce course concepts and guided simulations that allow for "hands-on experience" with the systems through an electronic tutor.

eHealth Education is considerably less disruptive than conventional training courses because the entire curriculum can be administered over the Internet at the customer's site, which allows users to participate without having to leave the office. Further, WBT allows clients to achieve cost savings through several means:

• First, there is no need to hire an instructor to lead the courses.

• Second, the programs are provided in a hosted computing environment and offered through a subscription arrangement, so there is no need to purchase software.

• Third, there are no travel expenses because users can take the courses from any remote location.

To further enhance user retention, eHealth Education includes automated processes for evaluation and feedback, and a learning management-based system for monitoring user progress. Additionally, each course is supported by a library of related resources and training programs and can be augmented by any documents that the customer wishes to add. Information in the library can be readily assessed through the program's search engine. Ongoing availability of WBT courseware also delivers a powerful tool to manage investigative site personnel turnover that occurs during a clinical trial process.

Knowledge Transfer and Investigator Relationship Management

Among the Community's most important attributes are its ability to support knowledge transfer and to serve as a vehicle for cultivating and maintaining investigator relationships. To facilitate these clinical research needs, the Community offers a range of resources including FAQ databases that allows users to be given privileges to read, write, or delete items. This allows sponsors to effectively manage the scope and the flow of information that is available to study personnel. FAQ databases provide a valuable repository for commonly asked questions related to a study, and can be easily expanded to include references and links to industry resources.

Discussion groups, an equally important feature, can be set up as "moderated," or "nonmoderated." Moderated discussions require the assignment of a "moderator" to review and approve all questions, and subsequent discussion threads to ensure the appropriateness of the information being communicated. Nonmoderated discussions are designed to offer more open participation in study related discussions. Lastly, the Community offers users the ability to organize and publish a variety of study-related information such as newsletters, forms, study documentation sets, and other important files. Any time updates are made to the discussion groups, the FAQ database or the study folders, the Community will signal the availability of new information via both e-mail and screen alerts.

Through these capabilities, the Digital ECG Community not only serves as a platform for information exchange, but it encourages increased coordination between clinical research personnel and ultimately strengthens overall clinical initiatives by linking all participants in value-added activities. Growing acceptance of the Internet as a business-operating platform for certain clinical research activities has made advanced solutions such as the Digital ECG Community possible. These systems provide the real-time information feedback and communication necessary to drive increased effectiveness of clinical research activities. Because the Digital ECG Community is a hosted solution, it is easy to deploy and software installation requirements are minimal. Also, advanced solutions providers are now able to provide systems, such as the Digital ECG Community, that deliver the 21 CFR, Part 11 and related regulatory compliance the clinical research industry has come to expect and demand.

CONCLUSION

Internet-based cardiac safety data reporting solutions, such as eRT's Digital ECG Community, provide tools that significantly enhance the ability of key trial participants to monitor progress of cardiac safety data collection and analysis in near real-time. The Digital ECG Community delivers an easy-to-use, secure, regulatory compliant environment for advanced decision support throughout the clinical research process. In addition to key cardiac safety data and associated digital ECG waveforms, the Digital ECG Community provides a comprehensive collaboration and communication platform to link all trial participants involved in cardiac safety aspects of a study. Users can access this web-based solution with appropriate authorization on a global basis. It can be quickly and economically deployed to support a single trial, a program, a therapeutic area, or an entire clinical development enterprise.

INDEX

355